Diet Recovery

Restoring Hormonal Health,
Metabolism, Mood and Your
Relationship with Food
By Matt Stone

A proud presentation of:

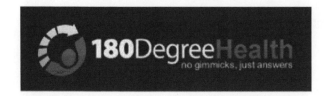

2

DISCLAIMER

The material provided here is for educational and informational purposes only and is not intended as medical advice. The information contained in this book should not be used to diagnose or treat any illness, metabolic disorder, disease, or health problem. If you have developed a serious illness of some kind, the complexities of dealing with that disorder are best handled by your physician or other professional health care provider, whom you should also consult with before beginning any nutrition or exercise program. Use of the programs, advice, and other information contained in this book is at the sole choice and risk of the reader.

Contents

6

About Matt Stone

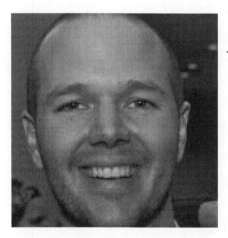

Hi, I'm independent health researcher Matt Stone. I am not the omniscient knower of all things, but I've spent the better part of the last decade immersed in the field of health research, and in that time I've made some key discoveries that are urgently needed by literally hundreds of millions of "dieters" worldwide.

What's emerged as my specialty over the "course" of my research, which has involved thousands of studies, over 300 books spanning an entire century, hundreds of health-related websites and blogs, close attention to the 100,000+ comments left at my blog, forum, and social media outlets, and personal communication with thousands of individuals from all walks of life, all ethnicities, and dozens of countries worldwide, is helping to guide people back to health from the devastation perpetrated by various popular diets.

In fact, in a world full of people seemingly on a quest for self-destruction through drinking, drugs, fast food, cigarette smoking, and otherwise abusive behavior, the people with the worst health that I've seen are not those that threw caution to the wind (although they ended up plenty sick, too). Nope. Those in the most dire circumstances were precisely the people who tried hardest to eat the perfect diet, live the perfect lifestyle, and otherwise intellectualized all their habits. Like fitness and nutrition authority Paul Chek said in a well-received talk given to the Price-Pottenger Nutrition Foundation, "If you want to see some really fat and/or sick people, go to a nutrition conference." Despite Chek's arrogance, there is some truth to that.

That's because all of the miracle health crusades out there are just plain dangerous – from the secret underground low-carb society that possesses the holy Atkins chronicles, to the high priests of the freakishly cult-like vegetarian movement, to the naïve, socially-dysfunctional, and scientifically-ignorant Paleo nutrition clan, to the food weighing calorie-phobic diet masters of the mainstream, to the pompous and self-righteous club of finishers of the ultimate litmus test of human stupidity – the 26.2 mile Moron-a-thon.

While nearly all of them serve up a healthy dose of apparent short-term benefits, and many are indeed highly beneficial on many fronts in comparison to pounding 2 liters of Pepsi daily while watching Jersey Shore marathons instead of running a marathon, they are all ultimately imbalanced, counterproductive if continued long-term, and dangerous to a human being who has convinced him or herself that the food (or rest) they need to rebalance their bodies is a villain.

One thing all of the above recommendations have in common is that they all reduce the metabolism (lower thyroid hormone production and utilization). Some, like marathon running or very low-calorie diets, more so than others. The metabolism is the centerpiece of our health, in charge of the proper oxygenation of our cells, the energy production that takes place in the mitochondria in every one of our cells, the health of our immune system, keeping our youthfulness intact for as long as possible, and a lot more. In fact, one popular book on the subject of hypothyroidism has a chapter on "Symptoms" that is over 80 pages in length. When every cell is influenced by the metabolism, there is really nothing that breaks down that doesn't somehow relate back to it.

There's a reason why, when people age, they become increasingly prone to store fat, they lose muscle mass, quickness, strength, and agility – and become much more prone to develop degenerative diseases. It's quite simple actually – they lose the full metabolic potential they had in their youth. Severe dietary restrictions, particularly of carbohydrates or calories as well as many other factors, all expedite the aging process due to their ability to obliterate a healthy metabolism.

"In some animal forms, at least, chronic undernutrition prolongs the natural life span. It has been suggested that the natural life span is fixed, not in time, but in terms of total metabolism or some function of the rate of living. But in man severe undernutrition makes him look, feel, and act prematurely old. There are also changes in basal metabolism and in sexual function which resemble those produced by age."

-Ancel Keys; *The Biology of Human Starvation*

Funny thing is, even Dr. Atkins, the top-selling weight loss author of all-time understood this – even as it pertained to his own diet (referenced by the phrase "this one" in the passage below)…

"Remember that prolonged dieting (this one, low-fat, low-calorie, or a combination) tends to shut down thyroid function. This is usually not a problem with the thyroid gland (therefore blood tests are likely to be normal) but with the liver, which fails to convert T4 into the more active thyroid principle, T3. The diagnosis is made on clinical ground with the presence of fatigue, sluggishness, dry skin, coarse or falling hair, an elevation in cholesterol, or a low body temperature. I ask my patients to take four temperature readings daily before the three meals and near bedtime. If the average of all these temperatures, taken for at least three days, is below 97.8 degrees F (36.5 C), that is usually low enough to point to this form of thyroid problem; lower readings than that are even more convincing."

In the pages that follow, I hope to lay out, as simply as I can, a few compelling reasons to quit dieting forever, and how you can go about rehabilitating your body from past diets, and your relationship with your body and food in general. There is no one-size-fits all, but for most it is not that hard of a process, no matter what your age, gender, or personal history. In fact, those with the most extensive history of restricted diets and who are substantially overweight tend to respond best.

Health Defined

"The physical energy of the adrenal type is seemingly inexhaustible, as is the nervous response of the sympathetic system, a result of perfect oxidation of phosphorous in the nerve tissue. Oxidation of carbon in the muscular system gives the adrenal type his great warmth. Thus, the temperature of his body is scarcely ever below 98.8, with hands and feet always pleasantly warm. As digestion and detoxication of food poisons depend greatly upon oxidation in the liver and intestines, it follows that the typical adrenal type, with his perfect oxidation, has thorough digestion. In fact, he may and often does boast that he can eat any and all kinds of food without discomfort. The exogenous uric acid products as well as the indoxyl compounds are completely detoxicated in the liver, do not accumulate in the blood, nor are they found in the urine."

"The skeletal muscles are well developed and have splendid tone. Fatigue is practically unknown to the adrenal type. His muscular endurance is spectacular. And the perfect tone of the involuntary muscles is evidenced by complete and rapid peristalsis, resulting in several bowel evacuations daily. He can dine on the most impossible food combinations imaginable with no evil results..."

"The quality of the blood is characteristic. A slight to marked polycythemia (more red cells than usual) occurs; leucopenia, or abnormal white cell count on the low side, is never noted. The blood, which is of a

rich, red color, clots quickly. Fatal hemorrhage seldom occurs. The immunity against bacterial invasion is spectacular. The typical adrenal type hardly ever becomes infected, even with venereal diseases…"

"A member of the adrenal-type group has a phlegmatic disposition — easygoing, jolly, slow to anger, never bothered with insomnia, fear or "cold feet." He will often go out of his way to avoid a quarrel. Customarily, he has a wide circle of friends because he is warm-hearted and surrounded by an 'aura' of kindly sympathy."

"Splendid circulation gives him warm, magnetic hands…"

"He never worries…His digestion is good and he is seldom constipated. It is possible for him to stand more treatments, operations and even more lung hemorrhages than any other type of patient. He is the patient most often discharged as arrested or cured. All the treatment necessary for his recovery is supplied by bed rest and fresh air."

I don't know of a more perfect representation of what the true health experience is than that — taken from Henry Bieler's *Food is Your Best Medicine*.

Although few of us will be able to ever get to that level of health no matter how or what we try, and it's important that we all have realistic expectations about how much we can advance our health by diet and lifestyle change alone, I've seen nearly everyone be able to take great strides toward that level of health.

Will restricting carbohydrates from your diet inch you closer to that state? No. Fats? No. Low-calorie diets? No. Hours on the treadmill? No.

Hopefully you can already see where this is headed. Instead of making the common error that most mainstream nutrition-minded people make — which is identifying your weaknesses and intolerances and catering to them with a set dietary "prescription," this is a program about having a real breakthrough. This is a digestive, immune system, and metabolic "strength-training" program. It's about stimulating your body to adapt to become better at the management of all the things we ingest, and face in life.

If you went to a personal trainer and said, "My upper body is really strong, but the problem is my really weak, skinny legs," you'd probably find the trainer putting MORE emphasis on your weak spot and working the weak spot harder. Although this isn't an exact parallel to what you're about to experience, that ain't too far off.

For example, cutting meat out of your diet can reduce hydrochloric acid production produced by your stomach and turn down several of the meat-digesting enzymes needed to properly dispose of ammonia and other by-products of meat digestion. Eating meat after being a long-term vegetarian can make you sick at first.

Most people that avoid carbohydrates and notice some immediate health improvements and weight loss are people with poor carbohydrate metabolism. In the absence of carbohydrates, glucose metabolism becomes increasingly worse from both a digestive and a metabolic standpoint. When they return to eating carbs they have their "carbs are the devil" beliefs reconfirmed, as they get foggy-headed, bloated, gassy, pimpled, fat, and have their cravings and hunger go wild.

Most people will eventually develop health problems on a low-carb diet (or low-fat diet, to pick on the fat haters too and anyone engaged in Macronutrient Warfare) – including even gaining a bunch of weight back that they initially lost, and they will eventually crave carbohydrates or find that a carb-free diet has become just too socially crippling. As I often say, "You can run from carbs, but you can't hide." A low-carb diet can even start to raise blood sugars to approximate diabetic levels! The real answer is to improve glucose metabolism and digestion, which is what this program will do. Same with fat digestion and fat burning, as well as being able to eat a high-calorie meal without gaining weight from it.

Even many food allergies and "intolerances" can be overcome as well, and these intolerances are yet another thing that pops up in the undernourished and overworked. If you don't believe food intolerances surface from lack of abundant nutrition, you should see what an anorexic goes through while trying to recover. They are hypersensitive to everything, can't digest or metabolize anything properly, have major glucose metabolism problems (severe reactive hypoglycemia), and are generally poisoned by food – hence why so few ever successfully recover. It's totally self-perpetuating, but so is Sherlock-Holmes-ing the crap out of your diet to figure out what you do and don't tolerate – a practice I've rarely seen lead to anything but a life sentence in dietary prison.

Anyway, I think you'll all find this to be really quite liberating. It's so liberating that I'm not wearing any pants right now.

Oh I'm funny, I should have mentioned that. Pardon, I TRY to be funny.

"If we added up all of the special 'avoidance' diets, no one could eat anything. Many people are ruining their health by avoiding too many foods."

-Ray Peat

A Few Words About My Research Style

I am often challenged about my research style, and called "unscientific" by the naysayers, of which there are many – to be expected when the ideas you promote, if true, undermine the credibility of nearly every major health/medical/nutrition movement on earth.

Today's standard for writing about health and nutrition, more than any other field of science, has become pitiful. It is expected that any claim you make must have a clinical trial to back it up or else it is as good as, in the words of R.J. Fletcher in the movie *UHF*, "a festering bowl of dog snot." It is assumed that clinical trials actually have some real basis, are reliable, and the conclusions that stem from such studies are totally infallible. In short, they convince the less educated, who don't understand the whole picture. And no study is done in the context of real life and any fool's experiential observation.

I think of using studies to back claims or hypotheses as being cheap – cheap to an almost infinite degree, taking something out of context and pretending it is supportive of your viewpoint. I've perused all kinds of things on Pubmed and other databases of scientific studies and papers. I've also experienced the psychology of coming up with an idea, doing a Google search, and finding my suspicion confirmed by umpteen different "credible" sources. It's awesome. Nothing feels more validating, and when you bring that idea to the public in a paragraph or article you're packing heat – heavy artillery that no one can argue against.

But over time as my thoughts and opinions have changed and been fine-tuned, I've seen that basically any thought that pops into my head can be confirmed by a long list of studies – from your industry standard double-blind, placebo-controlled, peer-reviewed golden boy to large, correlative epidemiological studies like The China Study (whose author pre-concluded that animal protein is the most vile offender in the diet – ha ha!).

Actually, let's look at the China Study, as that's a good example. The China Study was spearheaded by a strong vegetarian advocate – T. Colin Campbell. In the study, he looked at numerous Chinese provinces to find out what factor correlated most strongly with rates of heart disease, obesity, diabetes, cancer, etc. In this study, the strongest correlation between rising rates of degenerative disease was an increased intake of animal-source protein (according to him, but this has been formidably challenged by a young and very smart statistician named Denise Minger).

A bad researcher, and god-awful scientist, would see this correlation, jump for joy since it lined up with his preconceived beliefs, and shortly thereafter appear on a pedestal before the whole world to tell them of this great discovery while vehemently defending his position against those challenging him with contradictory ideas and data. That's exactly what T. Colin Campbell has done, gathering up other vegetarian-minded doctors and researchers as his wing men, and going on an anti-meat crusade. He's not interested in contradictory ideas, but instead fights off threats to the conclusion of the China Study (threats like, oh I don't know, the fact that nearly every society on earth eats lots of animal protein and several of those societies have no degenerative disease while others, eating the same amount of animal protein, have the highest rates of degenerative disease on earth) by saying something like (paraphrasing again):

"China Study… Bitches!"

These kinds of cheap tactics are used on all sides of the great health debate. Everyone is saying, "This study PROVES I'm right… Bitches!" Funny thing is, everyone is saying something different – some in complete opposition to one another, and each has a vast assortment of studies that they use as confirmation/ammunition against the infidels.

This same tragedy befell Ancel Keys, an excellent laboratory researcher, who looked at some rudimentary correlative data showing that countries that eat more fat had more heart disease than countries that eat less fat. This is what spawned the entire "fat causes heart disease" movement. To Keys it appeared simple, and he jumped to premature conclusions. There was cholesterol in the arteries of people who died of heart attacks, fat was shown in a few studies to raise cholesterol levels in the blood, and the citizens of Japan on a low-fat diet had less heart disease than other nations eating more fat.

The rest is history. Never mind that several of the countries that Keys deleted from that correlative study ate lots of fat and had fewer heart attacks than people eating far less fat (like France). Never mind that there are cultures eating an average of 355 grams of fat per day with no heart disease at all – far less than the Japanese, who happen to suffer from high levels of stroke, a disease with an almost identical pathology to heart disease.

Low-carbers? Well, don't even get me started with that. They've done a fantastic job at showing that insulin resistance and rising insulin levels are a key biomarker for virtually all degenerative diseases. I'll give them that. Their belief that carbohydrate ingestion causes that is one of the most easily-refuted hypotheses on earth. Traditional cultures eating very high carbohydrate diets had phenomenally low blood sugar and insulin levels – far lower than anyone on a low-carb diet, which is probably why those cultures had no heart disease, diabetes, obesity, and so on. I help people lower their insulin resistance and insulin levels routinely by having them increase the carbohydrate content of their diets.

Confused yet? Good. If you are not confused, then you have been seduced by one of the various cookie-cutter theories on Western disease, and the horrendous, evangelistic scientists that head up these religions. My own beliefs on macronutrients and disease are best described by this old saying of mine: "Fat causes disease? Carbs? What next, air?"

I on the other hand, am an excellent scientist in the true spirit of the word "science," and I know of no other source of health information that is taking a more purist scientific approach to unlocking the mysteries of nutrition and human health. My approach is not isolated, but broad, all-inclusive, and totally comprehensive. If I come to one conclusion, then I hold this conclusion's toes to the fire. I challenge it with every angle I can come up with. I am willing and eager to radically change my thoughts about something if I encounter information that gives me a more sophisticated viewpoint on the matter – or reveals variables that I had yet to take into consideration. I'm seeking to find the truth, and expand my knowledge – not prove that I'm right, and expand my dominion.

For example, if a study shows that people with the highest salt intakes have a 30% greater risk of developing hypertension, I make note. However, if the Kuna Indians living on islands outside of Panama eat tons of salt, and have absolutely ZERO cases of hypertension in every member of their population at any age, then the search deepens. Salt may be somehow involved in developing hypertension, but clearly, given that insight, it is not the primary causal factor behind developing high blood pressure. A more reasonable theory that could be birthed from such insights is that something in the Western diet screws up kidney function (I'm not making this theory, just throwing it out there to help you get the concept), and when Westerners eat salt, they are more likely to develop hypertension from it. And so the search continues.

Or let's say that the Pima Indians of Arizona have higher blood sugar and insulin levels the more carbohydrates they ingest – thus aging them faster and putting them at greater risk of developing diabetes, obesity, heart disease, and other ailments. Yet, diabetes and obesity was completely unknown to them when they were eating a diet consisting of 70% of their calories as carbohydrate in the form of wheat, corn, potatoes, squash, and beans – far more carbohydrates than they eat now. Clearly, this adds complexity, and telling them all to eat fewer carbohydrates lacks true scientific integrity and real, causal insight. For a theory to really be validated, it must pass through ALL of the many scientific fitness tests. It must not be refuted by history, epidemiology, observation, personal experience, common sense, and more.

My research style was best summarized by a long-time follower who did jump on board my choo-choo train of thought – to discover that yes, in fact, I really do pass everything I believe through a rigorous set of scrutiny and continue to seek out formidable challenges against those beliefs. Timmy writes:

"Matt Stone is not your run-of-the-mill health [writer]. Although he may sound rigid in his views, he is not only receptive to, but actually seeks out cognitive dissonance. His concern is not with maintaining and spreading blind faith in an idealized diet/lifestyle. Rather, he operates like a scientist, constantly updating and revising his theories in order that they conform more closely with reality. In line with his goal, his research has been expansive and open-ended. Although Matt does not have a medical degree — and therefore may not be able to wade through dense published medical articles with the same facility or level of comprehension as, say, Stephen at WholeHealthSource — he probably has developed a more comprehensive understanding of the underlying nutritional/metabolic theories advanced by nutritionists and doctors alike in the past century than just about any credentialed "expert" you will ever meet. He does this because it's his passion. He only charges money for some of his work because, huge dork that he is, this passion of his has kind of taken over his life. Guy's gotta make a living somehow.

Over the past three years, as he has gobbled through tombs of nutrition literature, his views have radically evolved. At each stage, he spoke as if he had finally attained nutritional enlightenment, only to change his mind a few months later upon exposure to conflicting information or new perspectives on old information. Some would view his inability to stick rigidly to a specific set of internally consistent dietary stipulations as vice, but I see this as his strongest virtue; it has enabled him to avoid the confirmation bias pitfall most nutrition researchers fall into. Over the past couple of years, his principal theories HAVE grown more stable, suggesting he has refined his ideas to the point where they are internally consistent with the preponderance of legitimate research…

I'm no evangelist for the 180 crusade. Matt Stone certainly doesn't have all the answers, nor do I expect he ever will, but he is a passionate researcher, a powerful thinker, and, in my opinion, a man of high integrity. I'd sooner take his advice than my doctor's any day."

Anyway, I thought it was important to address this before you go snooping around for unsubstantiated claims. I mean, why you would give any of my conclusions the time of day when Gary Taubes has over 100 pages of specific references to back up his claims while my references can be packed into just a few pages – and are mostly books, some dating back a century?

...Because those tactics are cheap, remove human logic and critical thinking and analysis from the picture, and dis-empower the reader. It's how people fall head over heels for short-lived, dead-end, dangerous, and narrow-minded health beliefs and approaches. If anything, I hope to educate and empower readers to think for themselves so they can avoid this seductive trap in the future, not brainwash them into total agreement. Or, more simply, this is what I'm trying to say – a comment I left on the 180 blog the morning of writing this:

"I don't rely on "cheap" tactics like using scientific studies to prove a pre-asserted hypothesis. Instead, I incorporate reasoning, logic, history, observation, and more.

That's what makes [180degreehealth] superior to other [health information] that relies on isolated studies that are fully citable....

Anyone can prove whatever they want. It's easy. I could "prove," via those mechanisms that carbs are the devil, fat is the devil, protein is the devil, grains destroy your digestive tract, grains are the ultimate food for digestive health, fruit is the devil, fruit is the salvation of mankind, dairy is the perfect food, dairy is atherogenic, dairy causes autoimmune disease, dairy cures autoimmune disease, fat makes you fat, fat makes you thin...

No wonder everyone else is so confused. I would be too if this is what I primarily relied upon to investigate the vast topic of human health."

Macronutrient Wars

The **Macronutrients**: Carbohydrates, Fats, and Proteins

Like a lot of people, I was easily excited by a lot of the low-carb biased research that I came across in the first couple of years of my health and nutrition research. I'm a natural contrarian, and with my background as a butter and foie gras-slingin' chef at some of the most absurdly expensive and over the top restaurants on earth, I fell right into the low-carb lair. I loved Weston A. Price's "butter is a health food" message. I couldn't wait, after eating a primarily vegetarian diet for years, to dig into some monster steaks and untrimmed pork chops. Some days I would just drink cream straight out of the container. Wow. I was in heaven.

And my initial results on a low-carb diet were amazing. In the past I had been one of those constantly-hungry guys. I had a serious sugar addiction, or so I thought. Those "low blood sugar" episodes seemed quite common, and I had the typical roller coaster ride that many on a high-carbohydrate diet report – and which the low-carb diet is powerful medicine for. So yes, low-carb was a life changer. What a difference. I lost my appetite, spontaneously grew muscle, started getting up at dawn with tons of energy without setting an alarm clock, had a constant and reliable mood for the first time in my life, and more. I thought low-carb was the greatest thing since sliced ham (not bread), at least at first I did (we're talking low-moderate carb, about 100 grams per day, not ketogenic low-carb or Atkins low-carb).

So I bit on the low-carb message hook, line, and sinker. It all seemed to make so much sense in the context of what I was feeling.

In particular, I bought into the low-carb theory on insulin resistance and how it develops.

For the newbies to the health and nutrition discussion, insulin resistance is a hormonal state in the body in which cells become unresponsive to the hormone insulin. To override the dysfunction, extra insulin is secreted to do the job. With this chronically-elevated level of insulin comes greater storage of ingested food into fat cells, and an inhibition of fat release from the cells to be burned for energy. Eventually, blood glucose levels tend to rise as well, particularly after meals. These are the baby steps on the yellow-brick-road to type 2 diabetes and serious weight problems.

The general belief about insulin resistance is that spiking insulin repeatedly, which happens every time you ingest a large quantity of food – particularly protein and carbohydrates, leads to the cells closing down and no longer accepting glucose. These big rises, according to the theories, and the greater the insulin rise, the more the cells become insulin resistant. You hear the phrase "wears out the insulin system over time" repeated frequently.

But this wasn't making sense with some of the new information I was reviewing, and my own personal experience. For starters, it is well known – totally irrefutable in fact, that gaining weight by force-feeding yourself, whether you are thin or fat, makes it increasingly difficult to gain weight the higher your weight gets. This makes no sense according to the low-carb theories. Their theory is a simple positive feedback system, in which the more you eat, the higher your insulin goes. The higher your insulin goes, the more insulin resistant you become. The more insulin resistant you become the hungrier you get and the more efficiently you store body fat. That's the theory. When overfeeding; however, whether it's with lots of carbs, lots of fat, or a mixture of the two – it doesn't work this way at all.

In fact, it is unmistakably a negative feedback system, in which the more you eat above your appetite, and the more sedentary you are to minimize the amount of calories you burn, the more the body fights back against this surplus by:

- Raising the Metabolism
- Decreasing hunger
- Increasing physical energy
- Increasing pulse rate
- Increasing body temperature
- Increasing the rate of lipolysis (burning fat for energy)

And the list goes on. These are all the homeostatic feedback mechanisms that regulate body weight kicking in. Whether thin or fat, virtually all humans share this same physiology. The more you eat above your level of appetite, the more difficult it becomes to continue gaining weight. Coming across this paragraph in Russ Farris's *The Potbelly Syndrome* was certainly an eye-opener as well, as Farris also challenged the belief that overeating and sedentary behavior leads to insulin resistance:

"Insulin resistance leads to weight gain, but most health professionals believe that the opposite is true. If obesity does cause insulin resistance, then we would expect people who are overfed to become more insulin resistant, but that is not the case. Researchers in Indianapolis overfed six slender, active, young adults for several weeks... Five of the six subjects became LESS insulin resistant!"

Oh I know what you're saying now – they were "slender and young." Old, fat people don't respond that way. If you thought that, you'd be wrong. ALL humans tend to respond that way. In fact, in my experience, the fatter a person is, the MORE difficult it is for them to gain weight above their weight "set point." Several overweight people have even begun losing weight immediately upon attempting to eat as much food as they can – albeit nutritious food.

"I must agree that eating like a fiend cuts out all cravings -and- I've lost 100 pounds over the last year eating like a fiend. The weight is coming off naturally and I'm never deprived and I don't waste hours at a gym. People think I'm lying to them when I tell them how I lost the weight. :)"

-Sasha

But let's back up for a minute.

As I came across more and more information suggesting that the low-carb theory absolutely couldn't be right, the more outside of the box I began to think. Think that carbohydrates cause insulin resistance? Well first off note that there are 5 billion thin people in the world, and about 99% of those people are eating a high-carbohydrate diet – typically 50-80% of total caloric intake. Also take note that there are nearly 500 species of primates, and most of those primates derive 70-90% of their dietary calories from carbohydrates without showing any signs of insulin resistance or metabolic syndrome. Next consider that there are several populations still left on earth today with no signs of insulin resistance. That means no documented cases of type 2 diabetes, no high blood sugars, no obesity – not even a single case of heart disease.

This is the health status of the Kitavans living on an isolated island in Papua New Guinea. Average blood sugar levels run between 60 and 70 mg/dl at any age. Carbohydrate comprises roughly 70% of their caloric intake. This is just one example. This has also been seen in relatively modern times amongst rural Zulu's, Ugandans, and so on.

Low-carbers make this out to be some kind of special adaptation that these people have to tolerate and metabolize carbs. Sorry Charlie. People of this same genetic lineage, when exposed to the Western lifestyle and diet, suffer from even MORE diabetes, insulin resistance, heart disease, and obesity – across the board. Clearly there's more to the story than the belief that carbs = insulin = obesity/insulin resistance/diabetes/death. Embarrassingly, it's whites of European descent that have the lowest obesity and diabetes rates on Western fare – who are the best adapted to an "obesigenic" diet, and it's typically whites of European descent rambling on and on about how humans are ill-adapted to carbohydrate consumption (with the exception of those genetic freaks in Kitava of course!). This is certainly what was found on the Pacific island of Kosrae…

"In 1994 scientists in Jeff Friedman's group examined blood samples taken in the course of Auerbach's islandwide screening of all 2,286 adult Kosraeans. Preliminary findings suggest that European genes inherited from randy New England whalers and other ethnically European visitors are, in Kosraeans, protective against obesity and diabetes. It appears that

the more genetically 'European' an islander, the less likely he or she is to be
obese or diabetic under the current conditions of plenty."

-Ellen Ruppel Shell; *The Hungry Gene*

Another example that I often bring up is the Pima Indians
of the American Southwest. There is much to be learned from
the Pima, as they have by far the greatest rate of insulin
resistance, obesity, and type 2 diabetes of any sub-population
on earth. The original theory was that they had "thrifty genes"
which made them more susceptible to food abundance. They
naturally had a physiology for fat storage to get through times
of famine. This initial theory has been debunked (but in some
ways remains very true – they certainly have very thrifty
metabolisms, and it is in large part hereditary, but I'm not going
to discuss that until later).

Low-carb author Gary Taubes was somehow able, through
a Houdini-like act of twisting logic, to pin this problem on
carbohydrates. Carbohydrates eh?

Just across the border there are Pima Indians living in the
mountains of Northern Mexico, the Maycoba, that are lean and
healthy – a night and day difference from their genetic twins
living in Arizona. Is it their low-carb diet that saves them?
Have the Pimas always subsisted off of a low-carbohydrate diet
until those darn carbs were introduced to them on the Indian
Reservation? Robert Pool reports:

"Researchers at the NIDDK in Phoenix have estimated that the
traditional Pima diet took about 70 percent of its calories in the form of
carbohydrates, 15 percent in protein, and 15 percent in fat. By the 1950's
the proportions had changed to 61 percent carbohydrate, 15 percent in

protein, and 24 percent in fat. In 1971 it was 44 percent carbohydrate, 12 percent protein, and 44 percent fat – a tripling of the fat content."

Don't worry, this is not a segue into a spiel on how low-fat diets are awesome – they aren't, not in today's society at least because low-fat diets make normal, satisfying food very fattening when it otherwise wouldn't be.   But you can clearly see it is not the carbohydrate, in and of itself, that is the chief culprit, as the staples of the healthy Maycoba and the healthy, obesity and diabetes-free traditional Pima were wheat, corn, potatoes, beans, and squash.

So yes, anyone who hasn't been seduced by low-carb biased half-truths about insulin, obesity, type 2 diabetes, and so on knows that carbohydrates are not the cause of insulin resistance and related health problems. Those that have moved beyond that conclusion usually blame food abundance and sedentary behavior for causing the diabesity epidemic.

This too, is a joke. Speaking of the Kitavans, Staffan Lindeberg, a Swedish researcher that paid these people a visit in the 1980's to thoroughly examine their health, diet, and lifestyle notes:

"It is obvious from our investigations that lack of food is an unknown concept, and that the surplus of fruits and vegetables regularly rots or is eaten by dogs."

Hmmm, some scarcity that is. Yet, when people in neighboring islands with virtually identical genetics are exposed to a Western diet and lifestyle, they develop obesity at greater rates than people elsewhere and are dubbed as having "thrifty genes." Makes sense to me. Wait, no it doesn't.

But why would one group of people, like the Kitavans, have unlimited food abundance and not become overweight while people in industrialized nations have obesity rates up to the stratosphere? That's really the bigger, more important question in the grand scheme of things. The main question in search of an answer is what makes one person eat more food than they burn through metabolic processes and exercise? Clearly there's something about the Kitavan lifestyle and diet that prohibits them from eating more than they use – or more precisely - storing more fat than they burn.

But make no mistake. If you think that the calories in-calories out equation can be consciously-regulated with willpower and discipline long-term, statistically-speaking you'd be very VERY wrong. The world's leading obesity researcher, Rudy Leibel, hasn't solved many things in his lifetime of obesity research, but he has come to one firm conclusion:

"We don't think body weight can be consciously regulated."

It can't. In fact, a 70-year old person with 70 pounds of body fat has stored only one peanut per day more than they have burned. No one can control a process so precise. It's like trying to increase your oxygen levels by breathing more. Cutting carbs, fats, or calories (dieting) is like trying to hold your breath. The longer you do it, the more your body resists it until you finally gasp for air – taking in more than ever to overcome the short-term deficit you induced.

"Diets all follow a similar pattern. By eliminating or severely restricting items from your diet, your body will, for a time, lose weight. You may lose weight quickly at first, but then the rate at which you lose weight

30

will start to slow. Eventually, you stop losing weight altogether. You find yourself in the unfortunate position of having to restrict yourself, count calories, or follow unnatural eating schedules, not to lose weight, but to simply maintain your current level of body fat. You feel like you're running on a treadmill that just keeps going faster. The longer you go, the harder it gets."

-Jon Gabriel; *The Gabriel Method*

Fat of course has been another scapegoat of the weight loss community. It has more calories so it makes you fat! This too, is false – not only as it pertains to weight but as it pertains to insulin resistance and type 2 diabetes.

When it comes to modern illnesses, there are no firm and consistent correlations between fat intake, carbohydrate intake, or protein intake. Fat, carbohydrates, and protein are called the macronutrients. I call the senseless masturdebating that goes on in the health and nutrition field "Macrontrient Warfare." Like tic-tac-toe in the movie *War Games* (those who have followed my work for a long time will have recognized that's about the most I've ever written without an 80's movie reference), the war cannot be won. Just when you think you find a correlation, something comes along to totally refute the idea.

Like the Chinese for example. They eat lots of carbohydrates, very little fat, and very little protein. The results of the famous "China Study" performed by vegetarian evangelist T. Colin Campbell and associates showed strong correlations between protein intake and heart disease/obesity/cancer/diabetes. The less protein consumed – particularly animal protein, the fewer the degenerative diseases. Wow! Way to go! Finally the answer!

Oops, travel to Mongolia just to the North and you'll find very little of any of the above-listed health problems resulting from their diet of mutton and full-fat milk. Travel even farther away to Kenya and you will see a tribe of people with ZERO documented cases of diabetes, obesity, or heart disease also consuming nothing but meat and milk – basically.

Fat intake is also highly variable. This passage by legendary nutritional mind Roger J. Williams points, once again, to factors far outside of any magical macronutrient ratio as being the root cause of modern disease. Of course, this passage could easily refer to the variability of carbohydrate content of the diets of "peoples of the earth free of heart disease (and insulin resistance, obesity, diabetes, etc.)":

"In an extensive review of the various peoples of the earth who have little or no atherosclerosis and are virtually free of heart disease, Lowenstein found that the fat intake ranged from 21 grams per day to as much as 355 grams per day. In both the Somalis and the Samburus of East Africa, the diet is from 60 to 65 percent fat (animal), and yet they are nearly free from atherosclerosis and heart attacks. While it might be argued that ethnic differences are involved here, population groups of wide ethnic variation have been reported who subsist on high fat, high cholesterol, high caloric diets while remaining virtually free of coronary heart disease.

"In the text we have mentioned the report by Mann and his colleagues of the Masai tribe who subsist on a diet excessively high in butter fat (and cholesterol), the fat constituting as much as 60 percent of the total calories consumed, yet are virtually free of cardiovascular disease. Gsell and Mayer report that the isolated peoples of the Loetschental valley in the Valaisian Alps of Switzerland habitually eat a diet high in saturated fat and cholesterol, high in calories, but evidence low serum cholesterol values and little cardiovascular disorders...

"It is clear, therefore, that adult males of widely differing ethnic stock can subsist on a high fat, high cholesterol, high caloric diet, and yet remain relatively free of cardiovascular disorders. Even if prevailing views are to the contrary, I think that the evidence points strongly toward the conclusion that the nutritional environment of the body cells — involving minerals, amino acids, and vitamins — is crucial, and that the amount of fat or cholesterol consumed is relatively inconsequential...

"A large amount of information, based upon carefully controlled scientific experiments, indicated very strongly that vitamin B6 is another key nutrient which is often present in inadequate amounts in the cellular environment of those whose arteriosclerosis is extreme. Experiments with monkeys have yielded clear-cut results. When they are rendered vitamin B6 deficient, they develop arteriosclerosis rapidly. When monkeys are fed diets supplemented with vitamin B6, they have much lower levels of cholesterol in the blood than when these diets are not supplemented. The animals on the supplemented diet eat much more food than the others, and since their diet contains cholesterol, they get far more cholesterol into their bodies. This does not matter, however; the extra vitamin B6 they get allows them to dispose of the surplus, with the result that their cholesterol blood levels are not as high as in those animals that consume less cholesterol."

It is certainly interesting that the Masai tribe mentioned above, engulfing a gallon of whole milk every day of their lives, have average serum cholesterol levels of roughly 125 mg/dl. Delusional low-fat biased researchers claim that they must have developed some kind of evolutionary adaptation to keep from turning that saturated fat into cholesterol. The Masai, as mentioned above, have no obesity, insulin resistance, or heart disease. Yet, when they move out of rural areas and into the city where they begin eating and living in the typical "Western" way, their cholesterol levels nearly double and they start suffering the same degenerative ills found in the rest of the world just like everybody else. Just like what happens to the Kitavans on a totally different diet. No special immunity. Sorry. Try again.

Okay, it's because in the city they don't exercise as much!

"The usual hypothesis that this may be due to differences in physical activity is doubtful, since men traditionally stop acting as warriors around the age of 25, and later their wives do most of the daily work."
                    -Staffan Lindeberg; *Food and Western Disease* (2010)

Crap. I can't use any of the mainstream or even alternative health and nutrition/lifestyle beliefs here. Guess we'll have to ditch them all.

Anyway, I included this chapter, not to make your head hurt, but to help you begin to overcome your diet phobias. If you're a seasoned diet veteran, and odds are if you're reading a book entitled *Diet Recovery* you probably are, there's a lot of reprogramming needing to be done. If some low-carb loser told you that eating carbohydrates will give you diabetes and are the cause of the obesity epidemic, you've been led astray, and it's probably undermining your health and sanity to live in low-carb prison.

If some mainstream doctor or news source has led you to believe that eating fat is going to raise your cholesterol (false), that cholesterol has something to do with heart disease (false), that saturated fat is REALLY gonna kill ya (false) hopefully you were reassured by seeing that some people ate 355 grams of fat per day with not only a lower rate of heart disease, but hardly a single case of heart disease at any age.

And don't even get me started on veganism, fruitarianism, etc. If you've been seduced by one of these self-deprecating, lean muscle mass-obliterating, libido-crushing, depression-inducing, family and friend-alienating food religions – well, may God have mercy on your soul.

Don't worry, I've fallen for just about all of them myself. The word "dipshit" comes to mind. Food-combining, all meat diets, low-fat vegan (for a very short time followed by a 15-pound fat gain), 30-day milk fasts, "cleanses," absurd amounts of the absolute worst kind of exercise – endurance exercise (think 140 mile bike rides and hiking 15 miles per day, 7 days per week), self-imposed starvation to the point where I literally lost my mind and some hair off the top along with it… and worst of all, the OCD mindset that accompanies "pinballing" between all these different dietary utopias is perhaps the worst symptom of diet disease.

But I'd like to think I have now moved past that phase. I've climbed that mountain and have taken thousands of people worldwide with me. Hopefully your baggage is packed (around your belly, hips, butt, and thighs), and you're ready to come with me. Not only can I help you take some big steps in overcoming your diet mentality, but I consider myself to be far and away the world's leading expert on rehabilitating the one thing that really does determine the level of your overall health, vitality, and resistance to disease both infectious and degenerative – your metabolism.

We don't have to do all these barbaric, socially-crippling, restricted diets to be healthy. In fact, every single one of them undermines our health and makes us weaker, softer, and often fatter than we ever would have been if we had just eaten the food and not tried so hard to "do the right thing." And they make us weaker specifically by reducing metabolic rate – which is without question after my decade of research the single biggest way in which a person can undermine his or her health. This was probably the cause of whatever health problem or "weight problem" you had to begin with, and dieting only made the root cause worse over time.

But you can be rebuilt! I think just about anyone can, and I've seen it all. This book will show you how.

You can start simply by realizing that your body needs protein, fat, and carbohydrates every single second of every single day from the time you are born until you die. Supply them from nutritious sources with religious fervor (instead of playing ping-pong back and forth between various diets that restrict something). Your patience here will have a payoff. Sorry no big discoveries in nutrition since the advice to "eat three squares a day." Our abandonment of this simple principle is our greatest wrong turn, but it's never too late to sell whatever stock you're invested in and go long on "Three Squares (TSQ)." Well, at least 3 meals. We can start there.

The Metabolism

The bottom line is that your metabolism is your bottom line. With age our metabolism starts its slow descent into oblivion. And that's precisely why, as we age, we become ever more prone to develop heart disease, cancer, type 2 diabetes, and other degenerative ailments. The secret is to protect and prolong the number of years your metabolism is at its highest. When you manage to do that, you keep a higher ratio of lean body mass to body fat, have greater functionality, more strength and mobility, more energy, and more zest for life in general.

Of course, some people are born with a slow metabolism right from the start. Actually, I've been increasingly led to believe that just about everyone in the modern world is born in a hypometabolic state – causing astronomical rises in allergies, food allergies, asthma, autism, autoimmune disease, early puberty, poor eyesight, and childhood obesity (just to name a few) – which is rising much faster than the rate of adult obesity.

And having a slow metabolism doesn't necessarily mean you're a fatty. The slowest metabolisms I've seen were in the highly underweight people who dug themselves into a deep, dark, vegan or low-carb tunnel (with body temperatures below 95 degrees F, yikes!).

But I assure you this really is a widespread phenomenon. Even the *New York Times* reported on how the global average body temperature is on a steady decline, putting out an eerie article entitled "Rethinking 98.6."

The basics work something kind of like this…

When metabolism falls, your sex hormone production falls (infertility, loss of sex drive, loss of period, erectile dysfunction, PMS). When metabolism falls, your youth hormone (growth hormone) falls, and you lose your ability to build muscle tissue, perform athletically, and you lose muscle tissue. When metabolism falls your rate of fat burning decreases and your body starts to manufacture more fat out of the food you eat. This causes a rise in triglycerides in your blood leading to insulin resistance (the precursor to metabolic syndrome and type 2 diabetes), increased appetite, increased storage of the food you eat into fat cells, and so forth. When metabolism falls you produce more estrogen (both men and women) and the opposing hormones testosterone and progesterone are produced in smaller quantities. This unopposed estrogen is a prime culprit in many cancers, osteoporosis, infertility (just like taking an estrogen pill as birth control), heart disease, autoimmune disease (which women suffer from much more often than men) and countless other conditions relating to estrogen's ability to deprive cells of oxygen and energy.

This of course is just the short list. When the mitochondrial energy production and respiration of every single one of your bajillion (rough estimate) cells is impaired, there is no end to how it can manifest in terms of real health problems and an overall lack of vitality. Here are some more specific scenarios…

Let's say you are a young woman not having your period. A low metabolism shuts down the production of progesterone, which is essential for menstruation. Bring the metabolism up and menstruation can reappear and become perfectly regular once again, which has happened consistently with more than a dozen women following some of the guidelines we'll cover later, including my own ex-girlfriend who failed to menstruate for a year at one point in her life (after running marathons and eating a low-carb diet). By the way, to avoid any confusion, "RRARF" refers to the name of my diet rehab program…

"Speaking of periods, I think mine have been regained by this diet. For about 5 years my periods were sporadic at best and the last year there was no period. Apparently if you don't have a period for 12 months or more you are considered to be entering menopause. I'm only 38 at the moment so definitely not prepared for menopause. I tried taking hormones previously without any success. My sex hormones were very low where they were supposed to be higher. My growth hormone was virtually non-existent. My endocrinologist had no answers for me other than I was getting older. Within 30 days of starting this diet, I got a normal period without any PMS or pain! Normally I'd be crippled by the pain in my lower back and pelvis. First 3 periods were also normal. Then the next few were getting lighter and shorter and this month it was late. About a week ago I stopped my thyroid meds in preparation for a blood test. Well guess what? One week after stopping the meds my period came back totally normal! So it seems my thyroid dose had become too high. This could all be coincidence of course, but it's looking pretty good for the RRARF way of life."

-Princess

Overcoming infertility is a consistent report as well, for the exact same reasons…

"Hey Matt, I've been following your work since probably Sep 2009 and I just wanted to write in with a little story and a thank you.

For reference, I am a 26 year old female, normal weight (5'7", 133 lbs.). I had been mostly paleo and lowish carb for many years. I started in my very early 20's for health reasons, not weight reasons, but all my old health problems were creeping back. I had always been fairly lax with my diet (hence the "mostly" paleo and the "lowish" carb), so I figured I just needed to tighten things up a bit.

To kick start, I decided to do Mark Sisson's Primal Challenge back in August 2009. Worst idea ever! I only got worse and added some new bad stuff into the mix, like extreme severe bloating. I called it my food baby because after eating I would literally look 7 months pregnant. Not getting what was going on, I got even MORE restrictive and decided to go meat-only for a week or two to sort myself out. Didn't even last 3 days on that. Also sometime in there (don't remember when exactly), my doctor diagnosed me as slightly hypothyroid with a TSH of 3.2 and put me on a low dose of Armour. I took it for 6 weeks and got my blood re-tested and my numbers were actually worse.

So at this point a few good things happened. After my 3 miserable days on meat only I found your website and Diana Schwarzbein's books. I finally had something to explain why my thyroid had gotten sluggish after all my years of "healthy" eating and how I could fix it.

I did Schwarzbein by the book for 2 weeks and saw modest improvements. Then I was hit with a freak random attack of ulcerative in October (which I've never had before or since, but let me tell you pooping blood and mucus is NOT FUN) and kind of reverted to my old ways throughout the holiday season.

I kept reading your stuff though, and back in the beginning of January I decided what the heck, I'll go for it. I don't know if I've specifically been OVER eating, but I have been making a concerted effort to not skip meals (something I used to do frequently) and I have been making sure I eat at least one starchy carb with every meal. I've also been avoiding sugar (even fruit mostly) and vegetable oils. I am eating a ton more grains, beans and dairy than I have in years.

Well I am one happy camper now, let me tell you! I think I gained a pound or three, but in the process I have regained a lot of health. My horrible bloat went away, my energy has gotten a little better (I've been very lethargic for awhile), my body temp has gone up a bit, I no longer get stomach aches/nausea, my bowels became regular (I used to joke that I had a shitty shitter), I haven't had a single headache since I started (I used to get several per week).

I could go on, but overall I used to feel like crap and now overall I feel pretty good. And the big one - after 18 months - EIGHTEEN MONTHS! - of trying and failing miserably (emphasis on the miserably), finally, this month, I was able to get pregnant! Coincidence? Probably not."

The above was written by a prolific and popular Paleo Nutrition blogger.

Or let's say you are constipated all the time and have heartburn every time you eat and feel bloated. When the metabolism rises food begins traveling through the digestive tract more rapidly. This causes less gas and bloating because less fermentation and putrefaction is taking place in the digestive tract. You are no longer having feces hang out in your lower bowel so long that those little turds become dehydrated marbles either – stools stay moist and pass quickly and easily. In addition, with an increase in metabolic activity the body produces more of the hormone gastrin, which turns your stomach into a furnace, burning up a big, mixed meal like it was nothing with no belching or heartburn afterward. I personally had heartburn for three years after every meal on every possible weird restricted diet you can imagine (aggravated the most by endurance exercise – hiking), but this went away within a week and hasn't returned following the guidelines coming up later in this book…

"For those that deal with constipation, I have been constipated my whole life and needed enemas just to go. I've done daily enemas for over 2 years now and by the 2nd week of RRARF I was going by myself once a day. Now for the last 2 weeks straight I not only didn't need an enema but am consistently going 3x a day on my own. The pride I now have as I leave the bathroom-well formed, good consistency, a joy that can be truly appreciated by the constipated.

-Sheri

Or hey, let's say you have hypoglycemia or you are not excreting toxic material properly in your liver. Thyroid activity exerts a lot of control over the functionality of your liver. For example, when metabolism falls as with excessive dieting or in anorexia, the liver loses its ability to store carbohydrate in the form of glycogen. Someone with a slow metabolism often suffers from terrible bouts of hypoglycemia after eating – either in the true sense (actual low blood levels of glucose) or in the pseudo sense (irritability, shakiness, nervousness, anxiety following meals – from the adrenals turning on for the emergency liberation of more glucose from muscle cells). Restore the metabolism and this clears up pretty reliably. There's no doubt it, at the very least, improves dramatically.

Or how about you are a type 2 diabetic or pre-diabetic with insulin resistance and have trouble clearing glucose out of your bloodstream. Increasing metabolic activity lowers stress hormones (cortisol) and decreases insulin resistance, improving glucose clearance (the ultimate sign of improved insulin sensitivity – meaning your muscle cells are responding to insulin and letting the sugar and amino acids come in). I first noticed this effect myself when I lowered my fasting and post-meal blood sugar substantially (26% in 30 days) and to near superhuman levels (fasting 67 mg/dl, 1-hour postmeal 75 mg/dl – even after 2 large baked potatoes). But I've seen this repeatedly, even in those who have gained weight (the supposed cause of insulin resistance according to the mainstream) and even in the most severe case of insulin resistance I've come across, such as that seen in a woman who has dieted for decades and has had multiple weight loss surgeries, Lisa…

"When I started reading 180DegreeHealth about a year ago my glucose was hovering dangerously in the 400-500 range. I was doing "low carb" at the time. After making adjustments in my diet to include starch in proportion to protein (with the fat intact) and eating to appetite my sugars are now in the 200s. Big difference. As I continue to heal I expect to overcome my Type II diabetes completely.

Matt's Rehabilitative Rest and ReFeeding (RRARF) has helped me to stabilize my moods, calm my appetite, reduce cravings, lower my blood sugar, grow back some hair, heal my digestive tract and feel better overall."

Anyway, the metabolism is central to all bodily functions. It is the grand master. Nothing that takes place in your body isn't directly impacted by it. That's not to say that some diet and lifestyle strategy is enough to miraculously cure all people's health problems completely. That's an unreasonable expectation for anything. But it is powerful, it does work to bring up the body temperature at least part of the way back to normal if not all the way to normal and above (I actually started a "Hot Chicks Club" for all the 180 women hitting 99.0 degrees

F or higher consistently during the second half of their menstrual cycle), and does so more effectively than even thyroid medication. Rises in body temperature of 3.0 degrees F in 30 days or less is actually common.

But since many of you have NEVER heard of this outrageously simple-sounding fundamental of all mammalian biology, and your doctor has never once said anything about your body temperature even if it was the same as that of a floating salmon, we'll continue to explore some of the connections between metabolism/body temperature/mitochondrial activity and the many facets of disease – including the one everyone is so freaked out about – metabolic syndrome and the belly fat that often accompanies it.

Needless to say these many connections compelled me to use my knowledge of food and simple biochemistry to craft a diet and lifestyle program to raise body temperature in the most efficient way possible. It's a multi-faceted approach to increasing mitochondrial activity and the metabolism in general – for disease prevention and reversal, greater infectious disease resistance, better digestion, greater overall vitality, and on and on and on. You'll hear more about it later. But let's just say for now that in theory I figured it should work. Its actual performance with real world health scenarios and its ability to bring body temperature up has been beyond shocking compared to what I theoretically thought might happen. It exceeded everything I ever thought possible, like I said – making even high-dose thyroid medication look like a joke in comparison.

Confirmation

There has been some pretty strong confirmation of the fact that mitochondrial activity/metabolism is really the kingpin in modern disease. Consider, for example, what was written by Stephan Guyenet, the driving force behind the truly groundbreaking website: www.wholehealthsource.blogspot.com. Pay particular attention to the fact that butyric acid (a type of short-chain saturated fatty acid) sped up metabolism, and therefore got these little rat bastards out of starvation mode – which had an appetite-suppressing effect, increased physical activity, and increased body heat production as all signs of their metabolic syndrome were reversed:

Susceptible strains of rodents fed high-fat diets overeat, gain fat and become profoundly insulin resistant. Dr. Jianping Ye's group recently published a paper showing that the harmful metabolic effects of a high-fat diet (lard and soybean oil) on mice can be prevented, and even reversed, using a short-chain saturated fatty acid called butyric acid (hereafter, butyrate). Here's a graph of the percent body fat over time of the two groups:

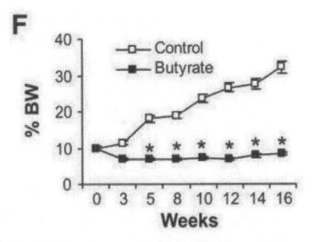

The butyrate-fed mice remained lean and avoided metabolic problems. Butyrate increased their energy expenditure by increasing body heat production and modestly increasing physical activity. It also massively increased the function of their mitochondria, the tiny power plants of the cell.

Butyrate lowered their blood cholesterol by approximately 25 percent, and their triglycerides by nearly 50 percent. It lowered their fasting insulin by nearly 50 percent, and increased their insulin sensitivity by nearly 300 percent*. The investigators concluded:

"Butyrate and its derivatives may have potential application in the prevention and treatment of metabolic syndrome in humans.

There's one caveat, however: the butyrate group ate less food. Something about the butyrate treatment caused their food intake to decline after 3 weeks, dropping roughly 20% by 10 weeks. The investigators cleverly tried to hide this by normalizing food intake to body weight, making it look like the food intake of the comparison group was dropping as well (when actually it was staying the same as this group was gaining weight).

Thanks to Stephan for this excellent post. It is without question the best blog post I read on the internet in 2009. To read the whole post, Google: "Guyenet butyric acid." Worth mentioning is the fact that, in traditional diets, butyric acid (and another important short-chain saturated fat... propionic acid) is supplied in greatest abundance by the fermentation of fiber (and what's called resistant starch) in the digestive tract – the very fiber that is removed from refined grain and refined sugar, hypothesized by Hugh Trowell and Denis Burkitt to be the predominant cause of most Western diseases. Like others, these men observed Africans with perfect health, completely free of most modern disease (heart disease, cancer, diabetes, tooth decay, constipation, diverticulosis, etc.) just like Cleave witnessed in the rural Zulu tribe, eating very high-carbohydrate diets built around unrefined plant foods such as grains, legumes, root vegetables, fruits, and vegetables.

I flippin' love the irony there – that the mainstream tells us all to eat a high fiber diet and avoid saturated fat, while fiber's health benefits are most likely attributed to the saturated fat that it is converted to in the digestive tract!

The other primary source of butyric acid is butterfat – the staple of the more or less disease-free people that consume no fiber whatsoever – the Masai tribe of Kenya. George Mann of Vanderbilt University found these people to be 100% free of heart attacks and obesity, even when consuming 3-4 sticks worth of butterfat daily. Coconut, rich in medium chain saturated fats, has similar properties – it shouldn't be a surprise that this is the staple fat of the Kitavans mentioned earlier in the book, as well as many traditional Pacific Islanders also once found (by Ian Prior, Weston A. Price, etc.) to have more or less outstanding health compared to modern standards.

Next in the confirmation lineup is the work of Broda
Barnes and others that monitored body temperature, and
treated patients with an endless array of health problems with
great success solely by increasing body temperature to the ideal
level. This is really the best evidence of the central role played
by the metabolism/mitochondrial activity as a whole. By
simply overriding the low metabolisms of their patients, with no
other means of treatment, many health problems fell into place.
Most promising is the huge drop in heart disease.

In fact, Broda Barnes, who closely monitored over 2,000
patients over 20 years, only had four patients have a heart
attack. Of those four, each was unique. One had just recently
begun seeking treatment from Dr. Barnes. Another was no
longer under his care. This represented a decrease in heart
attack incidence of well over 90% versus the rest of the U.S.
population at the time. Barnes, comparing his figures to people
in the Framingham Heart Study, the largest and most
comprehensive study ever done, noted that those in the study
were 75 times more likely to have a heart attack than one of his
patients. He noticed this by accident, as he was hearing from
other doctors and reading about the increased prevalence of
heart disease in medical journals, but as a practicing doctor, he
had only seen one cardiac event amongst his patients. This is
what led him to start keeping close track, and he documented it
all in the medical literature and later put his findings into a book
entitled, *Solved: The Riddle of Heart Attacks*.

*"One of my recurring objects of thought has been the slowness with which
raw knowledge is assimilated. For example, I have been thinking about
Broda Barnes's work on the prevention of heart disease with thyroid
extract. He did solve much of 'the riddle of heart attacks,' but recent*

48

statements by the Heart Association show that the dominant forces in the health business haven't learned anything at all from his work, which he began 50 years ago. His work is clearly presented, not hard to understand, and it is scientifically so sound that no one challenges it, at least not on the scientific level. It is ignored, rejected by people who choose not to be bothered to read it. How many people have died from heart disease, since his work first became available? (And how many more from cancer, tuberculosis, and other diseases he showed occur mainly among hypothyroid people?)"

-Ray Peat

This is a huge revelatory breakthrough, and the results of modern-day practitioners of Barnes's methods, although not flawless, echo those fantastic results — not just with heart disease, but autoimmune disease, allergies, asthma, chronic pain, constipation, and far too many other health problems to mention here.

One of the more recent developments was a study showing a seamless link between obesity in dogs and low body temperature. The two go together like peanut butter and jelly. At least that was what was reported by Dr. Roberto Refinetti in the *International Journal of Obesity*.

The Times of India summarized the study findings as follows...

> A University of South Carolina Salkehatchie professor has found that fat dogs have lower body temperature, suggesting that obese people may also be having cooler bodies.
>
> Dr. Roberto Refinetti, a professor of psychology and associate dean, studied the relationship between body temperature and body weight in lean and obese dogs.
>
> His findings showed that obese dogs have lower body temperature than lean dogs, and the difference in temperature is enough to account for weight gain.

Refinetti's study explored the theory that obesity may result from a less obvious reduction in energy expenditure: a reduction in body temperature.

The idea is that warm-blooded animals spend much of their energy generating heat to keep the body warm. However, some animals have body temperatures that are naturally lower and therefore do not need to use as much energy to stay warm.

The reduced body temperature would be sufficient to account for body weight gain over several months.

"Although not yet replicated in humans, these results suggest that human obesity may be caused by a small reduction in the temperature at which the body maintains itself," said Refinetti, who collaborated with researchers from the University of Messina in Sicily, Italy.

The study was published in the Aug. 10 issue of the International Journal of Obesity.

The actual study abstract, written in Nerdese, is…

BACKGROUND: Industrialized nations are currently experiencing an obesity epidemic, the causes of which are not fully known. One possible mechanism of enhanced energy efficiency that has received almost no attention is a reduction in the metabolic cost of homeothermy, which could be achieved by a modest lowering of body core temperature. We evaluated the potential of this obesity-inducing mechanism in a canine model of the metabolic syndrome.
METHODS: We compared the rectal temperature of lean dogs and obese dogs by (a) conducting cross-sectional measurements in 287 dogs of many breeds varying greatly in

body size, (b) conducting longitudinal measurements in individual dogs over 7-10 years and (c) tracking rectal temperature of lean and obese dogs at 3-h intervals for 48 consecutive hours in the laboratory.

RESULTS: We found that larger dogs have lower rectal temperatures than smaller dogs and that, for the same body mass, obese dogs have lower rectal temperatures than lean dogs. The results were consistent in the cross-sectional, longitudinal and around-the-clock measurements.

CONCLUSION: These findings document an association between obesity and reduced body temperature in dogs and support the hypothesis that obesity in this and other species of homeotherms may result from an increase in metabolic efficiency achieved by a regulated lowering of body temperature.

Anyway, there are certainly some connections there. And ol' Doc Refinetti is right that this body temperature connection has "received almost no attention." Emphasis on "ALMOST." I've certainly done what I could to highlight the connection. And I'm far from being the first to do so.

The Root Causes

This book isn't necessarily a book about dealing with health problems, although most readers will probably have some or many. It's not even about preventing heart disease, the leading cause of death in industrialized nations. It's more about taking a long, hard look at the destruction and devastation done originally by the modern human diet, and the subsequent and even more severe health consequences most have incurred by adding severe and often extreme dietary restrictions on top of it.

In this section I want to present some of the root causes of the low metabolism epidemic, which will give you a good mental framework for why the rehabilitation template is the way it is. We'll hit exercise too, as this is a very common place in which the majority of people do the worst kind of exercise ever for improving health and body composition – and then of course beat themselves up over their inability to lose weight or whatever, or find it mysterious when they develop autoimmune disease, asthma, food allergies, IBS and other digestive problems, and infertility when it is no mystery at all.

Piecing the whole puzzle together ain't easy, and I've gone into much greater detail already in my books *180 Degree*

Metabolism and *180 Degree Diabetes*. But it's important to get a little background here on the underlying reason why the global metabolism is plummeting and taking our general level of health, vitality, and leanness down with it.

Heredity

We know that most of the health problems we have, obesity and diabetes-proneness in particular, is something we owe primarily to heredity. Notice I did not say "genetics." Genetics implies that it is set in stone and immovable. That's simply not the case. In fact, most of what we inherit from our parents besides the basic genetic template that gives us two eyes, two ears, ten fingers, and ten toes is epigenetic – meaning that certain genes are turned on or off depending on the environmental cues given to the parents prior to your conception. Every event, every dietary choice, the air breathed and the water drunk effects this highly-advanced network of genes designed to prepare the offspring for the lifestyle and environment it's about to enter into.

Pretty cool if you know how to control some of those triggers, which I evidently do as the two sets of parents who have tried RRARF prior to conception have both reported their kids being exceptionally muscular and lean compared to standard references even in early infancy.

Aside from epigenetics, there is also a whole litany of known peri-natal impacts. For example, dieting prior to pregnancy, or even worse – during pregnancy, predisposes the kid to developing obesity and diabetes when it collides with the modern diet…

"They made the rather startling discovery that adult children of mothers exposed to famine during the first two trimesters of their pregnancy were 80

percent more likely to be obese as adults… From this, the researchers theorized that deprivation in the first two trimesters primed these famine victims for a life of scarcity. When food became plentiful after the war, this 'thrifty fetus' effect backfired, with obesity as the consequence. Later, scientists would also note higher rates of heart disease, diabetes, and other chronic disease and even mental illness…"

-Ellen Ruppel Shell; *The Hungry Gene*

Sweet! How many fat-paranoid moms were or had dieted prior to when you were born? I'm guessing a lot. Of course, this was part of their own war against their hatred for fat and their hatred for their own bodies. When you were born and became fat they of course forced you into weight loss programs, made you feel horrible, acted ashamed of you, and induced all kinds of disordered eating behavior (like restricted eating, known to increase the risk of obesity in adulthood as much as any known factor) – all the while activating your "thrifty gene" even more and making you fatter in incremental steps kind of like what happened with this anonymous 180 follower…

"Yesterday morning my waking temperature (under arm) was 95.9 degrees, this morning it was 95.6 degrees. This is pretty low I am guessing. So where do I go from here. My "fat" problems started when I was just about 5 years old and I was a little bit fat so my Mom rushed me to all sorts of docs that put me on low cal fat free diets. In the mean time, all I would drink was sodas and eat crackers and all those other "healthy" fat free foods. I know soda made me fat. So then I really blew up while yo yo dieting. When I was 13 I went on a year long 800 calorie a day diet and lost like 100lbs in a few months and then plateaued. After that year I gained all back and plus some. Many diets after that, always losing, then

gaining with some extra. At age 21, depressed as hell and weighing more than 300lbs, I became easily addicted to crystal meth and stayed there for 3 1/2 long miserable years. While most people lose weight doing meth, I gained weight. I finally quit and never turned back. After I quit it was a month long eating spree. Anyways, my weight at this time was 375lbs. I felt like a monster... I cannot budge from this weight. It seems my body will not let me. I even tried the Atkins diet for several weeks eating less than 20 g carbs a day and still did not even lose 1 pound. It's not like I don't try and work hard. When I diet I do not cheat, I work out, I do everything they say I should do and STILL nothing."

Don't worry, this person's in a much better place now – with a high body temperature, the inability to gain weight no matter what or how much she eats (a first important step), and has lost some weight but certainly not all of it. The main thing is that she feels better, is healthier, and on the right track. Improvement and incremental progress are the goals, not necessarily some fantasy about a utopian finish line.

Anyway, each of the following things we're about to cover influence your heredity if your parents were exposed to such things (like dieting, a nutrient-scarce diet, macronutrient restriction, and so forth), but also influence your metabolism in this lifetime and is under your control. But just know that you may have started out in life with one arm, maybe two, tied behind your back. Heredity is by far the biggest determinant of both health problems and obesity alike – studies of identical twins separated at birth show that heredity determines an estimated 80% of the outcome of a person's weight, but you have the power to change your heredity to a large extent. You have the power to turn off your "thrifty genes" and have a healthy metabolism. In fact it seems the more overweight a person is, the easier it is to turn the thrifty gene off and put a halt to weight gain.

Omega 6 Polyunsaturated Fat

A little over 100 years ago modern technology made it possible to start easily and affordably extracting lots of oil out of stuff that you wouldn't otherwise be able to – like corn and soybeans. With these being the biggest crops grown in the United States, getting the general public to embrace these oils was a very attractive thought to the business man.

Not only could these oils be used for cooking, and margarines and shortenings be made to replace butter and lard for baking and spreading on bread – but even more profitable was being able to use all of these oils in the newly-hatched food product industry. Right away, with such a huge potential market out there, the attempts to make these desirable over their competitors was on.

Of course, in the early 1900's in the United States, even the elderly had very low rates of heart disease, cancer, type 2 diabetes, and obesity. In fact, having a heart attack was a totally rare event at that time. And, coinciding with that, the top household fats used were lard, butter, and beef tallow (cow lard basically). Oils such as coconut oil and olive oil were also used at that time. Most of these fats are very low in polyunsaturated fat. Lard and olive oil contain about 10% of their fats as omega 6 polyunsaturated fat, and dairy fats (by the way, whole milk consumption was much higher at that time as well), beef, and coconut fat much lower than that (2-3% as omega 6). Anyway, we all know what happened. The lobby to replace these fats was highly successful even though it was slow going at first. But by the end of the 20th century the food industry managed to get Americans to increase their consumption of these seed oils by quite a margin. Between 1909 and 1999 according to the governmental data:

- Consumption of margarine increased 800%
- Consumption of shortening increased 275%
- Consumption of lard and tallow dropped 50%
- Consumption of butter dropped 72.2%
- Consumption of salad and cooking oil increased 1,450%
- Consumption of whole milk dropped 49.8%

Nice! Animal fat, dairy in particular (although we still love our cheese as much as ever), went out of style and was replaced by seed oils while a huge epidemic of heart disease, diabetes, cancer, obesity, and countless inflammatory conditions took place along with it.

Not that one can blame polyunsaturated fat for everything. I mean sure, we started driving cars during that time too, and watching TV, and using agricultural chemicals, and other massive changes. But when one takes a close look at the metabolic effects of polyunsaturated fat vs. saturated and monounsaturated fat, it becomes quite evident that these fats almost certainly play a role, if not a leading role, in the widespread epidemic of the "thrifty metabolism." I've even seen some studies floating around out there showing that in lab animals the greatest determinant in the development of obesity over time and even generations (as this has a transgenerational impact), was the ratio of saturated to unsaturated fat in the diet (more saturated, less obesity).

Why? First of all, polyunsaturated fats directly interfere with the function of the thyroid gland, as well as how the thyroid hormones can be taken up and utilized by the mitochondria in the cells. This interference can give a person, thin or fat, a slow metabolism with an endless array of consequences to go along with it.

Secondly, omega 6 is a precursor to the formation of inflammatory molecules in the body known to elevate several counter-inflammatory substances such as the "stress hormone" cortisol and Suppressor of Cytokine Signaling (SOCS-3). These factors rise in the presence of inflammatory molecules like Interleukin-6 for example, which is well-understood to rise in proportion to the omega 6 content of the diet – particularly in relation to the omega 3 consumption in the diet coinciding with that.

Okay your head hurts right? Good. Just know that the rise in Interleukin-6 means more inflammation, and the more inflammation that's produced the more SOCS-3 and cortisol is released to combat that inflammation. Why is this so significant? It's significant because of all the factors that have been studied when trying to determine what causes leptin resistance (the hormonal state that makes your body think it's starving, keeping your metabolism subdued and continuing to try to store fat even if you have way more than enough already), the closest ties are to these counter-inflammatory molecules.

Neato! Good thing we switched away from those pesky saturated fats and started gobbling up omega 6 polyunsaturated fat in quantities that our species has never done before. It's been quite a pleasure being a guinea pig hasn't it? Good news is, these polyunsaturated fats accumulate in our cells and tissues and have been for a century now – passed from generation to generation in a nice cumulative effect impacting every single cell and every single immune system reaction. Boo-ya! Yeah, I still say that.

So, this is most likely one of the root causes of the sluggish metabolism of modern man unlike what was seen in the past or is witnessed in many lean areas in the world today such as rural Africa. It takes many years to flush enough omega 6 out of the system to make any real difference. You may feel some benefits right away, such as more resistance to sunburn, clearer skin, and a little increase in body temperature by cutting them out now and replacing them with their antidote (unrefined starches, coconut, and dairy fat primarily), but don't expect any immediate miracles.

The biggest shift is simply switching out vegetable oils and margarine in your home kitchen with coconut oil and butter. Easy enough.

One tip on coconut oil: I would say for multi-purpose use, refined or expeller-pressed (as opposed to "virgin") is more likely to sit better with you. It's cheap as all get out, too. Many people don't like the strong taste and smell (and price) of the virgin oil, and the virgin oil often triggers some unpleasant digestive effects we'll call them. But the majority of coconut oil's benefits are derived from the large quantity of medium-chain saturated fatty acids that directly stimulate more metabolic activity (if you feel hot after eating it the first time and lose some blubber initially you are not imagining things), which are found in any type of coconut oil of any level of quality. But I wouldn't eat more than a couple tablespoons a day. It is, after all, a highly refined food. Nor would I blindly eat it if you are clearly not faring well on it after giving it a fair trial, and giving your body a decent chance to adjust and build up a tolerance for the food in question. That goes for any food you read about in any health book.

Dairy fat doesn't have the same content of medium-chain triglycerides as coconut, but it does contain more butyric acid than any other food. While the overall butyric acid content is pretty low overall (I think it's about 2.5% of the fat roughly), it's better than nothing. Butyric acid, if you had to pick one, is probably the most metabolically stimulating substance there is. While dairy fat doesn't contain enough to single-handedly make you catch fire with metabolic activity, it's important to understand the properties of butyric acid first, and then we'll move on to where, diet-wise, you can actually get a substantial amount of it in your diet.

Butyric acid actually facilitates the entry of T3, the active thyroid hormone, into the mitochondria where it does a sexy dance of sorts, excites the mitochondria, and makes it cheesily say something along the lines of "Is it hot in here or is it just me?"

This is why when rodents are bombarded with butyric acid as in the study pointed out by Dr. Guyenet, they have a drop in appetite, a drop in cholesterol (I'll explain this later), a drop in blood sugar, increased insulin sensitivity, an increase in physical activity, and a drop in body fat. No one told these rodents the virtues of eating less and staying in shape with some vigorous physical activity. They just simply had a drop in bodyweight set point, which is the only way to lose weight or improve health without the collateral damage of having your metabolism tank.

So where do we get this coveted butyric acid other than the trace amount in butter? Butyric acid is something we get primarily from the fermentation of fiber and resistant starch in the digestive tract. The digestive tract is built to feast on the fermentation of undigested plant matter into easily-absorbable short-chain saturated fatty acids (like butyric acid, but also acetic and propionic acids – by the way propionic acid is thought to reduce insulin resistance dramatically)

The best sources of fiber, and more importantly resistant starch which appears to be the perfect substance for producing short-chain fats, are:

- Beans
- Legumes
- Whole Grains including corn
- Root vegetables
- Plantains
- Bananas that aren't overly ripe (spotted)
- Hi Maize – a powdered resistant starch supplement

Nuts and seeds contain some resistant starch as well, but I wouldn't consider them optimal due to their extremely high content of omega 6 polyunsaturated fat. In fact, peanuts and Brazil nuts have the highest omega 6 to omega 3 ratio of any known foods. The only exceptions are the macadamia nut and the coconut, both of which do not contain the heat and light sensitive polyunsaturated fats in large quantity as an adaptation to the hot, sunny, tropical climate that they are adapted to (note, that's what your furless body that's cold below 60 degrees F is designed for, there are very few coincidences in nature, and mammals sharing our similar biological characteristics that live at higher latitudes and eat a lot of polyunsaturated fat just so happen to go into hibernation right after doing so – good for their circumstances, not so good for ours).

For added resistant starch, you can cool starches once they have been cooked, which decreases their absorption as carbohydrates and increases their absorption as short-chain fats. As I've laid out in my cookbook *180 Kitchen*, a simple salad comprised of beans and potatoes dressed with some homemade dressing is a great, convenient staple to take to work or whatever.

Let's finish this section by saying that seed oils such as corn, soy, canola, cottonseed, sunflower, etc. – by far the world's most commonly-used oils which are in flippin' everything (all fried foods, salad dressings, mayo and mayo-based sauces, restaurant-sautéed food, all packaged and processed foods), are a huge metabolism suppressor. Eliminating those from your diet and getting most of your fats from fish, red meat, coconut, and dairy products while also eating lots of high-resistant starch foods is a great antidote that may not magically solve everything, but should certainly help you make progress and protect your metabolism from experiencing so much age degradation. For a list of omega 6 content of some common foods, see Appendix II.

Oh, and one more thing since I promised to talk about it (cholesterol that is)... Isn't saturated fat supposed to clog arteries and cause heart disease and high cholesterol and all that? To fully convince you of the whole story it would take a separate book if this is your first exposure to the idea. For starters, just think long and hard about how easily an industry could highlight a certain perspective or hypothesis (the cookie cutter version the general public is spoon fed is called the "lipid hypothesis" by the way), shout it from the rooftops, get everyone eating cheap commodities instead of butter and other Holy things, and incidentally build up an entire cholesterol war with a multi-billion dollar cholesterol lowering medication industry accompanying it. It's like a 50 year-long Y2K scare that has permeated all facets of the food, restaurant, agricultural, and medical-pharmaceutical complexes.

That aside, consuming a lot of say, butter, can indeed raise your cholesterol level. This is how I believe it happens...

Cholesterol is the precursor to the formation of many of our hormones – like DHEA, testosterone, progesterone, pregnenelone, and so forth. What controls the conversion of cholesterol into these hormones? The thyroid gland does. If it is cranking out high levels of activity like it is supposed to, you convert LDL (the "bad" cholesterol) into these hormones at a high rate, keeping it from piling up in the blood. In fact, before the cholesterol test was used as a heart disease risk assessment tool, it was used AS A TEST FOR HYPOTHYROIDISM. When the metabolism is low however, cholesterol levels tend to rise, particularly the LDL to HDL ratio, which is precisely why cholesterol levels are a decent marker for a low metabolism. Note, in the Dr. Atkins quote mentioned earlier in which Atkins states that dieting shuts down thyroid function, one symptom is an "elevation in cholesterol." This also of course explains why, as people age and their metabolism lulls, cholesterol levels slowly tend to rise year after year (in industrialized peoples, that is).

"For many years deficiency of thyroid hormone secretion has been known to predispose to arteriosclerotic heart disease. In persons with a serious deficiency of thyroid hormone, the ability of the cells of the body to use oxygen is impaired. The basal metabolic rate is slowed in hypothyroidism, and the liver begins to make increased quantities of cholesterol and triglycerides. As a result the cholesterol and lipoprotein levels become elevated, and the risk of coronary heart disease increases... Subtle or marginal deficiencies of thyroid hormone, detected by measuring basal metabolic rate, are found to be widespread in populations with a high risk of arteriosclerotic heart disease."

-Kilmer McCully; *The Homocysteine Revolution*

"When a person's thyroid is functioning below normal, he or she makes fat much more quickly than it's burned, which drives up triglycerides, cholesterol, and LDL cholesterol. As mentioned earlier, hypothyroidism makes the liver and gallbladder sluggish, so that fat is not easily

metabolized and cleared from the body. Cells may be less receptive to taking up LDL, so that too much accumulates. When a person with healthy thyroid function becomes hungry and needs energy, the body is able to readily burn fat for fuel. Not so with low thyroid function."

  -Datis Kharrazian; *Why Do I Still Have Thyroid Symptoms?*

So, the problem is not the butter. Butter shouldn't raise cholesterol. Remember the Masai who eat the equivalent of four sticks of butter per day but have average cholesterol levels of 125 mg/dl? These are very hypermetabolic peoples, and switching them to a typical industrial diet lowers their metabolism (they add body fat on fewer calories – this has actually been studied, and I was turned onto this once again thanks to Dr. Guyenet), and they see big rises in serum cholesterol levels along with it despite huge decreases in saturated fat and cholesterol consumption.

  In short, heart disease is about your metabolism (which is why in the butyric acid study the rats saw a big drop in their cholesterol levels), not about saturated fat consumption, and one of the biggest keys to overcoming a sluggish metabolism is getting the industrial seed oils out of your diet in favor of saturated fats. In fact, as people age their total calorie consumption decreases, and their saturated fat and cholesterol intake gradually declines with it while blood cholesterol level gradually increases! You are not what you eat. You are what your body does with what you eat.

  Fix your metabolism, and your body is much more likely to process all foods like they are supposed to be processed.

  Heart disease also appears to be directly caused by a rise in an amino acid called homocysteine that is not metabolized correctly. What assists with the proper homocysteine metabolism, preventing this rise and even lowering homocysteine levels? Thyroid hormone of course.

The take home message here is metabolism, metabolism, metabolism – and polyunsaturated fats suck. If you can remember that you'll be well on your way. Did I mention they cause cancer and age your skin, brain, organs, and tissues faster?

"It is time for the housewife to make another decision. Can she afford to continue the unsaturated fats with their demonstrated toxicity and run the risk of cancer in her family? It was difficult to deny the members of the family their eggs, bacon, etc., but mothers have a way of achieving a desirable change. Now she has found that a mistake was made and she should be just as eager to reverse her stand and prevent some new tragedies. It will be hard to ignore the propaganda that the saturated fats cause heart disease. That propaganda will stop abruptly when the housewife passes up the unsaturated fats and fills her basket with cream, butter, eggs, lard, fat meat, and the other goodies which the family has been craving. The propaganda for unsaturates is perpetuated only by the vested interest of the manufacturers. The few pennies saved on the budget by purchasing cheaper margarines and oils may be a poor investment compared to the prolonged and horrible death from cancer. If the polyunsaturated fats are safe, let the manufacturers prove it on animals before a new plague develops from the false statements that unsaturated fats will prevent heart attacks."
"Everyone should have the privilege of playing Russian Roulette if it is desired, but it is only fair to have the warning that with the use of polyunsaturated fats the gun probably contains live ammunition."

-Broda Barnes; *Solved: The Riddle of Heart Attacks*

Stress and Inflammation

In the last section we discussed how, with the increasing production of inflammatory molecules, resistance to the hormone leptin can be induced in a roundabout fashion.

Hormones like cortisol, which are secreted in response to inflammation, trigger this effect. This is important because the hormone leptin sets the metabolism thermostat in your body, as it is master and commander of your thyroid gland. When your body is unresponsive to leptin, the system acts like it is starving. And it seems that stress and inflammation are the predominant root causes of leptin resistance, although the knowledge base on leptin is still in its infancy (the thing wasn't even discovered until 1994).

The thing about stress though is that it is non-specific. There is a general physiological response that takes place in reaction to any type of inflammation or stressor – mental, physical, or otherwise.

Common sources of physical stress include sleep apnea, infection, injury, arthritis, cancer, asthma, allergies of all kinds including food allergies, nutrient deficiency – minor or major, surgery and stored trauma from surgery and other traumatic past events, and dental decay and/or root canals (which are often not as sterile as your dentist thinks they are).

There are many environmental stresses as well. Watching television can apparently increase stress levels, bright lighting too late at night, irregular sleep patterns, loud noise, air pollution, food additives, pesticide residues, heavy metals, drug and alcohol abuse, many medications, and so on. They all contribute to the load.

Then of course are the mental and emotional stressors. Everything from the more direct things like anxiety, money worries, abusive relationships, and the passing of loved ones or divorce to the more nebulous such as feeling unloved by your parents, unappreciated at work, or not actively pursuing what inspires and interests you in life – these are all stressors.

Doesn't matter what the stressor is – any of them can contribute to a subdued metabolism, a tendency to gain weight, serious trouble losing weight, and an ever-climbing weight set point as you age. The physiological human response is the same, and triggers an increased release of cortisol – blocking thyroid function, wreaking havoc on the immune system including actually atrophying the thymus (our main immune system center) and interfering with leptin.

Of course, some stress is natural, normal, and unavoidable. It's impossible to live a life free of all of the above stressors, especially in today's modern world. It just sort of comes with being a part of 21st century society – a tradeoff for the many advantages we now have I suppose.

But the key to all these stressors and what unifies them all is the nature of the stress. It is CHRONIC. Acute stress actually strengthens us and has an overall stress-lowering effect, which is why many people find vigorous physical activity to be such a stress-reliever, vitality-enhancer, and inducer of weight loss and/or muscle gain. It's also why those who react to stressors with intense flurries of anger and emotional outburst tend to be less affected by stress than those who internalize and accumulate emotional baggage. But chronic stress, unlike acute stress, is a totally different animal.

In fact, I think the original pathway for chronic stress is chronic food deprivation – the reason why chronic stress can often trigger a chain reaction that activates the famine programs in our bodies. Increased appetite, emotional eating, binge eating, incessant cravings, compulsion for calorie-dense fat and sugar bombs, reduced desire for physical activity, poor muscle mass and strength, and propensity to store fat all tend to accompany a reduced metabolism/low body temperature, and you bet that chronic stressors can catapult many into such a state.

In fact, just recently I spoke with a personal trainer who was telling me that she really wanted to work specifically with the wives of military men on getting them to eat right and exercise properly. Seems that after the guys went off to war the women tended to slip away and binge on junk food and stay glued to the television all day, gaining weight and spiraling down. This is no coincidence.

Many people report getting an infection and gaining weight afterward, starting a new job and gaining weight, getting divorced and gaining weight (after the attempt at jealousy-inducing crash weight loss, lol), giving birth and gaining weight (this is a huge metabolic and nutritional drain that is the last straw for many women's metabolisms), and on and on and on. We know fully that sleep deprivation is one of the leading causes of metabolic syndrome, as is irregular sleep patterns. It's really endless.

Hope this isn't overwhelming. The main point of this chapter is to have a little compassion for yourself or others. Odds are some weight you may have gained at some point was due to one of many varieties of traumas. The last thing you would want to do is then starve yourself (the mother of all stressors) to get the weight off. That is simply the wrong approach when hoping to address the root problem.

Epigenetics has shown that the stressors your parents were exposed to at key times in the peri-natal period can influence your propensity to have a chronic stress-like metabolism as well (until you take action to turn those thrifty programs off).

It's important to understand the causal reasons for a low metabolism and some of the areas needing to be addressed for full recovery. This is one area that is highly personal and

68

individual, but also an area that much progress can be made –
particularly with mental stressors as the human mind wields
incredible transformative power when steered in the right
direction with thoughts that counterbalance polarized beliefs
and emotions. It's certainly worthy of putting on your radar
screen. Odds are you can trace every period of weight gain to
various stressful events, or illnesses, or medications, and so
forth – including restricted diets and the after-effects of
psychotic exercise regimens.

The refreshing news is that the simple dietary and lifestyle
changes laid out here can lower stress levels substantially, lower
cortisol levels substantially, and improve your overall response
to stressors – this is obvious as it is so effective at raising
metabolism. So there's hope for you yet!

Addiction

I have strongly been led to believe through my research that
addiction is a leading cause of a rising weight set point. If
you're wondering why you gain weight when exposed to the
sweet treats and salty crunchiness out there while others don't,
classic addiction neurochemistry may be highly involved.

We know that addiction proneness is highly dependent on
heredity. We also know that repeated exposure to substances
with an addictive quality can eventually flip the switch from
recreationally enjoying something to becoming pathologically
addicted to it.

Modern food is processed and manipulated in such a way by
food scientists that it can be quite addictive. The purpose of
one of these food "engineers" is to create food that evokes the
absolute maximum pleasure response in the human brain.
When they succeed, customers tend to suddenly find all other

food to be unpalatable, and need junk food to get the level of neural satisfaction their brains are in search of.

This may seem like a far-reaching concept to some. Others may be nodding their heads in enthusiastic agreement. Regardless of what you think when first introduced to this concept, I assure you that if you follow this rabbit hole deeply enough you'll arrive at much the same conclusions that I have.

For example, it's known that obese people have downregulated dopamine receptors in the brain compared to the lean. This is akin to turning up the volume on your stereo, and therefore having to shout louder to communicate with the person sitting across the room. When it comes to pleasure foods, the obese must eat more of the pleasure food in order to get the same level of neurological satisfaction. And it is self-perpetuating in nature – the more pleasure food you eat, the more numbed out the pleasure centers become, and the greater the spike you need to get the same sensation of satisfaction. Like I said, this is addiction pathology 101. This is how all addiction works, and the pleasure hit and the numbed receptors leave you feeling the opposite of satisfied in the absence of these pleasure foods, which most obese people find themselves needing a hit of every couple of hours (the constant sipping of Diet Coke comes to mind, with aspartame perhaps providing the most neural excitation of any substance due to its extreme sweetness).

There's no question in my mind that the needs of the pleasure centers in our brain are fully capable of trumping the messages of leptin, insulin, and other hormones that normally would regulate metabolism and appetite for a stable body weight. It could very well be that the neurotransmitters that dictate the feeling of satisfaction dominate all other biological and metabolic regulators, and that humans eat until the pleasure tank is full, not the digestive or metabolic tank.

It's not even the calories or fat or sugar in ice cream, cookies, brownies, sodas, chips, French fries, snack foods, and fast food mega meals that does it either. A person without this sensitivity is much more likely to self-regulate their weight without ever seeing a rise in weight set point. Plus, a lean person just isn't as likely to binge. The pleasure response kicks in much earlier. No 64 ounce cola required. A simple 12 ounce can does the job.

Studies in which lean and obese people are offered up both highly palatable (brownies, ice cream) and less exciting food (fruits, vegetables), the obese people always eat more of the palatable food than the lean and LESS of the less palatable food. Why? Because their standards are set higher with the numbing of the pleasure centers. Normal food can still give pleasure to a lean person, but it often requires something sweet, dredged in sugar, deep fried, or flavor-enhancer laden to interest someone with a higher weight set point.

Although I have little hard proof of such a theory, I'm almost completely convinced it is a legitimate factor based on how many unexplained phenomena it pieces together. For example, it easily explains why races of people with sudden exposure to white sugar, white flour, unlimited fats, and other modern junk foods as well as alcohol have an exponentially higher obesity and diabetes response and rate of alcohol abuse – such as that seen on the Pima Indian reservation and many Pacific islands. Living off of a sparse diet makes the reward centers in the brain more highly attuned and attracted to calorie-dense food for survival. This is an adaptation that is passed epigenetically as well as through peri-natal influences in order to prepare the next generation for the food environment it's about to enter into.

To survive, one must gravitate towards calorie dense food with great selectivity – turning up the nose to low-calorie foods in favor of that which ensures survival. This backfires when the food environment undergoes a radical shift from say, coconut, fruits, vegetables, root vegetables, and lean seafood – and takes a turn to include extremely calorie dense foods like white flour, white sugar, mutton flap (big slabs of lamb fat), oil, canned meats, sodas, alcohol, and snack foods. This just so happens to be the dietary shift that took place in the island nation of Nauru, the nation with the highest obesity rate (sorry U.S., U.K., Australia and others – you weren't even close, better luck next year).

This is just one connection. Another includes why rodents exposed to aspartame, saccharin, sucralose, or high-fructose corn syrup all spontaneously gain weight in an unrestricted food environment. They are all chemically unrelated, but they are all highly-sweet. The no-calorie sweeteners are much sweeter than the corn syrup, and they are also much more fattening than the corn syrup despite the absence of calories.

It also explains why lowering the calorie density or pleasure of one's diet induces spontaneous drop in appetite and a fall in weight set point. Ever try to eat nothing but boiled potatoes? How about nothing but meat? Give it a couple of weeks and you will hate food and have no appetite whatsoever (don't try this though or you'll just be priming yourself for rapid rebound weight gain when you return to variety, which you will have to eventually).

These are just glimpses into the dozen or so phenomena that can be linked to neurochemistry, pleasure, and weight regulation.

Anyway, expect to hear more from me as this idea continues to develop and unfold. There's simply no question that addiction plays into weight gain in some individuals, and your susceptibility is not your fault. Likewise, you have the power, by eating wholesome foods that are not cracked out by the food industry to seduce your reward centers, to normalize your reward centers and derive the same pleasure from natural, unadulterated foods while perhaps even seeing a spontaneous drop in your weight set point. Not only that, but the quantity of say, cheesecake or those villainous Doritos that it takes to satisfy you when you do have some will get increasingly smaller the longer you eat a wholesome, simple diet. You don't have to live imprisoned by intense junk food cravings. On the rehab program that follows, I've yet to see anyone not be able to at least improve and often fully overcome even lifelong junk food addiction.

As a final word on addiction, a personal trainer named Drew Manning has just intentionally gained weight eating junk food as a publicity stunt – and to learn how to go from "fat to fit." After gaining 70 pounds, this is what he says about his experience. Sounds to me like an addiction developed…

"All of these foods that I'm eating (sugary cereals, granola bars, juices, white breads, white pastas, sodas, crackers, chips, frozen dinners, mac n cheese, etc.) taste delicious. But then I feel like crap later on and I get hungry again and crave those same foods…

"I'm to the point where I feel lethargic and uncomfortable. I definitely feel "addicted" to these foods. In the beginning, I did not like soda, but now I can't go a day without, otherwise I'll get the headaches, bad mood, etc. Emotionally, it's taken a toll on my confidence level, even in my marriage. I don't like the way I look in public; nothing fits right; bending

over to tie my shoes or clip my toe nails has become so difficult. I've definitely taken those things for granted…

"I think the biggest thing I've learned is how intense and how real these food cravings are. I think a lot of people associate the word "addiction" with drugs and alcohol, but I do believe this addiction (to America's processed foods) is real and very similar. I know I'll never know exactly what it's like for every person that's overweight and I don't claim to, but at least I understand better than I did before when I never had to struggle with this. I hope to learn a lot more in the second half of my journey, from fat 2 fit."

Dieting

Dieting:

- *Slows the rate at which your body burns calories.*
- *Increases your body's efficiency at wringing every possible calorie out of the food you do eat so you digest food faster and get hungrier quicker.*
- *Causes you to crave high-fat foods.*
- *Increases your appetite.*
- *Reduces your energy levels (so even if you could burn more calories through physical activity you don't want to).*
- *Lowers your body temperature so you're using less energy (and are always cold).*
- *Reduces your ability to feel 'hungry' and 'full,' making it easier to confuse hungers with emotional needs.*
- *Reduces your total amount of muscle tissue.*
- *Increases fat-storage enzymes and decreases fat-release enzymes.*

-Linda Bacon; *Health at Every Size*

Well, it's no secret at this point how I feel about dieting. "Duck Fiets" has become a well-worn slogan of mine. I know of no highly-restricted way of eating that does not directly lead to a drop in body temperature in a large number of followers given sufficient time. I've seen body temperatures below 95 degrees F from both the low-fat vegan and the full-on zero carb carnivore side of the world of dietary extremism. But even with those who just had minor restrictions in carbohydrates, fats, or animal products the results were still capable of being near-catastrophic.

More importantly, on the subject of root causes, many people never would have had weight or metabolic problems if they didn't begin the diet practice in the first place. You don't have to be overweight to do a highly-restricted diet. You don't have to be genetically prone to develop obesity or metabolic problems either in order to develop obesity from excessive bouts with restrained eating. You can also be thin as a rail and have an ice cold metabolism. The starvation metabolism can be from either actual starvation or pseudo starvation – where your body acts as if it is starving, including making desperate attempts to store fat and/or binge eat.

I too watched my body composition fade away over the span of a decade as I repeated bouts of endurance exercise, restricted diets, attempts at cutting calories, and so forth. Like a typical dieter, with each round I lost both muscle and fat, and put back more fat than muscle and appeared softer, weaker, and pudgier by the time I returned to the exact same weight or a few pounds heavier. In fact, I'm an expert at raising the set point. If anyone wants to worsen their body composition, all it takes is a low-protein, low-calorie vegan diet and lots of endurance exercise punctuated by long sedentary breaks and junk food binges. Sure, binging on junk food and being sedentary will probably put some pounds on you, but much more if you do endurance exercise and a vegan diet to trim off muscle tissue, lower the metabolic rate, and prime yourself to store fat quickly before your appetite shuts down and metabolism speeds back up.

Anyway, never diet again. Do not believe the diet propaganda served up by highly polarized and short-sighted thinkers occupying various trenches in the popular diet battleground. There are no panaceas, no happily-ever-afters. Just ways in which you follow some strict and highly disordered form of eating until you:

1) Want to eat something else
2) Crave something else so badly you can't resist eating it
3) Develop health problems forcing you to eat something else

And when you do drop off the diet, you'll have a horrible time digesting and metabolizing the food or foods that you've omitted – whether it be simple calories or animal products or fats or carbohydrates. You can't win the diet musical chairs game, and the human body hates irregularity and diet "pinballing" as fitness mastermind Scott Abel so perfectly calls it.

Be realistic. This is the 21st century. To function as a member of society the right strategy to approach health is not to run from all the calorie-dense foods out there, or the carbs, or the fats – but build the absolute best and most resilient metabolic and digestive machinery you can. This book will show you how (we're almost there!). When you punish Thanksgiving and Christmas dinners without flinching or noticing the slightest change in your figure while everyone else around you gets bloated, passes out, and wakes up 10 pounds heavier on January 1st and panicked to starve it off, you'll feel quite empowered.

With the right metabolic machinery, you can get away with many things you never got away with in the past, tearing through food like a teenager without a waistline worry. This is not to say that you shouldn't still nourish yourself with quality, simple, fresh food. You should most of the time if you expect to sustain your health. But you will no longer live in a dietary prison with temptation and weight gain phobia lurking around every corner. You can return to society. Spend LESS time thinking about your diet. Worry LESS about what's going to be served at such and such's house. Leave the house without your special meals. Not panic when a group of friends orders a dessert for the table and passes you a spoon. You get the picture. This is freedom we're talking here. This is what *Diet Recovery* is all about.

Now it's time to find out how you can eat your way out of the Diet Dungeon.

Eat Your Way Out

Rehabilitative Rest & Aggressive Re-Feeding (RRARF!)

After three full years of exploration into what helps bring body temperature up most effectively, here's the best of what I've put together so far. Each person has his or her own subtle unique individuality, digestive function, and health history and status. For this reason, the details are certainly open to some personal experimentation. I have no interest in being a dogmatic ruler that tells you everything you're supposed to do at every waking moment and exactly what to eat. Don't turn this into another "diet" if you know what I mean. The customization of this basic template is up to you.

One thing I would discourage is over-thinking it and measuring this program up against what you think is and is not healthy. I'm not saying it is healthy to eat as much food as you can every day while sedentary. This is just a temporary strategy to perform one very specific task – increase mitochondrial activity, which seems, from my research, to be more healing and more central to excellent physical function than any other thing one could focus on. And to get out of a hole, it takes a set strategy. After that you can sorta eat whatever you want. I eat much more like a "normal" person than a health guru that's for sure.

With that, here are the basic guidelines for getting started:

1) Make a general assessment of your overall health. Do you feel good? Is your morning body temperature at least close to ideal (98 degrees F or higher first thing upon waking up)? Do you have digestive problems like bloating or heartburn? Do you get drowsy throughout the day? Are your emotions erratic and unpredictable? Do you have cravings that are very strong, and feel uncontrollable at times? Can you make it through the day without any addictive substances like caffeine or alcohol to prop you up or make you feel at ease? Do you have a lot of belly fat or a big 'gut'? Do you have allergies? Trouble sleeping? Acne? High blood pressure? A lot of aches and pains including frequent headaches? Menstrual problems? Sexual dysfunction? Hair loss? Low energy? Manic energy? You get the picture.

2) If you suffer few or none of the above problems, continue living your life and remember to eat quality, nutritious, real food the majority of the time, never starve yourself, do any extremely restricted diets, and so on. If you suffer from several of those problems, and your body temperature is considerably lower than normal, it might be time to start giving more to your body than you ask in return. After all, you are not fully well, and disease and dysfunction of all kinds is typically not cured through hard work and depriving yourself but by doing the opposite – flooding your body with the tools it needs to repair and rehabilitate itself.

3) The next step is to begin eating better. Eat to appetite three times per day. Meals should be wholesome and hearty. If you are a long-time caffeine abuser, Day 1 is not the time to

stop cold turkey. Take it easy on yourself. Nourish yourself well and keep your physical activity low to moderate (walking, stretching, light yoga), and keep high intensity exercise to short bursts only, if you do any hard exercise at all. Go to bed earlier if you can. Take naps if you are tired. Don't fight yourself. Just listen and obey – more so than you ever have before. Your body knows what it needs. It is not a lazy pile of junk that sabotages itself. No more jogging or extreme exercise. Save that for when you have recovered if that really sounds fun to you. Just chill. Every day is spa day.

Once you've eaten well for a while, and have been resting up, it may be time to think about going full-RRARF for a while, intentionally shooting for a calorie surplus for an extended period of time.

4) Once you are done RRARFING and your body temperature has been restored, it's best to start incorporating exercise back into your program, eating only to appetite but not actively trying to overfeed, and generally continuing a healthy and "clean" diet free of most refined foods – without causing yourself some kind of social anxiety over it or letting it dictate your entire life. Yes, eat the birthday cake – even the kind with propylene glycol in the frosting.

The guidelines for following RRARF are simple. You are basically trying to create a state of *Nutritional Superabundance* within your body. Surplus baby, of vitamins, minerals, amino acids, sugar, fat, sleep, rest – everything basically.

To follow it properly, the best set of advice that I have devised so far is as follows:

1) **Take a month off from exercise.** The only exception would be to do some light walks that don't cause you to

become overly winded, some stretching, some sunbathing, and other easygoing things. Just don't overdo the duration of your physical activities. This is a particularly important step if you have a low body temperature and have a long history of exercise fanaticism. I love exercise too, I've hiked over 10,000 miles in the last 14 years, but it can wait, and it should wait if you've been a slave to your jogging shoes or local gym going at it too hard for too long. Please rest up. Your physical conditioning can be restored just as quickly as it is lost. Be prepared, if you are an exerciser taking a break, to be tired, groggy, grouchy, achy, irritable, and perhaps even ill from stopping your exercise routine. These are all signs of your adrenals commencing their much-needed vacation. Healing doesn't always feel good. In fact, really good healing feels kind of like a hangover. Like you feel when you "oversleep," and this feeling often lingers for up to several weeks on this program.

2)   **Start each day by eating as much food as you desire, plus a little extra, ideally within 30 minutes of waking up in the morning.** Many people are not "breakfast eaters." This can be one key reason for some people's entire metabolic problems. Break the fast after sleeping as quickly as possible. You get far more metabolic mileage out of that first hour after waking than at any other time of day, and this is an essential time to supply glucose to your system and shut down the early morning load of stress hormones. Eating a good breakfast can be life changing. Seriously. The best breakfast to eat is one comprised of mostly carbohydrate foods, and little heavy food like meat. This may make you crash at first, and get hungry. But this should pass as you recover. Fruit, toast, juice, muffins/waffles/pancakes/breads, fried potatoes or yams, rice, fruit smoothies, any kind of grain porridge, the occasional dry cereal – these are all excellent. But try to

emphasize the carbohydrate at the morning meal, and don't hold back at all.

3) **As soon as you feel inclined to eat again – eat again!** See how easy this is! Eat until you do not desire another bite, potentially eating slightly more than you desire. Make sure each feeding you eat to fullness. No snacking. No light meals. If you eat 3 meals by noon, fine. Eat until you are deeply satisfied each time though. That is key. You do not have to force lots of unwanted food down your throat. That will ruin the whole experience. Eat as much as you can enjoy plus a few bites for good measure.

4) **Get extra sleep.** Take naps if you get tired, and go to bed as close to sunset as possible. In other words, go to bed early. If this doesn't fit into your schedule somehow, make sure you get AT LEAST 8 hours of sleep per night. The 180 follower who completely committed to RRARF and had the quickest and most dramatic response to it claimed, between naps and sleeping at night, to have slept between 12 and 14 hours per day! She was coming off of caffeine, cigarettes, tragically undereating of poor foods, and overexercising all thrown in together. She's like a new woman now. Clean, strong, nourished, and "losing weight while still eating more food in one day than I used to have in three."

5) **Don't Overhydrate.** This is often completely overlooked in other metabolism-related programs. The lower your metabolic rate, the less fluid one can tolerate. It's best, until you get your metabolism up, to eat a lot of foods that aren't too watery and be careful about chugging too many beverages. How many fluids should you take in daily? That is an unanswerable question with all of the variables that affect our fluid needs at any given time. If you meet anyone

who can answer that question for you, run away quickly. The best way to determine how many fluids you should consume is simply the concentration of your urine. Your urine should be yellow, and you should urinate once every four hours or so during the day and none at night. It should be consistent, and you shouldn't have strong sudden urges or episodes where you urinate several times in an hour or two. If your urine is very clear and you find yourself having to urinate frequently, avoid ALL plain water and tea, drinking only small quantities of milk and fruit juice (preferably lightly salted) until this problem resolves itself during the course of metabolic rehab. When my metabolism was at its lowest, I would urinate 3-4 times per hour just from eating a bowl of oatmeal!!! Frequent urination and night urination is a sure sign of a less than ideal metabolism.

6)   **Minimize mental and emotional strain, within reason.** You probably know yourself well enough to know what triggers that excessive mental noise. Most will have to go to work as usual during this period. That's okay, but try your best not to take it home with you or get too bent out of shape with various work crises. This is a good frame of mind to take to work with you anyway, but really psyche yourself up to be non-reactive and protective of your emotional energy and stress during this time. Don't get fired for being incompetent, but be mindful of your stress levels and know when to back off and let it go. RRARF is a great time to do relaxing activities such as reading, meditating, getting massages, listening to music, or whatever gives you peace of mind. Remember – every day is spa day!

The Specifics of the High-Everything Diet

"Just as your body became a fat storing machine because of your habits (reduced caloric intake) you can just as easily instruct it to become a fat

burning machine. The first and most critical step in losing fat is to prepare your body for the task ahead by raising your metabolism as high as you can. For the majority of us, this is accomplished by (take a deep breath ladies) gradually increasing your caloric intake—in layman's terms, eating more!"

-Ric Rooney; *Secrets of a Professional Dieter*

I created RRARF to reiterate that this process is not just a diet, but a comprehensive mind/body/lifestyle protocol. But the "high-everything diet" in its purest form is what is used as the food component of it. You can eat whatever you like, but I believe that the most important fundamental aspects of the diet is that it is comprised of mostly wholesome, unrefined, unadulterated foods and contains plenty of fat, a lot of carbohydrates, a lot of calories, and sufficient protein. In other words, "high in everything."

Certain aspects are worth mentioning in terms of specifically cranking this up to increase metabolic activity. The reasons for each of the following guidelines is discussed in great detail in my other books. Long-winded reasons aside, I believe the most potent version of the HED1 to be:

1) **Rich in saturated fats, particularly short and medium-chain triglycerides found in greatest abundance in dairy fats and coconut.** Butyric acid, as we discussed earlier, has great potential to raise the metabolism, and milk and ice cream would be the ideal source from the feedback I've gathered so far – so long as you have a good tolerance for it. Sour cream is my favorite for savory dishes, and fatty cheeses like my favorite – Fromager D'Affinois, are

---

[1] By the way, sorry about my love affair with acronyms like RRARF and HED. I used to work for the government.

totally fair game. Coconut is the best source of medium-chain triglycerides, and coconut milk and fresh and dried coconut are my favorite sources of MCT's. Beef would be the third choice if you have a dislike or exhaustively-confirmed intolerance to the above. Chocolate is another rich source of saturated fats, and a totally acceptable food for refeeding. You don't have to overdo it on the fats, and if one had to choose between a very high-fat diet and a very high-carbohydrate diet for raising mitochondrial activity – the high-carb version usually outperforms, but I think it depends on where you're coming from. If you are coming from a low-fat diet, you probably need more fat at first. If you are coming from low-carb, you probably need way more carbohydrate and less fat at first.

2) **Rich in unrefined carbohydrates.** Starch is a great tool for increasing metabolic activity, as almost all of it metabolizes into glucose or short-chain fatty acids – both being the almighty metabolism stimulators. Root vegetables, corn, and rice tend to be the best tolerated overall. Potatoes and yams are the best friends of the HED freak. Corn and corn products (cornmeal, corn tortillas) are fantastic. Rice, white or brown depending on what you fare best on, is at the top of the list as well. Amaranth, quinoa, buckwheat, and other "out there" hippie-ish grains are also top choices. Grains like whole wheat, oats, barley, and rye are also fine, but, perhaps ironically, experience has shown me that refined grains usually treat people better than whole grains during recovery and in general. Refining grains, while it does remove important nutrients, also removes the polyunsaturated fats in the grain. As long as your diet is rounded out with plenty of nutritious, unrefined foods I don't think you have much to worry about. Beans and legumes in theory should be the best with their amazingly high content of fiber and resistant starch, but also can be a

digestive nightmare. Personalize it to your preferences and limitations, but don't be afraid to challenge yourself a little. This is about getting better at handling problem foods, not just continuing to avoid your weaknesses forever. If all goes well you should find many sensitivities as well as starch-induced gas and bloating clearing up as metabolism rises.

The simple sugars – from fruit, dried fruit, and juice, and sweeteners like blackstrap molasses, honey, and maple syrup (and of course that found in ice cream and gelato) can also help people out a lot. There were years of masturdebating about whether it was preferable to get most of your carbohydrates from starches or sugars, and in actuality there are tremendous individual differences here. Be open and experiment freely. I know we've all received a heavy helping of scary information about sugar, but as my experience grows I find sugar, above all other energy sources, to often be the key to unlocking many frozen metabolisms.

3)   **High in calories.** You don't have to feed yourself to the point of being uncomfortable and gagging, but the calorie is a powerful weapon in the battle to increase metabolic activity. Eating a lot of nutritious calories, if you are already overweight, is often not as fattening as you would envision either. Appetite often falls off a cliff with the slightest increase in metabolism – as fat stores are liberated and flood the body with surplus energy. Some even lose weight instantly upon eating to appetite or even beyond appetite of exclusively whole, nutritious foods – including one woman who has lost over 100 pounds now "eating like a fiend" in her words. If you are underweight – be prepared to gain, which is a good thing. The good news is that at least 25 percent of those gains will be lean body mass – and not fat. Even better news is that once your body stores all the

fat it desires you are at a much higher level of your hormonal and genetic potential for building muscle mass and burning body fat. Gaining fat is often the first essential step in achieving the most impressive physique you are capable of constructing for both males and females. Do not count calories and do not pay attention to scale weight, ever! It is meaningless. I'm leaner at 190 pounds than I once was at 160 pounds after wasting away from endurance exercise.

4)   **Low in polyunsaturated fat.** While I believe that omega 3 polyunsaturated fat like that found in the greatest abundance in flax seeds and coldwater fish may even have a positive role to play in increasing the metabolism, I am also aware of the dangers of consuming too much. But you don't have to consume a lot of omega 3 to get some of the potential benefits of these fatty acids, because omega 3 competes with another type of fat – omega 6 polyunsaturated fat. In other words, you can reduce your omega 6 fatty acid consumption and get more from your omega 3's, negating the need to supplement your diet with fish oil or some other nonsense, when doing so has many potential negatives such as excessive lipid peroxidation (yes, it's as bad as it sounds). Then you get the benefits of omega 3 without the drawbacks of excessive omega 3 intake. Nuts (except for macadamia nuts), seeds, peanuts/peanut butter, liquid oils (except for macadamia oil), poultry fat (goose, duck, chicken), and pork fat are the biggest contributors to your daily omega 6 load. You don't have to be paranoid about these foods, but eat them very sparingly. This too, has great potential (over the long-term) to increase metabolic activity. A chart of omega 6 content of common foods can be found in Appendix II. Most of your dietary calories should be coming from sources with less than 5% of calories coming from omega 6 polyunsaturated fat, such as beef, lamb, fish, cream, coconut, beans, yams, rice, and potatoes.

5) **High in protein (but not TOO high).** Broda Barnes was a firm believer that consuming too much protein was really draining on the metabolism, particularly if calories were limited. He stated, "It has been clearly established that a high protein diet lowers the metabolic rate, [therefore] symptoms of hypothyroidism will be aggravated…" This may not be true on a calorically-superabundant diet, but protein is not used for metabolic fuel in the same way fats and carbohydrates are – making them preferable to protein. As calorie consumption increases, less protein is needed to maintain muscle mass as well – as little as 30 grams per day for an adult male (although I recommend much more for overall health and satisfaction). Plus, protein is found in all foods, and the more overall food you eat, the more protein you get – whether you eat meat, fish, and eggs or not. Last but not least, animal-source protein contains anti-thyroid amino acids in much higher proportions (methionine, cysteine, tryptophan). For this reason, portions of meat, fish, eggs, cheese, and poultry should probably be on the small side. I usually eat meat a few times a week. If you are drinking some milk as part of your approach, you don't need any supplemental meat at all, and RRARF can certainly be done as a vegetarian with milk or eggs, starches, fruits, legumes, and vegetables. There are vegan success stories, but the "carnage" greatly outweighs the success on a long-term basis. So that is a roulette game I don't recommend for extended periods of time.

6) **High in Salt.** Salt is a powerful metabolism stimulator. You don't have to get too carried away with it, but your food should be pleasantly salty, something salty should appear at every meal and snack, and all the food and fluids you take in should be counterbalanced with at least a little salt. This is not a permanent prescription, but salt is very therapeutic for

raising metabolic rate. Eat enough and you might actually feel uncomfortably hot, with burning-hot fingers, toes, and ears. You can read a lot more about salt's role in metabolic rate in my bestselling book *Eat for Heat: The Metabolic Approach to Food and Drink*.

A list of common food choices on a truly purist version of the HED would be something like the following:

Rich Protein Sources:

- Salmon; canned, frozen, or fresh
- Halibut
- Trout
- Cod
- Bass – any kind
- Snapper
- Sardines
- Other fish
- Skinless chicken
- Skinless duck
- Skinless turkey
- Cottage cheese
- Hard cheese – like cheddar or parmesan
- Rind-ripened cheese – like Brie
- Blue cheese
- Unsweetened yoghurt
- Milk; prefer raw milk, but am not a raw Nazi
- Jerky without additives
- Beef sausage or bacon
- All cuts of beef

- Pork – preferably on the leaner side; I personally wouldn't recommend eating much pork
- Ground beef, turkey, chicken
- Lamb
- Game meats
- All beans and legumes
- Eggs

Carbohydrate

- Potatoes; any variety
- Sweet potatoes/yams
- Carrots
- Turnips
- Parsnips
- Beets
- Rutabaga
- Celery root/celeriac
- Other starchy root vegetables
- Cornmeal porridge/polenta
- Fresh corn
- All beans and legumes
- Oatmeal
- Hot buckwheat cereal
- Amaranth
- Quinoa
- Brown rice
- White rice – basmati is the best (different type of starch in it)
- Homemade air-popped popcorn with coconut oil
- Bread
- Crackers
- Pasta

- Corn tortillas
- Tamale dough (Masa)
- Fruits – tropical are the best
- Juices – like orange juice, grape juice, apple juice, grapefruit juice, pineapple juice
- Coconut water
- Blackstrap molasses
- Honey
- Maple syrup
- Milk, kefir, and yoghurt

Fats

- Coconut milk
- Fresh or dried coconut
- Beef fat/tallow/suet
- Fatty cheeses
- Full-fat milk
- Half n' half
- Cream
- Sour cream/crème fraiche
- Macadamia nuts
- Macadamia nut oil
- Olives
- Olive oil
- Very fatty cuts of beef and ground beef
- Fatty fish (like salmon)
- Bone marrow
- Chocolate
- Whale blubber (just kidding – making sure you're still reading this)

Oh yeah, you should eat some vegetables, too. You don't have to panic about meeting a certain quota though. In fact, many vegetables, such as kale, bok choy, cabbage, broccoli, and cauliflower, contain powerful anti-thyroid substances. So eat some vegetables sure, just don't force yourself to eat them to achieve some kind of Popeye awesomeness. If you want forearms like that, I would eat lots of carbs and protein and masturbate excessively.

For extensive recipes and cooking instruction, you will enjoy my book *180 Kitchen: 180 Tips, Recipes, and More*. It's very important that your food tastes good and is enjoyable. In fact, that's probably THE MOST important factor of all. For this to work, you need a surplus of calories, and to get a surplus of calories you must be eating food that you enjoy.

A SAMPLE DAY

So what the heck do ya eat? For starters, I wouldn't even call it *"The High Everything Diet"* if I were you. That was just a term coined to describe it because nothing major was restricted. Your diet shouldn't have a name or be something you can tweet about using the # sign. If you, in your chronic dieting ways must name it, it should be your first name, followed by an apostrophe s, and the word "Diet." So for example, what I eat is referred to as "Matt's Diet." If your name is Jean Claude Van Damme, then what you eat is called "Jean Claude's Diet," and probably consists mostly of metal chards and King Cobra filets. If your name is Shooter McGavin, then you probably eat pieces of shit like Happy Gilmore for breakfast. My diet is different every week and depends on what I feel like eating, what's on sale, what I'm sick of from the week before, etc. Today (and yesterday) was definitely a full-fledged RRARF day which included:

- 9am – 2 bowls oatmeal with 4 bananas, 1 pint half n' half, 2T molasses
- 12pm - 6oz. ground beef with its fat and yams and pinto beans
- 2pm – 1 pint milk with 1T molasses and 1 more bowl of oats
- 7pm – ½ lb. turnip greens, 2 baked potatoes, bowl of fresh fruit

I don't eat like this all the time, but my temps had fallen slightly and 2-3 days of eating like this has been enough to clear and soften my skin, make me fiery hot from head to toe, plump up my muscles, jolt me with jittery energy – I can't stop fantasizing about exercising as I write this, and deepen my sleep. YOU eat what YOU think sounds awesome and satisfying, and that will change every week. No more diet plans. Nothing but main courses from here on out.

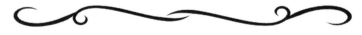

MAXercise

First of all, we've got some myth-busting to do. It's generally thought that exercise raises metabolism. Some forms, like the one you are about to discover generally does. Some exercise is metabolically-neutral, like easy walking, stretching, or light yoga. But most common exercise today slows down your metabolism. How many calories you burn is not your metabolic rate, but your total energy expenditure (TEE). TEE may rise with endurance exercise, but resting metabolism PLUMMETS severely.

Pay attention to how exercise impacts your actual body temperature, including the type discussed in this section. If you notice your first-thing-upon-waking body temperature falling, stop doing it. I don't recommend doing any difficult exercise at all for the first month, including what we're about to discuss. But eventually you will want to become physically active and train your muscles and cardiopulmonary system once you are healthy enough to do so. There is no question that exercise, done consistently, intelligently, and with great enjoyment, is one of the greatest enhancers of health, vitality, and functional longevity.

Although there have been some truly genius breakthroughs in our understanding of exercise physiology over the past few decades, and there are some true pioneers out there disseminating truly magnificent information, most are still caught in the quagmire of exercise beliefs that are like, SOOOO 1984.

Richard Simmons never had a nice body folks. And mimicking "his" style of workout or anything approximating it isn't gonna do much for ya. While it's nice to spend your days moving and on your feet doing light exercise, including but not limited to sweating to the oldies, most of the research points to acute bouts of vigorous, challenging physical activity as providing the most benefit. Steady-state, low to moderate intensity cardiovascular exercise, or what the ridiculously-ripped fitness model and trainer Paula Owens calls LSD (long, slow, distance), certainly looks detrimental when viewed through the metabolism lens. Paula writes:

"One must exercise for long duration and often in order to burn any amount of fat with LSD. This is how long distance runners maintain their slim physiques. However, when a runner sustains an injury and is unable to train their metabolism spirals down. This leads to increased body fat over time."

"LSD exercise is problematic because it causes cortisol to rise unopposed by the growth-promoting hormones, testosterone and growth hormone. This creates a physical stress response to your entire body. Prolonged release of cortisol, whether from long-term physical, mental, or emotional stress, or the wrong kind of exercise, atrophies your muscles, nerves and brain cells. This may explain why standard aerobic exercise is not effective for optimal body composition and why marathon runners exhibit frail bodies devoid of muscle. The duration - not the

intensity - of the exercise is the most significant issue in regards to
cortisol. Chronic over-secretion of cortisol causes a weakened immune
system, a decrease in lean muscle, hair loss, thinning skin, infertility,
inability to grow nails and a decrease in concentration and
memory. Excess cortisol kills brain cells, including those in the
hippocampus, where the brain processes emotions. Excessive cortisol
production can also deplete serotonin levels causing depression."

Okay Paula we get it, jeez! Settle down. Lady's got some issues!

Basically what Paula is getting at is that your body adapts to endurance exercise in counterproductive ways from a metabolic point of view.

For starters, the chronic rise in stress hormones causes an extreme fall in basal metabolic rate. After a summer of hiking for example, my body temperature fell from 97.9 F to 96.2 F. During endurance exercise you lose lean body mass as well, which can further slow your metabolism down (although, like I mentioned earlier, isn't quite as straightforward as many people think). You also, when doing long duration exercise at a moderate pace, burn mostly fat for energy instead of glucose. This ensures that your body, when given the chance (like when you stop doing it or take a break), will store back a bunch of fat to help fill the fat tank – particularly around the abdomen. You also store a bunch of fat in your muscles called intramuscular fat, which blocks the delivery of glucose and amino acids into your muscle cells to keep them from growing or expending energy efficiently. This is of course, insulin resistance.

With all this you see a big drop in testosterone and growth hormone like Paula mentions. This favors, once again, a drop in athletic performance and capability, prevents fat loss, and accelerates the aging process. There is really nothing good about endurance exercise as far as its effect on your body composition and health. And we're not just talking marathons. Even athletes that train for a 1-mile race undergo many of these adaptations – looking like stick figures. That's not the body you want to build underneath your fat or you'll never burn it off. You simply won't have the hormonal firepower to do so.

All of these changes should sound familiar. These are all the physiological adaptations to inadequate food/calorie restriction/dieting.

But these are of course the right adaptations to this type of exercise. When going long distances, your body needs to be more efficient. This means using less oxygen and fewer calories to do the same activity. To do this, the body induces a state of severe hypothyroidism, and is why you often see female runners become infertile and stop having their periods and develop autoimmune disease and such in response to endurance athletic training.

But efficiency is just one adaptation the body can undergo. I liken it to turning your body into an economy car designed to hold up better on the road and get better gas mileage (calorie mileage). But you can go all Ferrari, too, it just takes a different set of stimuli.

"By doing those kind of activities you actually 'ask' your body to make those changes. And in response, it does. You can train your body to make any kind of change you want."

-Al Sears; *P.A.C.E.*

So forget what you think about exercise. It can be fun – and is extremely fun when you notice immediate, tangible, and substantial improvements from doing the right kind of exercise. The right kind of exercise is one of the biggest tools out there for making real physiological adaptations that get your body to lose fat and gain muscle automatically and spontaneously (any gender, any age). So let's talk about what that is.

I coined the termMAXercise, partly because I'm a dork, partly because I love acronyms, but mostly because coining something makes me seem really cool.

It means Metabolic Adaptation Xercise to help remind you that exercise is something you can do as a tool to trigger a certain set of metabolic adaptations to the training itself. You may only do this type of exercise for a few minutes twice a week, but the hormonal changes, if you trigger them successfully, work 24 hours per day 7 days per week. That's why hormones are so much more powerful than playing around with calorie intake and calories burned through exercise.

The acronym MAX also helps to remind you of how you achieve that adaptation, and that is through short bursts of MAXimum effort.

It's really quite simple. In a quick flurry of exercise (someone recently referred to it as "spazzercise"), you take your heart and lungs to their cardiopulmonary maximum – encouraging them to adapt to become bigger, stronger, and more effective. This is not something that requires a lot of time. This is not something you do every day. You do not need to go to a gym (although some of the equipment can be helpful and give you more variety). You are just trying to encourage your body to get better and more powerful and explosive. The rest – the improvements in health, increase in growth hormone and testosterone (in both males and females – don't worry ladies this won't put hair on your chest), the improvements in insulin and leptin sensitivity, fall of stress hormones, increased production of anti-inflammatory hormones... and the corresponding rise in metabolism, increase in lean body mass, and decrease in body fat… all falls right into place.

It is also safe unlike what you might think at first blush. While you should always consult with your doctor to make sure you don't have a heart condition before doing this kind of exercise or any other, the bottom line is that this type of exercise, with its increase in cardiopulmonary strength and capacity, is one of the secret weapons against aging and degenerative disease. At least that's my impression of it so far.

I'll try to keep my explanation of it as simple and straightforward as possible so that you can be turned loose and ready to give it a try right away as your new prioritized form of exercise – the rest can be up to you, whether it's weight training – which will be made much more effective by this type of exercise, calisthenics, yoga, Pilates, tennis, golf, walking, hiking, cycling, professional napping or sunbathing, or other forms of recreation – it is solely up to you and what sounds enjoyable and fulfilling.

MAX effort means MAX effort. While you may not be able to give a max effort right away, you should start building towards that destination. A max effort for a 350-pound 63-year old may be walking up a flight of stairs without stopping. Hey, maybe that's not even possible. But the point of the training is to push your cardiopulmonary system to the point where you simply can't continue for another second. It's getting into this new turf that forces the body to adapt to become better at handling these difficult situations.

After you have pushed yourself to a MAX effort, you pay attention to your own biofeedback (your breathing and pulse rate), and when you have recovered to the point of being able to breathe in a fairly relaxed manner with your mouth closed, you go for another round. 2-10 rounds of this can be performed depending on your comfort and overall fitness level. Total exertion time, meaning the amount of time you are actively engaged in a MAX effort outburst (not including rest/recovery time), should be no longer than 5 total minutes to avoid using fat as a fuel source for the activity, and 2-3 minutes of total exertion time is plenty for me.

You want to use almost 100% glucose to fuel this activity, which is one of the things that separates POWER activity from EFFICIENCY activity like jogging. This unclogs the entire glucose metabolism system enabling your body to start storing amino acids and glucose from the food you eat into muscle where it is converted into energy, heat, and muscle – it also tends to have an appetite-suppressing effect when your carbohydrate reserves are finally able to be topped off in this way – which is not possible when you are insulin resistant because you are unresponsive to the hormone that stores all of that energy into the muscle cells to begin with.

The ultimate type of exercise would be about a 100-200 meter sprint, but sprinting is very dangerous in terms of joint damage, muscle pulls, and other injury. Sprinting is also way too advanced for an older person with a lot of excess weight that stands to gain the most from doing this type of training. For a beginner, Elliptical machines, stationary bikes, and bodyweight exercises are the three best options.

Before we go any further, I must reiterate that the key is relying on your own biofeedback. Only you can know when you've really gone to your cardiopulmonary max and cannot continue. And recovery time is highly variable. Actually, recovery time is probably the best indicator of overall cardiovascular fitness. But this is why traditional interval training of 30 seconds on and a minute off, or some other narrow window of recovery is not applicable to an out-of-shape person. You have to progress it at your level and work on getting better. Likewise, if you are already really fit and want to expand your fitness, the standard exertion periods and recovery windows of typical interval training may not be challenging enough to push you to your MAX effort.

Plus with set interval periods, the more you do them, the easier they get. You don't want it to get easier! Ever! The idea is to keep pushing yourself to the MAX no matter what your fitness level.

Only you can know your MAX effort, and your max effort depends on what day it is, what time of day, how you feel, what you've eaten, how long it's been since your last workout, and all kinds of other unknowns that set time periods of exertion and recovery and heart rate targets cannot take into consideration. This is your own personal fitness improvement program, and only you, listening to your own body and knowing when you are challenging it to a new level of intensity it's not equipped to deal with, can decide both your exertion and recovery times.

And you must have progress with the program to have long-term success with it. Progression is key with all forms of exercise, and you will not progress doing the same routine over and over again. You have to be going beyond your prior thresholds routinely, switching up exercises that you use to test your MAX, and all the while staying highly attuned to your own progress. Easier said than done perhaps, but no set batch of guidelines can do as much for you as you can do for yourself. The goal, as a reminder, is to increase how much you achieve in your MAX efforts, and steadily improve your recovery time – needing less and less recovery the longer you move forward with the training.

Don't let me fool you into thinking it's easy though just because it's short. It's grueling. Brutal. But after you've given it some time and see what it can do for your overall levels of strength, fitness, energy levels, and body composition you'll see what all the fuss is about. I hope you will at least. There are no one-hit wonders out there that work magic on everybody. That's for sure. But this is worth some self-experimentation, and would be even if it didn't change your body composition a lick (and you really must ignore the scale with this exercise, as it's totally possible to lose 20 pounds of fat without the scale moving an inch due to increases in lean body mass and stored glycogen).

Try MAXercise on a stationary bike at first if you have one. Get on and warm up for a couple minutes, pedaling slowly but enough to get your heart rate up slightly. Make sure the level is giving you plenty of resistance and doesn't feel like you're just waving your feet in the air with nothing pressing back against them. Then…Explode!

In a mad flurry pedal as hard and fast as you absolutely can for 10 seconds. Then pause and return to slow pedaling. Feel how your heart thumps in your chest and notice that your breathing is elevated. For some, this 10 seconds may wipe you out for the rest of the day. That's fine. We all start somewhere, and the farther you are from being a superhero, the more ground you stand to gain by making progress with your explosive capabilities.

If the 10 seconds didn't kill you, continue to pedal until your breathing starts to become relaxed almost like normal and you feel pretty rested. This may take 30 seconds. This may take 3 minutes. It doesn't matter, but you should be paying attention to know where you are starting at in the two most important categories – how long you can go at full speed, and how long it takes you to recover. When you feel rested, go again for 20 seconds at the fastest speed your legs can generate.

Then repeat and pay attention once again to your biofeedback. How did you do that time? Almost lose a lung? Were you sucking wind so hard that the toupee of the guy in front of you is caught in your windpipe? If not, 20 seconds probably isn't quite your MAX effort.

Anyway, continue this until, instead of counting seconds on the clock, you are going until you reach what you know, when being honest with yourself, is your physiological limit. When you get there, it's a "different" experience (don't eat too much before you try it!), but this is what actually causes your body to adapt and change towards all the desirable things you're looking to achieve through exercise, but never could by jogging in the past because you were hormonally pissing into the wind while you did it.

It doesn't matter whether this is 8 seconds or 2 minutes. You shouldn't even be watching the clock. You should be going all out for as long as you can, and then stopping when you get there. When you get there, it's important that you rest to a decent level of recovery. Get off the bike if you have to and walk around. Sip some water. Focus on your breathing and try to keep your mouth closed and suck air in through your nostrils. This calms you and improves your recovery time – and opens up the nasal passages like a champ.

When you have recovered to a level of comfort, but not full relaxation, get back on the bike and go at it again to the same point of exhaustion and repeat. Maybe you only muster up the courage to do 2-3 rounds the first time, but over time work on progressing this. For example, you could do 2 rounds for a month, then add a round every month until you are doing 10 rounds with each workout. That would be some serious progress, but it's doable. One way or another, keep making it harder and harder and harder (not longer though), by mixing it up and somehow keeping it just as challenging as it was on day one. Remember, the point of this exercise in a nutshell is pushing yourself to new levels. This, by definition, requires that you keep making progress and reaching new limits each time.

That's all there is to it. Now, that may be a little boring for some, and I don't recommend just doing the bike every time although it is one of the better instruments for reaching your cardiopulmonary maximum safely in a short period of time (Elliptical machines are the best) – but there's an infinite number of ways you can make it more fun, interesting, diverse, and challenging. And you should because, like I said, introducing new challenges and adapting to them is one of the most important, if not THE most important key of all physical training.

For example, let's say after 2 months on the bike you are so bored you're contemplating suicide. Switch to an elliptical machine. This is actually much better at challenging your cardiopulmonary max than the bike. The bike, in fact, has limitations. The thing with the bike is that you are using primarily your quadriceps muscles and that's about it. This is a big muscle no doubt, and it causes a lot of air-sucking and heart thumping – but often the leg muscles fail before your lungs and heart are maxed out. An extreme example of this in action would be to squeeze a tennis ball with your hand over and over and over again until your forearm muscles failed to contract. This is called muscle failure. By the end of doing this you wouldn't even be out of breath. So exercises that work just one muscle can cause muscle failure long before you reach your cardiopulmonary threshold, and this threshold is really the impetus for building more fast twitch muscle fibers, creating more lactic acid, using the heart muscle anaerobically, and all the things that work synergistically to increase growth hormone secretion and stimulate adaptive responses.

The elliptical machine is superior to a bike because you are using not just your quadriceps muscles, but also your hamstrings, glutes, biceps, pectorals, and upper back – especially if you are really trying to push and pull hard on the handles. In this instance you are creating more blood and oxygen demand by engaging more muscle simultaneously, and your heart and lungs are taxed much more than they would be on a bike or just doing bodyweight squats or pushups. Some gyms also have mountain climber machines that would be perhaps even better than an elliptical, as you climb with both your hands and legs while in place.

Anyway, you get the picture.

For those looking to enhance athleticism and maybe build more mobility, agility, strength, and muscle – especially after undergoing several months of serious cardiopulmonary conditioning from the introductory stuff on the cardio machines, you can also circuit through various functional exercises and create absolutely absurd demands on your cardiopulmonary system, although it takes much longer to reach your maximum threshold time-wise. Still, this can be awesome, and remove the need for you to go to a gym completely (although, like I said, gym equipment is awesome for fun and variety).

The type of exercises one might do would be to jump up in the air as high as you can until you are about to collapse. But since this is just the leg muscles working, you collapse into a pushup position and peel off as many pushups as you can. When you are maxed out there you might pump your knees from that pushup position for more core work and to squeeze the last few drops left in your legs and chest. You will probably find your MAX in this third position about 2 minutes into the set. This is much more draining and challenging than just hitting the cardio machines, and you might find 3-4 sessions of this, with a different set of exercises each time for a full body workout, enough to make you puke in the garbage can before all is said and done. But the cardio machines do have the advantage of being simpler and safer and allowing you to reach your MAX much more quickly like a sprint. Certainly superior for entry level exercise.

You can also work some weights into this as well if you like. Olympic lifts and kettlebell exercises, which are all the rage right now, engage the entire body and put you at your threshold really quickly. Just make sure you are truly reaching your MAX by finishing with something like bodyweight squats or squat jumps at the end of each round for extra insurance. Same goes for doing standard weightlifting exercise. A bicep/tricep/squat jump circuit repeated three times through without rest with descending amounts of weight each time is a killer. The theme is the same. Work as many muscles of the body as possible so that you reach your cardiopulmonary MAX before you reach muscle failure. Or, put another way, take a muscle group to failure and then switch to another muscle group immediately to further your level of total oxygen depletion.

For more creative stuff along these lines, and serious body development, the Innervation and Metabolic Enhancement Training developed by Scott Abel is as good as it gets. I recommend trying out some of his many "blasts" available to watch for free on YouTube at www.youtube.com/scottabelcoaching

While there are dozens of great contributors to our understanding of physical exercise on health, metabolism, muscle development, strength gain, cardiovascular fitness, and all the things that exercise is used for – there is absolutely no doubt that Scott Abel has the most thorough, comprehensive, and expert understanding of the big picture of how movement of all types and varieties affects the human body.

But that's enough of that. I don't want to turn off any newbies while trying to impress the gym nerds. I'll leave that up to those who specialize in training elite athletes like Scott. All I mean to do here is show you that there is a way to use exercise to get results unlike the lame and ineffective stuff you've tried in the past – from aimlessly lifting weights with no program or strategy (a step in the right direction, but that's about it) to running marathons (26.2 miles in the wrong direction). It has nothing to do with how many calories you burn doing it and everything to do with your body and its hormonal profile changing to work with you, instead of against you. No matter how hibernatory or thrifty your metabolism is, I think you will be pleasantly surprised at how your body rises and adapts to the challenges you present it with. Especially after you have taken measures to restore and repair your metabolism with *Diet Recovery* and properly support your physical activity with lots of carbohydrates, calories, and sleep for proper refueling.

One important rule of the training is to never do it two days in a row, and do it at least once per week. The ideal would be to do it three times per week, every other day, with total exertion time between 2 and 10 minutes. On your off days, and the rest of the day on your training days, you can do whatever else you like. Play Frisbee. Go dancing. Lift weights. Even go jogging if that's something you actually enjoy. You'll find that the training supports you in whatever endeavors or sports you participate in.

For more on the general ideas behind the formation of MAXercise – but remembering the importance of your own biofeedback, I highly recommend watching a demonstration of Phil Campbell's Peak 8 exercises done by Dr. Mercola. Just consider yourself warned about Mercola's short-shorts. Peak 8 has regimented exertion and recovery periods that may be too hard for many people and too easy for elite athletes. Again, you have to adjust for individuality and also keep making them harder and harder to keep making progress. But the concept is very straightforward and about as complex as a redneck's turn-ons (Daisy Duke, fake breasts, beer). What I like is that the exertion period is at maximum speed and is very simple and easy to follow – one problem Mercola had with Sears's PACE program evidently. http://bit.ly/y7cwbv

Dr. Mercola's results have been unmistakably good though – for a 56-year old dude doing 8-12 minutes per week of this type of exertion, you can't be too bummed about this dramatic body composition change: *"So far I've lost 13 pounds of fat and gained over 10 pounds of muscle."*

A good read on the topic is *PACE*, by Al Sears. Sears does a great job at stressing the need for listening to your own biofeedback in determining how to best perform the exercise, and has a lot of compelling evidence for why expanding your lung capacity and cardio output is such a health protector and secret to aging well.

Anyway, don't underestimate the power of smart exercise. And this exercise is invigorating – not draining and spine-crushing like many other forms of exercise, which is a great bonus.

And as far as exercise is concerned in general, see what you can do to purge your mind of your prior conditioning. As humans, we often have a lot of mental baggage that eclipses our natural human desires. One of those desires is to move our bodies in invigorating and playful ways on a daily basis – just like the family dog, without mental baggage, is always up for a round of Frisbee or a jaunt around in the woods. But, in an effort to salvage our self-esteem many of us have labeled those more athletic than us as "dumb jocks," and exercise as something that only those inferior narcissistic knuckleheads engage in.

A lot of us also accumulate tons of mental baggage after having viewed exercise as "work" and something that "burns calories" – or maybe, like myself, exercise was something I did to earn self-esteem or exalt myself over those less athletically gifted. These are all human interferences with the true calling of our bodies to move, play, be challenged, and be invigorated in movement, expression, sport, and life in general.

Or maybe in the past you just overdid it, or did the kind of exercise that really broke you down and undermined your health and vigor. Or exercised in a calorie or carbohydrate deficit. That will make anyone come to resent exercise. It happens to the best of us.

Spend some time scrutinizing why you feel the way you feel about exercise if it is resoundingly negative. I assure you that your health and well-being can only be positively impacted by reconnecting with your body's true innate desires to be active and useful. Take it real slow if it's been a while! You'll make yourself sick if you don't!

And exercise with no goal in mind other than to improve your health and live a better life. Those are not finite, and keep you moving forward forever. Weight loss is not a goal, it's either something that happens or doesn't happen as a result of living, eating, and moving in smarter and healthier ways. But whether you attain the figure you've always dreamed of (keeping in mind that your dream to attain this figure is due primarily to media poisoning and the flaunting of unrealistic and unobtainable goals that dominate our head space from birth to death for no good reason other than to force us to minimize ourselves compared to anorexic people whose life is a living prison), or you simply get healthier and enjoy your life more, either way you win. What matters is that you are healthier and enjoy your life more. I assure you from my own experiences that you can be one ripped m'fer and still hate every minute of your life. It's not about how we look. It's about how we feel, and feeling good has a lot more to do with healthy practices and attitudes than it actually does a cosmetic change.

If you disagree that is fine. In fact, I would agree with you on that, but then we'd both be wrong!

Food Rehabilitation

"You can hardly talk about health and taking care of yourself without discussing nutrition. But our experience has shown us that if a healthy relationship with food is not in place first, it's difficult to pursue a truly healthy diet. If you've been a chronic dieter, the best nutrition guidelines can still be embraced like a diet."
-Evelyn Tribole and Elyse Resch; *Intuitive Eating*

This book, as much as it is about restoring your metabolism, it is equally about restoring your relationship with food. After going through a long and arduous journey through diets, you may find it hard not to analyze the calories on your plate, think about how many carbs or fat grams are on it, or wonder what's in the pizza you're enjoying with friends on a night out (the antithesis of a relaxing and HEALTHY carefree evening). You really have to let go. We know from countless studies at this point that the very concept of restrained eating often leads to binge eating and long-term weight gain. While we all should intend to nourish ourselves with primarily quality food that has nutrients in it (what a concept!), there's a fine line that almost every veteran dieter crossed ages ago, and it's important to come back across that line.

"Overall, more than seventy-five studies have been conducted to examine the effects of various situations that disturb the restrained eater's self-control. The results are consistent: Restrained eaters react to emotions and external cues in a nearly totally opposite manner of unrestrained eaters. Emotions such as depression, anxiety, anger, fear, and excitement or disinhibitors, such as alcohol, cause a restrained eater to overeat. Conversely, they turn off the appetite of an unrestrained eater. As long as things go well, the restrained eater can maintain control. But if anything gets in the way or changes, she can't maintain that control. The reason is clear: Restrained eaters don't rely on the normal signals of fullness to regulate their eating, so there are no brakes in place."

-Linda Bacon; *Health at Every Size*

Like I hinted at earlier, this program is intended to strengthen your digestion and metabolism, expanding the foods you "tolerate," and expand your dietary freedom – not to mention get your appetite and metabolism on the same team so that you regulate your weight effortlessly and naturally like a healthy person. So you will find that you can eat like so and so and not notice any ill effects from it. So that's exactly what you should do. You should go to restaurants with friends, you should join the family in eating dessert at Thanksgiving, and you should be able to have a juicy burger at a restaurant, covered with a white flour bun, without zapping that burger with psychological distress.

Generally speaking, what you do habitually is everything. What you do on occasion is inconsequential, and living a good, fulfilling, and healthy life goes far beyond what a "perfect diet," whatever that is, can give you. A diet really can be so healthy it destroys your health – and more importantly, the overall quality of your life. You simply must stop attaching utopian happily-ever-after fantasies to various ways of eating. People will try to seduce you with all kinds of "sure things" against disease or weight "problems," but when you feel the urge to check them out, slap yourself in the face. If you have a longstanding dieting problem, you should probably never read another health or diet-related book again (except the ones that reinforce body acceptance, non-dieting, and other helpful things instead of distracting messages), just like someone with a heroin problem probably shouldn't shoot up again. You've already spent way too much of your mind energy and time on intellectualizing and controlling everything you put in your mouth, and you've got a lot of missed life to catch up on.

If there is such a thing as a healthy relationship with food it is quite simple. Food is something you eat to fuel and nourish your body most of the time. Food is not something to use for satisfying emotional longings, boredom, or as a target of your primordial desires to commit sin (violate what you've decided in your mind is "right").

I mean, you can know that French fries are cooked in oxidized, omega 6-laden vegetable oil and that they aren't the healthiest thing to eat. But having a desire to live life dangerously and be a bad boy or bad girl doesn't need to involve a trip to the drive-thru for a Supersize Order. I eat French fries every now and then. It's no big deal. I don't have one and then say, "Ah, F$#% my diet I'm going to eat 4 pounds of fries and hey, since I've already blown it I might as well keep the momentum going and drink a case of beer and eat a half gallon of ice cream while I'm at it."

"One of the classic studies involved fifty-seven female college students at Northwestern University. The students were led to believe that the goal of

the study was to evaluate the taste of several ice cream samples. The actual purpose of the study was to determine how diet thinking might affect eating after drinking milkshakes. The women were arbitrarily divided into three groups based on the number of eight-ounce milkshakes given (none, one, and two shakes). After drinking the shakes, the subjects were asked to taste and rate three flavors of ice cream. They were allowed to eat as much ice cream as they wanted and 'taste-tested' in private to guard against self-consciousness. The researchers saw to it that ample ice cream was provided so that substantial amounts could be eaten without making an appreciable dent in the supply!

Here's what happened. The nondieters naturally regulated their eating; they ate less ice cream in proportion to the amount of milkshakes consumed. The dieters, however, displayed a dramatic opposite behavior. Those who drank two milkshakes ate the most ice cream — a 'counterregulation' effect. The researchers concluded that forcing the dieters to overeat or 'blow their diet' caused them to release their food inhibitions. With inhibition banished, restraint was eliminated and the dieters overate the ice cream."

-Evelyn Tribole and Elyse Resch; *Intuitive Eating*

If you file foods into absolute good and bad categories and grade yourself on how many "good choices" you make versus "bad choices," then you are still plagued by the diet mentality and are doomed. I mean really doomed. There are no forbidden foods. Speaking of forbidden foods, what happened when God told that Adam dude not to eat the forbidden fruit? That was probably the first thing he did! Don't "forbidden fruit" your dietary choices. If you want *Sour Patch Kids*, you can eat them. If you think ice cream is bad, you should literally fill your freezer with it and eat it until it becomes neutral. Work on this stuff. Challenge your dietary demons. There's a huge payoff if you do, and really learn to frigging chill out and stop being such a Nazi about everything.

When you actually arrive at this state of dietary Zen, then you actually are at a point where you can begin to choose things to put into your mouth because they are nutritious, because of how you know they will make you feel, and because you have a nourishing, loving relationship with yourself. You'll never, ever arrive there by diligently avoiding foods that you want. In fact, the name of the game and the entire premise of this program is to do everything in your power to convince your body that fats, carbohydrates, protein, calories, and nutrients are all present in complete and total abundance. It's this reinforcement that thoroughly convinces even the most deep-seated thrifty metabolism that it's okay to burn energy at the optimal rate, and there is no longer any reason to store excess energy in the body. If you don't believe that there is truly magic in this psychological shift, read *The Gabriel Method* by Jon Gabriel and get back to me.

In fact, I strongly believe that a hoarding mentality can create hoarding physiology. Most of our weight is managed within our brains in the hypothalamus. Why wouldn't our thoughts be able to give us the mother of all placebo/nocebo effects? One of my 180 followers actually claimed to once be able to put on four pounds just by eating dessert. But of course, it's this "Ah screw it, I never get to eat this. It'll be months before I have another slice of cake" psychological noise that instructs the body to say, "Oh, big brother is about to eat something that he never gets a chance to eat. It could be months until we see this food again, we better hold on to it."

Rules are meant to be broken, so for a long-term sustainable approach to a healthy diet, don't make rules. The guidelines in this book are meant to get your metabolism restored, and once restored, you move on, just eating a diet that satisfies your every need and that you can stick with. You decide what you eat, not some douchebag health guru like me. I can report on what I think is healthiest, but ultimately it's up to you to interpret it, customize it to your liking, implement the ideas you find useful, and trash anything you find to be unsustainable or unrealistic.

A healthy diet and a healthy relationship with food is something that is cumulative and spans decades. I might not advocate endurance exercise, but I certainly advocate endurance healthy eating. Stick with it and make it realistic for the long haul. Speaking of exercise, it's much healthier to exercise once per week for 20 years than to ping pong between exercising five days per week on some unsustainable workout program for one year and then get burned out and not exercise at all for another year before picking up the same program you got burned out on the first go around. Same principle applies to your eating. Make sure your diet and lifestyle is something that you love and want to continue for life. If you feel that way about it, you've found the healthiest diet for you. Make the diet fit your life. Don't change your life around to fit your diet. Don't let the diet take over your life. Let it play a supporting role in your life, helping you to feel better and have more energy for the things you would love to do and experience.

My number one tip…

No matter what you've read, no matter what you've heard, no matter what you've experienced…

Make a conscious point to actively ENJOY every bite of the stuff that you've conditioned yourself to believe is unhealthy with intense focus every time you decide to eat it.

This simple practice completely changed my life, and led to my first experience with sustainable healthy eating years ago — before that I would eat all organic rabbit food 6 days per week while exercising 5 hours per day and then binge on Krispy Kreme doughnuts (my body's last-ditched effort to save me from starvation), but that's another story.

Seriously. Eyes closed with every bite of chocolate cake. Play with that frosting as it slowly melts between the tip of your tongue and the roof of your mouth. Feel your tongue move across your front teeth like a wiper blade clearing off the crumbs. Make it blissful, not another "I shouldn't" diet moment or round of binging and hoarding. I promise it works.

This rule applies to just about everything in life. Always be on your own team. Guilt is far more unhealthy than any Krispy Kreme doughnut I've ever eaten. And repressing your true human urges and desires is a great way to pervert your true human urges and desires, not only binging on junk food, but molesting children, cheating on your spouse, and about any twisted sickness you can imagine. Life is too short not to love who you are as hard as you possibly can — not letting anyone, especially yourself, convince you that you are wrong for who you are.

Body Image Rehab

"If you want to live a long and healthy life, you don't need some fad-diet-guru-optimization-lifestyle book to tell you how... You already know the answer. It can be summed up in four words: Eat right and exercise... The hard part, the part you will probably resist with everything you've got, the part that could turn your world upside down (in a good way) is the part where you stop hoping to lose weight. That hope has nothing to do with health or with living a long and happy life and even less to do with real hopefulness. Wishing your weight would change is about conformity and self-hatred and insecurity and prejudice, and everything that's designed to bring you down."

-Marilyn Wann; *Fat! So?*

This is a mother of a topic, but I wanted to mention something about it briefly, as this is often the core problem behind a dieter's constant misadventures. Before you even begin this program, you should be ready and willing to lose weight or gain weight, and be comfortable with whatever results from feeding your body everything it needs in abundance you get. Some people gain some weight and some health from following this program, others lose some weight and gain some health following this program. I assure you the gaining of health far exceeds any changes you experience in body composition in the first couple of months, which, in the grand scheme of things, is totally inconsequential.

We have a global fat phobia and hatred that, when considering the well-known hereditary component driving our increasing body fat, this hatred is akin to the most overt racism, gender bias, or discrimination based on sexual orientation. In 20 years, I predict that fat discrimination is not something that is just taken for granted as a fact of life the way it is today. While it's far-fetched to think that society will come to truly appreciate fatness and view it as beautiful the way it does the slenderness of say, Salma Hayek (Hey Salma, you left your toothbrush over at my house last night. I'll bring it over later!), there's definitely a body "acceptance" movement going on out there and it will continue to grow.

Anyway, just like the long, slow, patience-heavy process of diet rehab, so too is body image rehab a "process." This brings up an important point that it would be criminal not to mention. Remember that taking 2 steps forward and 1 step back is progress. But the perfectionism that lies at the heart of many disordered eaters and self-loathers, instead of viewing 2 steps forward and 1 step back as progress, tends to make one see the 1 step back as an abysmal failure, throw in the towel, and give up. Actually, 36 steps forward are often all toppled with 1 small step in the wrong direction.

What I'm saying is, with both diet and body image rehab alike, there will be some relapses. You can view these relapses as personal failures and quit the process altogether, or you can actually take a wiser perspective and see how much ground you've covered, pause, assess, and continue moving forward. This is called being resilient, and it's a much more difficult quality to cultivate than perfection in many areas.

I don't have any words of wisdom to cling to other than some of my other writings, such as this article which is a must-read if you have long-held body image issues (as any dieter does)…

Google: "Weight Fixation: Waist of Time"

But one thing I know for sure is that the game of trying to improve your life by trying to get your body to look like a supermodel is not a game that can be won. The pursuit of wanting to look better, not only isn't finite with no destination, the more time and effort you dedicate to it, the more obsessive you become. The system that preys upon our desire to fit a certain image is built around trying to fit an ideal that is unobtainable. And trying to perpetually obtain the unobtainable is a waste of time. No matter what you accomplish, you'll be left wanting. If it's not your fat that's making you feel bad about yourself, it will be your hair, your nose, a mole behind your ear, or some other nonsense.

"This logic promises that when the weight-obsessed individual finally achieves a certain weight, she will be satisfied with the appearance of her body. But this is a false promise. An eating-disordered culture functions by making people deeply dissatisfied with their appearance, no matter what that appearance happens to be."

-Paul Campos; *The Obesity Myth*

The only way to win that game is to try hard to stay out of the game entirely, putting your focus on what you want your attention to be focused on and a lot of practice (and resilience) to keep from getting dragged back into body image obsessiveness.

So whatever goals you have with any health pursuit begin and end with only one goal – using health information to help better facilitate your own personal goals, dreams, and aspirations. That's it. That's what health information is for. If you happen to lose weight being good to yourself great! If not, great! Either way, you don't need to lose weight to fix a weight problem. I know very few who fixed their weight problems by losing weight.

"Decades of research – and probably your own personal experience – show that the pursuit of weight loss rarely produces the thin, happy life you dream of. Dropping the pursuit of weight loss isn't about giving up, it's about moving on. When you make choices because they help you feel better, not because of their presumed effect on your weight, you maintain them over the long run."

-Linda Bacon; *Health at Every Size*

The bottom line? Your purpose here on this earth is a lot grander than obsessing over your diet and body. If you keep obsessing over your diet and body you are likely to drown out the signals pointing you to what that purpose really is. Enough already.

Which brings me to one final tidbit I'll leave you with… The belief that being fat is unhealthy is false. In fact, in the United States, at age 70 and above, those with Level 1 obesity (BMI of 30-35) have the lowest rates of degenerative disease and greatest longevity statistics, particularly if you are physically fit and don't cycle your weight (meaning yo-yo diet).

"Contrary to almost everything you have heard, weight is not a good predictor of health. In fact a moderately active larger person is likely to be

far healthier than someone who is svelte but sedentary. Moreover, the efforts of Americans to make themselves thin through dieting and drugs are a major cause of both 'overweight' and the ill health that is wrongly ascribed to it. In other words, America's war on fat is actually helping cause the very disease it is supposed to cure."

"There is no good evidence that significant long-term weight loss is beneficial to health, and a great deal of evidence that short-term weight loss followed by weight regain (the pattern followed by almost all dieters) is medically harmful. Indeed, frequent dieting is perhaps the single best predictor of future weight gain."

-Paul Campos; *The Obesity Myth*

Conclusion

What to expect…
The first thing you should expect to feel is doubt. You
think, "Me? Eat not just how much food I want to eat but
MORE than I want to eat and this is somehow supposed to
make me healthy and not balloon up to 600 pounds?" I know
it sounds sort of crazy in the 21st century in a country like the
United States of Anorexica, but the bottom line is that modern
people are sick, we are getting fatter and fatter as we interact
with the modern food environment, and all the information and
data we have on trying to achieve "intentional" weight loss
through any number of diets, exercise programs, and forms of
restraint is not only ineffective, and not only does it worsen our
health both physically and psychologically, but actually makes
us fatter than we would have otherwise been if we had never
bothered to try them.

*"The only other large study to look into the question of the health effects of
intentional weight loss – the Iowa Women's Health Study – produced
some rather extraordinary data in regard to the assumption that trying to
get thin is the appropriate 'cure' for the 'disease' of above-average weight.
The Iowa study is particularly striking, in that it featured no less than 108*

different statistical comparisons, based on age, initial weight and health status, and cause of death. In seventy-nine of these comparisons, intentional weight loss was associated with higher mortality rates. By contrast, the number of comparisons in which intentional weight loss ended up being associated with lower mortality rates was zero. This is especially significant information, given that the Iowa study is one of only a few studies that have distinguished between intentional and unintentional weight loss when measuring the effects of weight loss on health..."

"Simply put, dieting causes the condition it's supposed to cure. Most people who diet would be happier, healthier, and thinner if they never dieted."

-Paul Campos; *The Obesity Myth*

The power of eating enough to fully satisfy appetite on a consistent basis is very strong. Do not underestimate it. The psychological and physical aspects of completely making an about face on your relationship with eating is even more powerful than that however.

Consider the fact that, as a chronic dieter, it becomes ingrained time and time again the idea of forbidden foods. These forbidden foods we label as "treats" that we are to consume in moderation or else! Then we proceed to follow a diet program that creates an escalating desire to eat the forbidden foods on both a physical and psychological level. Even if these restricted diets would work, they are really just hypothetical – because we live in the real world in a very unique food environment and the psychological complexities of advertising, cooking shows, health claims, and more make following a restricted diet more or less impossible. Today's modern food environment and body image-obsessed environment requires unique weaponry that no weight loss-oriented diet could ever offer with reliability.

What RRARF does is completely change your relationship with food. The idea of "treat" just means that food becomes associated with pleasure with a Pavlovian conditioning. And rules are meant to be broken. But when you intentionally eat a little MORE than you want to eat, and do so religiously for an extended period of time, eating becomes a heck of a lot less pleasurable. This might sound like a bad thing, but really it just removes the psychological noise getting in between you and your natural appetite signals.

Then eating becomes what it is – eating. No longer is it a sin to eat, there are no more "treats" because eating when you are stuffed already isn't pleasant or rewarding at all. It's like offering a drowning man a glass of water. You also lose all those food inhibitions that primed you for binging and hoarding when you finally did have a break in your willpower and bulldozed a bunch of cake. It takes the focus away from food and forces you to find pleasure elsewhere. I used to be a former chef. I lived for food and cookbooks, and cooking shows were like porn to me.

But magic happens when you purposefully stuff yourself silly, overcome your food fears and the horrible phobia you may have of giving in to your body's inner hunger, and just step aside to let your body do the calorie accounting. It is much better at it than you are. I promise you that. When you look at the sensation of hunger like you would a fire in your living room (Quick, put it out immediately!!!), and prioritize keeping your tank full of the carbohydrates, fats, protein, vitamins, and minerals with the intention of setting a personal best for getting fuel into your body every day, life is just totally different.

"You may already know that the conventional 'solution' to being overweight – low-calorie dieting – doesn't work. But you may not know why. It is for this simple yet much overlooked reason: for the vast majority of people, being overweight is not caused by how much they eat but by what they eat. The idea that people get heavy because they consume a high volume of food is a myth. Eating large amounts of the right food is your key to success."

-Joel Furhman; *Eat to Live*

You won't believe how many mood swings and aches and pains and dips in energy levels and digestive problems and so forth have been related to your insufficient food intake and restricted eating patterns. Cravings? I was a sugar fiend my whole life. Some days I'd eat a whole pound of chocolate. Couldn't have sugar in my house or I'd eat it all within 24 hours. In less than a week of actually eating well for once I was finding half-eaten chocolate bars going stale already that I totally forgot about! Imagine having chocolate in your house and not even remembering it's in there. I know how it is, and it doesn't have to be that way. This program addresses both the mental and physical aspects of cravings, binge eating, etc. The key is really going for it and taking the concept of eating hard very seriously. It takes tremendous discipline. Eating a little less than you want and skipping meals when you're busy is much easier than this. But don't get the wrong idea. It is incredibly fun to eat, eat, eat, and eat some more after years of dieting. There's nothing quite as refreshing.

If you are wondering if it will really work or not to bring your metabolism up, you need not. The success rate for bringing the metabolism at least somewhat higher if it's low (but not necessarily making you catch fire) is damn near 100% as far as I know. It works on a basic biological level.

But like I said, have realistic expectations for it. I know I've hyped it up to sound pretty sweet, but not everything will miraculously heal. I didn't go from not being able to read a book two feet from my nose to 20-20 vision just because I ate well. You shouldn't expect miracles either. But many things do change and improve – from fertility to sex drive to dropping blood sugars, triglycerides, and blood pressure to allergy disappearance to skin health to digestion to muscle growth to re-growth of hair to increased hair and nail thickness and shine to any number of minor and sometimes major health improvements. And like I said, the crazy thing is that some people even lose fat doing this, particularly the severely obese.

The program is not about weight loss of course, but something much greater. And you are very likely to lose fat over the course of a year or so after rehabilitating your metabolism. No matter what you eat after you finish the program.

As you start out, remember that you are challenging your metabolism, your glucose metabolism, your digestion, and more. This does not feel good!!! Headaches, skin breakouts, brain fog, severe drowsiness after meals, out-of-control hunger – particularly if you are coming off of a low-carb diet, heartburn and other digestive glitches – these are all normal in the first week or two. But just when you think you are poisoning yourself with all this food something pretty cool happens. You start to notice improvements in how your body handles everything. Instead of running from all these problem foods and big, heavy meals you experience your body rising to the challenge, making use of the tools you've given it, and functioning much, much better.

So be prepared to be challenged and have to muster up some resilience and persistence. This is not all fun and games.

It's like trying to get back in shape after years of couch surfing. You get tired. You get sore. You ache. But it makes you stronger. You'll see.

I don't want to encourage you to look for ways out or be timid about the program, but if the concept is too overwhelming you can always try overfeeding for just a portion of the day. I'm confident that the morning hours are the time to do this. Maybe eat a normal breakfast upon waking and eat a full-size meal two hours later, a normal lunch, and then just go along with your day as usual. Saturating your body with food early in the day is a great way to be fueled, with your mind off food and feeling strong and stable.

Or maybe it's more convenient just to have food available to munch on all day at work. Just munch all day on food that you like while working at your desk or whatever your job may be.

That's how I got started with all this actually. I had grown tired of restricted eating and inflicting guilt upon myself every time I failed to adhere – so I just vowed to eat every time I wanted to and promised to enjoy everything I ate instead of burdening myself with feelings of guilt, shame, and resolve to make up for it in the future. So at work I always brought a bunch of cheese, salad, nuts, fruit, and dried fruit to eat. I ate something literally every hour for the whole eight-hour shift and never let my mind judge me for it.

This was slightly fattening compared to doing the same thing but with steak and potatoes - probably because of the anti-metabolic properties of all the polyunsaturated fat in the nuts and seeds I was eating. But we're only talking a few pounds in several months of doing this practice, so this is all details really. There was definitely a difference when I switched to meat, fat, vegetables, and starches eaten in the same manner though. Knowing what I know now I'd have to say a diet of meat or milk, beans, root vegetables, grain porridges, whole fruit, and greens with a little added coconut is probably ideal at getting your low metabolism and high appetite to trade places.

I should also bring up timelines and transitions. In truth, there is no beginning and end to the RRARF concept. It's more about getting your appetite and metabolism in synch together. No one truly stuffs themselves against their will for very long. It's incredibly difficult and would be just as much of an eating disorder to constantly eat when you don't want to as to constantly not eat when you want to. Rather, you slowly transition into eating a more relaxed diet and take your head out of the game. It's about helping you graduate to looking at your diet like a healthy person does – with less attention to details and more attention to what sounds appealing and to your natural appetite and satiety mechanisms. Easier said than done for a chronic dieter, but Diet Recovery will at least point you in the right direction. Ultimately, it's up to you to solve your own diet "case." I can only give you a few major clues but can't guide you the rest of the way. Good luck Sherlock.

Anyway, I hope *Diet Recovery* will significantly contribute to you recovering your metabolism, your mood, your health, and your life in full. I hope you stick around with me for years to come to see where this health and nutrition investigation leads. It gives me great pleasure and fulfillment to be able to spend my days bringing it to you and keeping your minds captivated as the young and immature sciences of human health and nutrition unfold.

Best of luck to you and your health. If you ever remember one thing from me, remember to use whatever health and nutrition information you come across to improve your life overall. I see far too many people trying too hard, and becoming too paranoid about trying to be perfect. The end result is a hot mess. Don't go there. The perfect diet is the one that fits your life, not the one that fit the life of some fabled healthy tribe somewhere!

Actually, if you remember two things remember that. If you only remember one thing, let it be…

EAT THE FOOD!

Appendix I

As a former Broda Barnes worshiper, I used to recommend taking armpit (axillary) temperature first thing in the morning just like he had his patients do, with a target of 97.8 to 98.2 just like him as well. But I'm all grown up now and have ideas and experience of my own. Take the temperature wherever you want, just be consistent. Good morning-temperature targets are 99 butthole, 98.6 oral, 98.0 armpit. I don't know anything about ears and foreheads and vaginas and stuff. I'm old-school I guess. Later in the day temperatures should rise above that.

Armpits are weird though, so I'm kinda steering people away from that now. Sometimes the left and right armpits are a full degree different. That doesn't scream accuracy to me. So go oral, rectal, or vaginal. Man that's fun to write. Here are the best times to gather useful temperature data:

- Take one temperature first thing upon waking (good way to track how your resting metabolism is changing in response to your interventions).
- Take another temperature about a half hour after each meal (helps you determine what time of day you tend to need more calorie-dense food, and also how to structure food and

fluids to give them the net-warming effect – as your temperature should always rise in response to food… if it doesn't you're either strung out on adrenaline and crashing – which will go away so stick with it, or your meal has too many fluids in proportion to calories and salt).

• Take another right before you go to bed (if it crashes right before bed, probably a good idea to regularly eat a tasty snack about a half hour before you go to sleep, like a dish of ice cream and something salty like a few handfuls of popcorn).

Do this for a few days, and then just start taking a morning temperature for a while to make sure it is trending upward. It doesn't move in a straight line. It goes up and down and up and down – but generally you should see it moving in the right direction in a general sense.

Women should know that when you start your menstrual cycle your temperatures will drop by about .5 degrees F. Don't be alarmed by this or discouraged. This is normal. After ovulation, your temperature should jump up and be slightly higher than the ideal temp targets listed above.

To make sure your temperature readings aren't artificially low, I recommend warming up your thermometer in your hand or something warm first. You don't want to stick a cold thermometer somewhere or the thermometer itself will actually lower the temperature of the area you are testing.

Once you have warmed up the thermometer to close to body temperature, put it in the testing orifice, then let it sit for at least a half a minute or longer. Then turn the digital thermometer on (a cheap Vicks digital thermometer is as good as any) and get a reading.

If you catch yourself taking more than just a few temperature readings during the day, or taking your body temperature every single day beyond the first few weeks as you start experimenting with this, you might want to throw away your thermometer. It's a useful tool. It's not a license to become obsessive.

After a month or so you should start to know your body metabolically. You should know what having a perfect temperature feels like and when to eat a little more, when to rest a little more, etc. You shouldn't really need a thermometer anymore other than to just check in every once in a while to see if you've fallen off the deep end.

That is all. Have fun.

Oh wait, one more tip. If you use the thermometer in your butt, don't take an oral reading with it right after, heh heh. Or leave it lying around where your kids might pick it up and check their oral temperatures out of curiosity.

Appendix II

Omega 6 content of common foods by percentage of total calories:

Omega 666 – the most Evil omega 6 powerhouses (over 50%)

- Grapeseed oil 70.6%!!!
- Corn Oil 54.5%
- Walnuts 52.5% (oil is 53.9%)
- Cottonseed oil 52.4%
- Soybean oil 51.4%

Very High Omega 6 sources (20-50%)

- Sesame oil 42.0%
- Pepitas 34.5%
- Margarine 27.9%
- Pecans 26.9%
- Peanut Butter 22.5%
- Pistachios 21.3%

High Omega 6 Sources (10-20%)

- Chicken Fat 19.5%
- Almonds 19.1%

- Canola oil 19.0%
- Flaxseed oil 12.9%
- Cashews 12.6%
- Duck Fat 12.2%
- Bacon Grease 10.2%
- Lard 10.2%

Moderate Omega 6 Sources (5-10%)

- Olive oil 9.9%
- Goose Fat 9.8%
- Avocado 9.4%
- Chicken with skin 9.0%
- Olives 7.4%
- Bacon 7.0%
- Eggs 6.8%
- Pork chops 6.2%
- Popcorn (Air Popped) 5.8%
- Oats 5.6%

Low Omega 6 Sources (2-5%)

- Corn 4.7%
- Chicken Liver 3.7%
- Sunflower Oil 3.7% (High oleic variety- others are very high in omega 6)
- Butter 3.4%
- Beef Tallow 3.1%
- Cocoa Butter 2.8%
- Cooked carrots 2.7%
- Macadamia Nut oil ~2.5%
- Brown rice 2.5%
- Cream 2.2%
- Beef liver 2.1%

- Grassfed Beef 2.0%
- Whole wheat flour 2.0%

Extremely low Omega 6 Sources (Less than 2%)

- Coconut oil 1.9%
- Prime rib 1.8%
- Whole milk 1.8%
- Half and Half 1.8%
- Ground Beef 1.6%
- Macadamia Nuts 1.6%
- Chicken without skin 1.4%
- Lamb 1.4%
- Cheese/Brie 1.3%
- Corn grits 1.2%
- Beets 1.2%
- Coconut Milk 1.1%
- Seal Oil 1.1% (to satisfy the curiosities of those with an Eskimo fetish)
- Foie gras 1.1%
- Palm Kernel Oil 0.8%
- White rice 0.7%
- Sockeye Salmon 0.5%
- Yams 0.4%
- Potatoes 0.3%
- Halibut 0.2%
- Shrimp 0.2%
- Clams 0.2%
- Canned tuna 0.1%
- Blue crab 0.1%
- Lobster 0.1%

When you look at how much tastier the bottom of the omega 6 chart looks than the top, is it really a problem to redefine the term "healthy fats" and load up on great seafood, macadamia nuts, lamb, brie, half and half, prime rib, and potatoes fried in coconut oil?

I assure you I have no problem (non-fiscally-related) trading those foods for peanut butter and grapeseed oil.

I hope this serves as a great reference for years to come for those interested in lowering their cellular levels of omega 6 polyunsaturated fat.

And keep in mind that this says nothing of the free radical damage done to our bodies by omega 6 fats, which is a whole other problem with rich omega 6 sources like solvent-extracted vegetable oil that this doesn't even address.

As you attempt to use this chart, keep in mind that these figures show the % of calories as omega 6. The total, in order to be within a range that can have a significantly positive influence over your systemic levels of inflammation, your body temperature, and your weight should be no greater than 2% of calories – ideally about 1%. 2% of calories is roughly 6 grams per day on a normal diet. 1% is 3 grams. While intentionally eating a super-caloric diet in attempt to expedite a rise in body temperature, even more diligence is needed, as 2% of calories from omega 6 on a 4,500 calorie diet is 10 grams of omega 6 – which I think is probably far too much to expect the best results – although it's still only about half of the average intake for an American male (yikes).

You can instantly see, especially considering the likelihood that carbohydrate is the most metabolically-stimulating type of food (assuming nutritional needs for fat and protein are met), that a fairly high-carbohydrate diet built around root vegetables and seafood is perhaps the ultimate low-omega 6 diet. Interestingly, the Kitavans, a group of Melanesians studied by Swedish researcher Staffan Lindeberg, have been found living to old age without a single case of heart disease, diabetes, obesity, asthma, acne, or any of the other prevalent diseases found in other parts of the world. Their diet contains absolutely nothing that is more than 2% omega 6, consisting almost solely of fish, yams, coconut, and fruit – oh yeah, and they chain smoke ☺

This is a great testament, in my opinion, of the protective power of a low omega 6 diet built around whole, unprocessed, and fresh foods. The ultimate human diet? Who knows, but it's certainly better than doughnuts, French fries, and peanut butter. On such fare, even something as basic, natural, and essential as sunlight is enough to give us skin cancer. The word unprotective (not an actual word, but you know what I mean) certainly comes to mind. Whaddya expect when the hot, bright sun hits heat and light-sensitive fatty acids?

References

The assertions made in *Diet Recovery* are a comprehensive culmination of conclusions pieced together, in part, by a thorough and critical examination of the following books, websites, and articles (although this is most certainly just a partial list):

Abrahamson, E. M. and A. W. Pezet. *Body, Mind, and Sugar.* Avon Books: New York, NY, 1951.

Agatston, Arthur. *The South Beach Diet.* Rodale: New York, NY, 2003.

Allan, Christian B. and Wolfgang Lutz. *Life Without Bread.* Keats Publishing: Los Angeles, CA, 2000.

Appleton, Nancy. *Stopping Inflammation.* Square One Publishers: Garden City Park, NY, 2005.

Appleton, Nancy. *Suicide By Sugar.* Square One Publishers: Garden City Park, NY, 2009.

Atkins, Robert. *Dr. Robert Atkins New Diet Revolution.* Avon Books, Inc.: New York, NY, 1992.

Aziz, Michael. *The Perfect 10 Diet.* Cumberland House: Naperville, IL, 2010.

Bacon, Linda. *Health at Every Size.* Benbella Books: Dallas, TX, 2008.

Barnes, Broda. *Hypothyroidism: The Unsuspecting Illness.* Harper and Row: New York, NY, 1976

Barnes, Broda. *Solved: The Riddle of Heart Attacks.* Robinson Press: Fort Collins, CO, 1976

Barnes, Broda. *Hope for Hypoglycemia.* Robinson Press: Fort Collins, CO, 1978

Bass, Clarence. *Great Expectations.* Ripped Enterprises: Albuquerque, NM, 2007.

Bennett, Connie. *Sugar Shock!* Berkley Books: New York, NY, 2007.

Bieler, Henry. *Food is Your Best Medicine.* Random House: New York, NY, 1965.

Brownstein, David. *Overcoming Thyroid Disorders.* Medical Alternative Press: West Bloomfield, MI, 2008.

Burkitt, Denis, Hugh Trowell, and Kenneth Heaton. *Dietary Fibre, Fibre-Depleted Foods and Disease.* Academic Press: London, 1985.

Campos, Paul. *The Obesity Myth.* Gotham Books: New York, NY, 2004.

Challem, Jack. *The Inflammation Syndrome.* John Wiley and Sons, Inc.: Hoboken, NJ, 2003.

Chilton, Floyd H. *Inflammation Nation.* Fireside: New York, NY, 2007.

Cleave, T. L., *The Saccharine Disease.* Keats Publishing: New Canaan, CT, 1974.

Cleave, T.L. and G.D. Campbell. *Diabetes, Coronary Thrombosis, and the Saccharine Disease.* John Wright & Sons LTD.: Bristol, UK, 1969.

Colpo, Anthony. *The Fat Loss Bible.*

DesMaisons, Kathleen. *Potatoes Not Prozac.* Fireside: New York, NY, 1998.

DesMaisons, Kathleen. *The Sugar Addict's Total Recovery Program.* Ballantine Books: New York, NY, 2000.

Dufty, William. *Sugar Blues.* Warner Books: New York, NY, 1975.

Ellis, Gregory. *Dr. Ellis's Ultimate Diet Secrets Lite.* Targeted Body Systems Publishing: Glen Mills, PA, 2003.

Enig, Mary. *Know Your Fats.* Bethesda Press: Silver Spring, MD, 2000.

Farris, Russell and Per Marin. *The Potbelly Syndrome.* Basic Health Publications: Laguna Beach, CA, 2006.

Fife, Bruce. *Eat Fat Look Thin.* Healthwise: Colorado Springs, CO, 2002.

Fife, Bruce. *The Coconut Oil Miracle.* Avery: New York, NY, 1999.

Fuhrman, Joel. *Eat to Live.* Little, Brown and Company: New York, NY, 2003.

Gabriel, Jon. *The Gabriel Method.* Atria Books: New York, NY, 2008.

Galland, Leo. *The Fat Resistance Diet.* Broadway Books: New York, NY, 2005.

Gedgaudas, Nora. *Primal Body – Primal Mind.* Primal Body – Primal Mind Publishing: Portland, OR, 2009.

Johnson, Richard J. *The Sugar Fix.* Pocket Books: New York, NY, 2008.

Keys, Ancel et al. *The Biology of Human Starvation.* The University of Minnesota Press: Minneapolis, MN, 1950.

Kharrazian, Datis. *Why Do I Still Have Thyroid Symptoms?* Morgan James Publishing: Garden City, NY, 2010.

Kolata, Gina. *Rethinking Thin.* Farrar, Straus and Giroux: New York, NY, 2007.

Langer, Stephen E. and James F. Scheer. *Solved: The Riddle of Illness.* McGraw Hill: New York, NY, 2006.

Lindeberg, Staffan. *Food and Western Disease.* Wiley-Blackwell: West Sussex, UK, 2010.

Lipton, Bruce. *The Biology of Belief.* Elite Books: Santa Rosa, CA, 2005.

Macfadden, Bernarr. *The Miracle of Milk.* Macfadden Publications: New York, NY, 1924.

Martin, Courtney E. *Perfect Girls, Starving Daughters.* Free Press: New York, NY, 2007.

McCarrison, Robert. *Studies in Deficiency Disease.* Henry Frowde and Hodder and Stoughton: London, England, 1921.

McCully, Kilmer S. *The Homocysteine Revolution.* Keats Publishing: New Canaan, CT, 1997.

Morris, Richard. *A Life Unburdened.* New Trends Publishing: Washington, D.C., 2007.

Murray, Michael. *The Encyclopedia of Healing Foods.* Atria Books: New York, NY, 2005.

Paula Owens. *The Power of 4.* Paula Owens: USA. 2008.

Page, Melvin, and H. Leon Abrams. *Health vs. Disease,* The Page Foundation, Inc., St. Petersburg, FL 1960.

Peat, Ray. *Progesterone in Orthomolecular Medicine.* Raymond Peat: Eugene, OR, 1993.

Peat, Ray. *Generative Energy.* Raymond Peat: Eugene, OR, 1994.

Peat, Ray. *Nutrition for Women.* Raymond Peat: Eugene, OR, 1993.

Peat, Ray. *Mind and Tissue.* Raymond Peat: Eugene, OR, 1993.

Peat, Ray. *From PMS to Menopause.* Raymond Peat: Eugene, OR, 1993.

Pekarek, Martha L. *Freedom from Obesity and Sugar Addiction.* Wheatmark: Tucson, AZ, 2007.

Philpott, William H. *Victory Over Diabetes.* Keats Publishing: New Canaan, CT, 1983.

Pool, Robert. *Fat: Fighting the Obesity Epidemic.* Oxford University Press: New York, NY, 2001.

Porter, Charles Sanford. *Milk Diet, as a Remedy for Chronic Disease.* Burnett P.O.: Long Beach, CA, 1916.

Price, Weston A. *Nutrition and Physical Degeneration.* Republished by the Price-Pottenger Nutrition Foundation: La Mesa, CA, originally published in 1939.

Reaven, Gerald. *Syndrome X.* Fireside: New York, NY, 2000.

Roberts, Seth. *The Shangri-La Diet.* G. P. Putnam's Sons: New York, NY, 2006.

Rooney, Ric. *Secrets of a Professional Dieter* (eBook). www.PhysiqueTransformation.com

Ross, Julia. *The Diet Cure.* Penguin Books: New York, NY, 1999.

Schmid, Ron. *Traditional Foods are Your Best Medicine.* Healing Arts Press: Rochester, VT, 1987.

Schwartz, Bob. *Diets Don't Work!* Breakthrough Publishing: Houston, TX, 1982.

Schwarzbein, Diana. *The Schwarzbein Principle.* Health Communications, Inc.: Deerfield Beach, FL, 1999.

Schwarzbein, Diana. *The Schwarzbein Principle II.* Health Communications, Inc.: Deerfield Beach, FL, 2002.

Schwarzbein, Diana. *The Program.* Health Communications, Inc.: Deerfield Beach, FL, 2004.

Selye, Hans. *The Stress of Life*. McGraw-Hill: New York, NY, 1976.

Sears, Al. *P.A.C.E.* Wellness Research and Consulting, Inc.: Royal Palm Beach, FL, 2010.

Sears, Barry. *Enter the Zone*. Regan Books: New York, NY, 1995.

Sears, Barry. *The Age-Free Zone*. Regan Books: New York, NY, 1999.

Sears, Barry. *The Anti-Inflammation Zone*. Collins: New York, NY, 2005.

Sears, Barry. *Toxic Fat*. Thomas Nelson Inc, 2008.

Shell, Ellen Ruppel. *The Hungry Gene*. Atlantic Monthly Press: New York, NY, 2002.

Shomon, Mary J., *The Thyroid Diet*. Harper Resource: New York, NY, 2004.

Sisson, Mark. *The Primal Blueprint*. Primal Nutrition, Inc.: Malibu, CA, 2009.

Starr, Mark. *Hypothyroidism Type 2*. Mark Starr Trust: Columbia, MO, 2005.

Talbott, Shawn. *The Cortisol Connection*. Hunter House: Alameda, CA, 2007.

Taubes, Gary. *Good Calories, Bad Calories*. Alfred A. Knopf: New York, NY, 2007.

Tribole, Evelyn and Elyse Resch. *Intuitive Eating*. St. Martin's Press: New York, NY, 1995.

Wann, Marilyn. *Fat! So?* Ten Speed Press: Berkeley, CA, 1998.

Weil, Andrew. *Eating Well for Optimum Health.* Harper Collins: New York, NY, 2000.

Wiley, T.S. *Lights Out: Sleep, Sugar, and Survival.* Pocket Books: New York, NY, 2000.

Yudkin, John. *Sweet and Dangerous.* Bantam Books: New York, NY, 1972.

Websites:

www.raypeat.com
http://nutritionscienceanalyst.blogspot.com/
www.stopthethyroidmadness.com
http://thescientificdebateforum.aimoo.com/
www.wholehealthsource.blogspot.com
http://www.youtube.com/user/WellnessResources
http://www.youtube.com/user/GabrielMethodVideo
www.omega-6-news.org
http://blog.cholesterol-and-health.com/
www.westonaprice.org
www.carbsanity.blogspot.com
www.weightology.net
www.sethroberts.net
www.junkfoodscience.blogspot.com

Specific Article and video titles with accompanying URLs:

"Why We Gain Weight: Adiposity 101 and the Alternative Hypothesis of Obesity"
http://www.dhslides.org/mgr/mgr060509f/f.htm

"Depressive Symptoms, omega-6:omega-3 Fatty Acids, and Inflammation in Older Adults"
http://www.psychosomaticmedicine.org/cgi/content/abstract/69/3/217
"Suppressor of Cytokine Signaling-3 (SOCS-3), a Potential Mediator of Interleukin-6-dependent Insulin Resistance in Hepatocytes"
http://www.jbc.org/content/278/16/13740.full.pdf
"Sugar: The Bitter Truth"
http://www.youtube.com/watch?v=dBnniua6-oM
"Eluv Live Interview with Dr. Ray Peat"
http://eluv.podbean.com/2008/10/10/eluv-live-interview-with-dr-ray-peat/
"Obesity: 10 Things You Thought You Knew"
http://www.youtube.com/watch?v=Qk4UKD00aOo&feature=channel
"The Ghost in Your Genes"
http://video.google.com/videoplay?docid=1128045835761675934#

Suggested Reading

180 Degree Metabolism by Matt Stone
The Gabriel Method by Jon Gabriel
Health at Every Size by Linda Bacon
The Obesity Myth by Paul Campos
Perfect Girls, Starving Daughters by Courtney Martin
Hypothyroidism: The Unsuspecting Illness by Broda Barnes
The Cortisol Connection by Shawn Talbott
Hypothyroidism Type 2: The Epidemic by Mark Starr
http://wholehealthsource.blogspot.com

About the Author

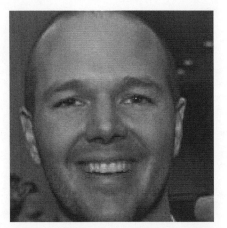

Matt Stone is an independent health researcher and author of fifteen books on various health-related topics. He launched an independent investigation into health in 2005, and has since been exploring a wide range of health fields - from general physiology and nutrition to areas as diverse and specific as psychoneuroendocrinology. His investigation has yielded many great, practical insights and simple tips on how regular people can make substantial improvements in their health - for the purpose of both improving or eliminating specific health problems and preventing some of the most common ailments in the modern world. Most of his research has drawn him towards metabolic rate and how many basic functions (digestion, reproduction, aging, immunity, inflammation, sleep) perform better when metabolic rate is optimized.

Made in the USA
San Bernardino, CA
22 March 2014

Praise for

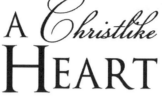

A *Christlike*
HEART

"If you want more light in your life—the light that comes from the word of God and His prophets—you should read this book. By focusing on the word heart, the Squire brothers not only lift and inspire, but more importantly they motivate us to be more devoted gospel learners, more enthusiastic about studying the Book of Mormon, and more eager to testify of its truthfulness to our family and friends. The mark of a good book is the degree to which it increases the reader's desire to be a better person. *A Christlike Heart* passes this test in every way."

—RUSSELL T. OSGUTHORPE, former Sunday School
General President (2009–2014)

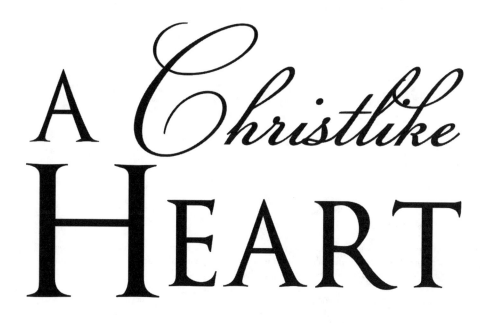

A STUDY
of the HEART
in the
BOOK
OF
MORMON

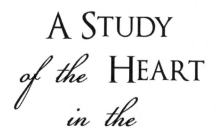

DEREK SQUIRE   RYAN SQUIRE

CFI
An imprint of Cedar Fort, Inc.
Springville, Utah

ISBN 13: 978-1-4621-2346-9

Published by CFI, an imprint of Cedar Fort, Inc.
2373 W. 700 S., Springville, UT 84663
Distributed by Cedar Fort, Inc., www.cedarfort.com

LIBRARY OF CONGRESS CATALOGING-IN-PUBLICATION DATA

Names: Squire, Derek, 1980- author. | Squire, Ryan, 1976- author.
Title: A Christlike heart : a study of the heart in the Book of Mormon /
    Derek Squire and Ryan Squire.
Description: Springville, Utah : CFI, an imprint of Cedar Fort, Inc., [2019]
    | Includes bibliographical references and index.
Identifiers: LCCN 2018056047 (print) | LCCN 2019001555 (ebook) | ISBN
    9781462129843 (epub, pdf, mobi) | ISBN 9781462123469 (perfect bound : alk.
    paper)
Subjects: LCSH: Christian life--Mormon authors. | Book of Mormon--Criticism,
    interpretation, etc. | Pride and vanity--Religious aspects--Christianity.
    | Emotions--Religious aspects--Mormon Church.
Classification: LCC BX8656 (ebook) | LCC BX8656 .S68 2019 (print) | DDC
    289.3/22--dc23
LC record available at https://lccn.loc.gov/2018056047

Cover design by Wes Wheeler
Cover design © 2019 Cedar Fort, Inc.
Edited by Valene Wood and Sydnee Hyer
Typeset by Kaitlin Barwick

Printed in the United States of America

10 9 8 7 6 5 4 3 2 1

Printed on acid-free paper

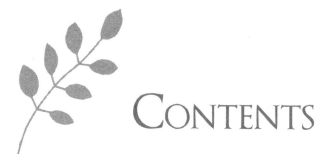

CONTENTS

CONTENTS

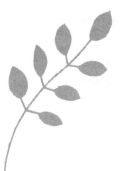

PREFACE

While the Book of Mormon has long been for us an area of intensive personal study, we consider ourselves normal, run-of-the-mill members of The Church of Jesus Christ of Latter-day Saints. We would like to think we are fairly representative of Church membership everywhere in our love for the Savior and His gospel. We are quite happy to be along for the ride on the "old ship Zion," rubbing shoulders with so many good and faithful members.[1] Like countless others, we simply love our Savior, Jesus Christ, and are trying every day, in so many imperfect ways, to become better disciples of Him.

We are two brothers with similar educational and career backgrounds. We each have a bachelor's and master's degree in accounting, and our careers have thus far been spent as CPAs, healthcare administrators, and business owners.

We also share one other thing in life as brothers: a fiercely captivating and burning passion for all things Book of Mormon and its testimony of Jesus Christ. We each fell in love with the Book of Mormon at around the same time of our lives, when we were teenagers together. It was then that we came to study the prophetic promises of President Ezra Taft Benson to those who would undertake a serious study of the book. He taught, "There is a book we need to study daily, both as individuals and as families, namely the Book of Mormon. It is the book that will get a person nearer to God by abiding by its precepts than any other book. President

[Marion G.] Romney recommended studying it half an hour each day. I commend that practice to you."[2]

This prophetic instruction forever changed the course of our lives. Before we experimented on the words of a prophet, our Book of Mormon study could best be described as casual and irregular, more driven by finishing a chapter and the turning of pages than with bothering with what we could actually learn or apply in our lives. We came to know shortly after making a concentrated effort to study the Book of Mormon that this practice would have a more profound spiritual impact on our lives than anything else we could do. Neither of us has ever felt a period of sustained and significant spiritual growth in our lives that wasn't accompanied with a regular and focused study of the Book of Mormon.

It was our love of the Book of Mormon that led us to focus on the role of our hearts in the great plan of mercy. Derek had a very distinct impression to write this book about the heart in July 2016. Since that time, the idea has been the subject of many conversations between us. We feel strongly that this book can bless each of its readers thanks to the doctrines taught by both Book of Mormon and latter-day prophets. We have an ardent desire to impress upon people's minds the importance of yielding our hearts unto God, sanctifying ourselves, and coming nearer to Him. These matters of the heart are laid out with greater clarity in the Book of Mormon than anywhere else.

Combined, we have read the Book of Mormon over 150 times, with many of our favorite portions read and studied hundreds of times. We have studied numerous commentaries, articles, and online observations about various topics in the Book of Mormon. So much has been written that has blessed our lives, enlarged our memories, and expanded our hearts.

Though we enjoy studying the Book of Mormon, our testimonies are not founded upon any knowledge or familiarity with its various writing styles, literary tools, stories, geography, or historical context. Our love of the Book of Mormon and our testimony of its truth have come from the Spirit, which has been carried into our hearts through the effect that sustained study has had in our lives.

Waves of pure knowledge have washed over us, and the Spirit has come into our lives like the return of the tide when we have sat down to a serious study.

Like so many others, we have received personal revelation and pointed inspiration for our lives through the study of that book. We are told Nephi and Lehi (sons of Helaman), and many of their brethren were able to receive "many revelations daily" (Helaman 11:23). As members of the Church of Jesus Christ, we too should strive for this blessing of receiving many revelations daily! God is no respecter of persons, and we all are invited, encouraged, and even summoned to partake in that revelatory process.

The Book of Mormon has changed and continues to change our lives. Every day we study, we feel a greater motivation to do a little better, work a little harder, be a little kinder, and draw closer to Christ. Our interactions with family and friends are softer and gentler. Our eye becomes less focused on the things of the world and more single to the things of God. Each time we study, our hearts grow a little more sanctified and holy. Our perspective on life grows sharper and clearer, accompanied by a greater self-awareness of thoughts, words, and actions. The Spirit distills faith, hope, and charity upon our souls through that book, and the appetite for further gifts of the Spirit grows within us.

We love the Book of Mormon for how it changes our lives and inspires us to seek after good things in our daily journey. If we will have the faith, diligence, and patience to nourish the word, it will become a great and mighty "tree springing up unto everlasting life" (Alma 32:41). It is our greatest desire that our readers will be given their own insights and understanding as they study the heart in the Book of Mormon. We hope that all may see that revelation and inspiration are not only possible, but also necessary in the lives of "regular" members of the Church. It is through this revelation and inspiration that we will be given ways to draw our hearts nearer to our Lord and Savior, Jesus Christ.

INTRODUCTION

Elder David A. Bednar said, "The Book of Mormon is our handbook of instructions as we travel the pathway from bad to good to better and strive to have our hearts changed."[1] This quote perfectly captures our purpose in writing this book. We believe that studying the Book of Mormon will motivate us to change our hearts to be more like our Savior's more than any other book of scripture. It identifies more conditions and diseases of the heart than any other book of scripture. It also provides more examples and teachings on changing the heart than any other book of scripture. The Atonement of Christ is the means by which our hearts can truly be changed from bad to good to better. The Holy Ghost is the agent through which the Atonement can work within us to make these changes. We will focus on this process repeatedly as we study various conditions of the heart that we either want to eliminate from our hearts or develop within our hearts.

Our hope in writing this book is to help each of us consider ways to develop our hearts to be a little bit more Christlike and to then act on those truths. Our focus will be on testimonies, stories, and experiences that illustrate and emphasize the teachings concerning the heart found within the pages of the Book of Mormon.

Throughout this book, we will use phrases such as "we need to change our hearts" and "we have to develop our hearts." We recognize these phrases could be read to infer that the ability is within us to change or improve our own hearts. While such phrases are used to improve the flow of language, please know our intent is to assume a complete dependence on divinity. Heavenly gifts of growth and progress can only come to us through grace. All change for the better, each gift of development, and every good thing that comes into our hearts comes only in and through the Atonement of Jesus Christ and His grace.

Mormon observed, "Nevertheless they did fast and pray oft, and did wax stronger and stronger in their humility, and firmer and firmer in the faith of Christ, unto the filling their souls with joy and consolation, yea, even to the purifying and the sanctification of their hearts, which sanctification cometh because of their yielding their hearts unto God" (Helaman 3:35). Purifying and sanctifying our hearts through the Atonement of Jesus Christ will be the ultimate focus of this book. This sanctification of our hearts is preceded by yielding our hearts unto God. Yielding *all* of our hearts—*every piece*!

The Book of Mormon does a marvelous job illustrating various conditions of the heart we may experience. It also lays out the requirements to access grace sufficient both to overcome the diseases of the heart as well as to acquire and develop spiritually vital virtues of the heart. Furthermore, it teaches us how to assess, educate, train, and purify our hearts.

President Russell M. Nelson said, "The heart of the plan of salvation is the Atonement."[2] Elder Jeffrey R. Holland provided additional clarity when he explained, "Mercy, with its sister virtue forgiveness, is at the very heart of the Atonement of Jesus Christ."[3] In writing a book about the heart, we would be remiss if we didn't focus greatly on the heart of the plan of salvation—the Atonement of our Lord and Savior, Jesus Christ, and the heart of the Atonement—the mercy granted and available to us through that divine gift. President Henry B. Eyring discussed the need for the Atonement to be "working in the hearts of the members" of the Church.[4]

But how exactly do we get the Atonement to work in our lives? President Henry B. Eyring taught, "Now [here] is a fact you can act on with confidence. You can invite the Holy Ghost's companionship in your life. And you can know when He is there, and when He withdraws. And when He is your companion, you can have confidence that the Atonement is working in your life."[5]

President Eyring's quote provides powerful clarity on how the Atonement of Christ actually works in our lives. Even though our mortal comprehension of the Savior's Atonement will always be imperfect and lacking, there are key principles that will lead us to greater light and knowledge. One of these key principles is understanding that His Atonement is working in our lives when we are feeling the companionship of the Spirit.

The Holy Ghost acts as an agent of the Savior's Atonement. He is a purifier and a sanctifier. He can remit our sins as we "apply the atoning blood of Christ" in our lives (Mosiah 4:2). What a glorious blessing! When we feel the Spirit, we can have the peace of knowing the Savior's Atonement is working within us.

Why focus on the Book of Mormon's teachings on the heart in particular? Elder Craig C. Christensen said, "Written scripture, especially the Book of Mormon, brings us to believe in God and 'be reconciled unto him through the Atonement of Christ, his Only Begotten Son'" (Jacob 4:11).[6] We can access the power of the Atonement of our Savior more effectively through the Book of Mormon than through any other book!

While the New Testament is the most prolific book of scripture we have detailing the earthly life and ministry of our Savior, Jesus Christ, the Book of Mormon is the greatest book of scripture we have declaring the Atonement of Jesus Christ. The Book of Mormon brings this single most significant act of all of history to the forefront of our gospel study. We learn of Christ's purpose in performing the Atonement, the blessings associated with His Atonement, and the manner in which we can draw on its power in our own lives.

The Book of Mormon details many stories of prophets and others who accessed the power of the Savior's Atonement to overcome challenges, bondage (both physical and spiritual), and weakened, sickened hearts. The Book of Mormon is the great convincer that Jesus is the Christ, that He atoned for our sins, and He made it possible for us to return and live with Him again.

A lawyer confronted Jesus in Jerusalem and asked Him what the greatest commandment was in the law. Jesus responded, "Thou shalt love the Lord thy God with all thy heart, with all thy soul, and with all thy mind. This is the first and great commandment" (Matthew 22:37–38). We find it significant that Jesus would say that we must love Him with all our heart first. Jesus wants our hearts to turn and draw near unto Him. He invites us to find ways to purify and sanctify our hearts that we may become more like Him and be allowed to enter His presence someday.

Elder Marvin J. Ashton said, "When the Lord measures an individual, he does not take a tape measure around the person's head to determine his mental capacity, nor his chest to determine his manliness, but He measures the heart as an indicator of the person's capacity and potential to bless others."[7]

The Book of Mormon has 442 references about the heart! That is almost one reference of the heart per page in the Book of Mormon! This is more than quadruple the frequency per verse of the New Testament and more than double the frequency of the Old Testament. Book of Mormon prophets clearly saw the role of the heart and its powerful imagery as a central focus in relation to our Savior, Jesus Christ. Isn't the gospel nothing more than a call to change our hearts from our fallen state in which we are "carnal, sensual, and devilish" to a state of sanctification and purification through the Atonement of Christ? (Alma 42:10).

In this book, we will study different uses of the word *heart* in the Book of Mormon in an effort to develop our hearts in ways the Lord desires. The Lord taught Samuel, "For the Lord seeth not as man seeth; for man looketh on the outward appearance, but the Lord looketh on the heart" (1 Samuel 16:7). That is both a comforting and encouraging message as well as a very sobering and straightforward warning. Our time, energy, and efforts need to be anxiously engaged in the development and conversion of our hearts.

Elder Gary E. Stevenson said, "Imagine for a moment . . . what if there was a way to measure the condition of one's heart in a spiritual context, as outlined in the scriptures? How would we do? What would the 'heart monitor' say to us if it were monitoring our spiritual hearts? It seems if we profess to be disciples of Jesus Christ, then His love must be written in our hearts."[8] Our Savior will indeed measure our hearts when we are judged. The Book of Mormon in particular shows us how to prepare for that day by assessing the condition of our hearts.

This book will be divided into three parts. The first section is concentrated on the most significant diseases of the heart that can come upon us, namely hardheartedness, pride in our hearts, and having our hearts set upon earthly riches and treasure. This section commences with a chapter on how Satan attempts to use his "devices" to cultivate these diseases and destroy our hearts (Alma 30:42).

The second section focuses on heart conditions and practices that relate to the personal conversion of our heart. We will study the mighty change of heart that each of us needs to begin our spiritual journey back to our Heavenly Father. We will examine the practice of pondering spiritual things in our hearts. Pondering in our hearts will lead to increased personal revelation upon which our testimonies must be built. We will also learn about being lowly in heart. If we are not lowly in heart, we are not sufficiently humble and teachable. Accordingly, we will not progress in our knowledge of the gospel because we will not allow the Spirit to instruct us. We will then discuss the consequences of the thoughts, intents, and desires of our hearts, and what the Savior expects of converted Saints in this regard.

The third section centers on the sanctification of the heart and virtues of the heart that are necessary to keep temple covenants and receive exaltation. The Book of Mormon teaches us in somewhat subtle ways about temple covenants. It is evident from studying the heart in this great book of scripture that prophets were pleading for us to be worthy of going to the temple, to enter into and keep sacred covenants, and to sanctify our hearts. In this section, we will study the virtue of a broken heart and a contrite spirit as it relates to the law of sacrifice. We will examine the virtue of being pure in heart and its connection to the law of chastity. We will discuss the virtue of following Christ with full purpose of heart and the associated law of consecration. We will also explore Malachi's prophecy of turning our hearts to both our fathers and children, and how this practice can make temple worship more meaningful and bind our families together.

There is a natural progression from overcoming the diseases of the heart, to the conversion of the heart, to having a sanctified heart worthy of entering the temple of our Lord and one day receiving exaltation. Our journey here on earth was not intended to be a casual one, and the path is strewn with struggles and challenges. The prophet Joseph Smith's counsel succinctly sums up our mission on the earth. He said, "Search your hearts and see if you are like God."[9] We cannot afford to ever give up on the effort and work involved in this search. The Savior is ready and willing to provide us a new heart free from earthly stains if we come unto Him and accept His grace and mercy.

It is our desire that you will find joy in the journey to understanding your own heart as you look to draw it nearer to our loving Savior. Sweet blessings await those that sincerely try to follow the Savior. We can access the power of the Savior's Atonement every day of our lives. The Holy Ghost will accompany us on this journey and will provide us with added sanctification and strength in this pursuit.

At the end of this book, in Appendix A, there are three tables we have constructed concerning the references of the heart in the Book of Mormon. These tables show how often the heart is mentioned in the Book of Mormon by topic, by prophet, and by book, respectively. We only show topics that are mentioned at least three times in the first table.

As former CPAs, we love analyzing and examining information. We believe thorough scrutiny of information can give us greater understanding and insights into prophets and what they most frequently emphasized. We can discover patterns that we did not know existed before. We can also see the prominence each particular subject has in the Book of Mormon.

More than any other goal, it is our hope that you will feel the Spirit as you read and ponder the Book of Mormon's messages of the heart. Through the companionship of the Spirit, we can be inspired in small ways to begin to change our hearts, become more sanctified, and draw nearer to our loving Savior. It is our desire that the Lord will consecrate our efforts as we turn our hearts unto Him, so that someday we can stand before Him with confidence as He measures our hearts!

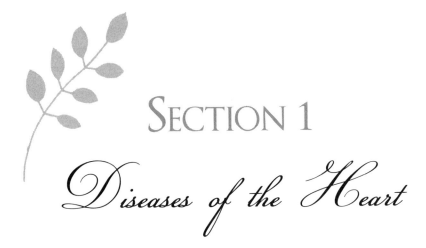

SECTION 1

Diseases of the Heart

The majority of references to the heart in the Book of Mormon focus on various diseases of the heart. The Book of Mormon speaks of the diseases of the heart for which we need to repent, diseases that we must eliminate from our hearts in our journey forward. It also provides illumination on the ways that the adversary and the world will work to inflict these diseases upon us.

Over the next four chapters, we will study the methods and techniques that Satan and the world use to sicken and weaken our hearts. Studying the manner in which the adversary tries to attack our hearts will help us better recognize his strategies and devices and will enable us to overcome and rebuke his advances. We will then discuss the three main diseases of the heart mentioned in the Book of Mormon that afflict the natural man, namely hardheartedness, pride in our hearts, and having our hearts set upon worldly riches and treasures. Book of Mormon prophets felt it was particularly critical that we learn about these diseases of the heart and the effects they can have on us. These three diseases alone comprise 144 references of the heart in the Book of Mormon—almost one-third of the total mentions of the heart in this book of scripture.

In these chapters, we will also study different ways we can overcome each of these diseases and be healed through the Atonement of Christ—to go from bad to good, and good to better—along this journey of mortality. By internalizing the words of these prophets, we can gain power over our own hearts to the point that Satan will eventually have no power over us because of our righteousness (see 1 Nephi 22:15, 26; Ether 8:26).

The process of developing a more Christlike heart is best described by Elder Bednar. He said, "The journey from bad to good is the process of putting off the natural man or the natural woman in each of us. In mortality we are all tempted by the flesh. But we can increase our capacity to overcome the desires of the flesh and temptations through the Atonement of Christ."[1]

It cannot be overemphasized that many of the prophets from the Book of Mormon were shown the temptations of our day and knew intimately, through divine revelation, the struggles we would face. Book of Mormon prophets focused on these diseases of the heart with great intensity of purpose. It is by divine design that these particular diseases of the heart are mentioned so frequently in a book of scripture meant specifically for us in our day. It follows that we must closely examine our hearts and consistently perform the treatments necessary to overcome any diseases that may afflict our hearts.

The idea of conquering these diseases of the heart may feel overwhelming at times. As humans, we are not perfect, nor will we achieve perfection while on this earth. However, we should have joy in the journey and rejoice in our progression, no matter how sluggish or imperceptible it may be.

If you focus on working to improve even one action suggested in this book, then it has been worthwhile for us to write it. The miracle of the purification and sanctification of our hearts is possible for those with patience, diligence, and desire! Again, such sanctification and purification are possible only through the enabling power of our Savior and His atoning sacrifice. We will only be given new hearts through His mercy and grace.

Chapter 1

SATAN STIRS UP THE HEARTS OF MEN

Satan uses a variety of methods, or devices as the scriptures often refer to them, to overtake our hearts. There is some captivating imagery in the Book of Mormon describing how Satan has success in stirring up the hearts of men to anger and all manner of iniquity. There are numerous examples of the adversary attempting to influence the hearts of men in one fashion or another. He works tirelessly to weaken our hearts with invasive, infectious diseases that, if invited in, will take over our hearts. His ultimate goal is to break our hearts and destroy us in the process.

Satan will utilize whatever strategies necessary to introduce disease into our hearts. He stirs up our hearts, places evil designs in our hearts, leads away our hearts, takes possession of our hearts, has power over our hearts, rages in our hearts, and takes hold upon our hearts. There are 26 such references in the Book of Mormon. If you further add in all of the other references in which people, due to Satan's influence, are attempting to do these same things to others, there are over 50 references!

We have all felt Satan's pull on our hearts. He tries to bring us down and tell us we cannot change for the better. He whispers to

us that we cannot accomplish the things that we have been foreordained to achieve. We take great solace in Elder Neal A. Maxwell's
words, "We can be comforted to know that God, who knows our
capacity perfectly, placed us here to succeed. No one was foreordained to fail or to be wicked. When we have been weighed and
found wanting, let us remember that we were measured before and
we were found equal to our tasks."[1]

In discussing Satan's techniques and strategies, it is comforting to remember that he cannot take control of our hearts without
our invitation and consent. Joseph Smith taught, "The devil has
no power over us only as we permit him. The moment we revolt at
anything which comes from God, the devil takes power."[2]

Mormon taught, "The power of the devil . . . comes by the
cunning plans which he hath devised to ensnare the hearts of men"
(Alma 28:13). Satan is continually trying to fill our hearts with
pride, wickedness, bitterness, and hardness through his deception. He is constantly working to ensnare our hearts to be set upon
riches and the treasures of the earth. The First Presidency in 1942
described Satan thus: "He is working under such perfect disguise
that many do not recognize either him or his methods. There is no
heart he would not break, no soul he would not destroy."[3]

Dividing asunder all the cunning and snares and wiles of the
devil, the Book of Mormon sounds a voice of warning that Satan
is actively trying to get hold over our hearts (see Helaman 3:29).
President Brigham Young said, "The men and women, who desire
to obtain seats in the celestial kingdom, will find that they must
battle with the enemy of all righteousness every day."[4] There are so
many weapons that the adversary employs in this daily battle, but
we have also been given means with which we can put off the devil
and keep his destructive rot from entering into our hearts.

It is easy to appreciate the power of the Book of Mormon when
you identify the distinctive ways prophets describe various conditions of the heart and the diverse ways in which Satan works upon
our hearts. Had Joseph Smith written the Book of Mormon, it
would have been much easier for him to use a single concept or
description regarding how Satan works on our hearts, and then

repeatedly use it. Instead, various prophets in the Book of Mormon walk us through subtle and unique differences in each description of the heart.

This nuanced and dynamic language about the heart is a convincing testimony to us that Joseph Smith did not write this book. Various prophets of old, influenced by their own personalities and experiences, wrote as directed and inspired by the Holy Spirit. Jesus Christ Himself searched the Nephite record and expounded all things unto the Nephites that were contained in the scriptures. He then commanded that additional things be added to the record that He saw were missing (see 3 Nephi 23:8–13). The Book of Mormon should be read within this context—that prophets called of God were inspired by the Holy Ghost to include things in the record. The Savior also personally commanded that certain things be written and recorded. It is truly our Savior's book for us.

HEARTS STIRRED UP TO ANGER

When Jesus came to visit the Nephites, He warned them that Satan would try to stir up their hearts to anger. Jesus warned, "For verily, verily I say unto you, he that hath the spirit of contention is not of me, but is of the devil, who is the father of contention, and he stirreth up the hearts of men to contend with anger, one with another. Behold, this is not my doctrine, to stir up the hearts of men with anger, one against another; but this is my doctrine, that such things should be done away" (3 Nephi 11:29–30).

What does it mean to stir up? While stirring in regard to baking speaks of the ingredients we are mixing together, there is another definition that provides greater clarity in relation to the heart. The phrase *to stir up* means to cause someone to feel a strong emotion and a desire to do something.[5] Satan will work hard to corrupt emotions and desires in our hearts. It is then up to us how we respond to his beguiling invitations. We can go along with what Satan tries to place in our hearts and become angry and contentious, or we can diffuse these emotions and desires and bring peace to our hearts. We can allow the adversary to stir our hearts to anger or iniquity, or we can allow the Spirit to stir up within our hearts a remembrance of Jesus Christ.

Elder Lynn G. Robbins said, "The verb *stir* sounds like a recipe for disaster: Put tempers on medium heat, stir in a few choice words, and bring to a boil; continue stirring until thick; cool off; let feelings chill for several days; serve cold; lots of leftovers."[6]

This verb, *to stir*, is mentioned well over 50 times in the Book of Mormon. In almost every case, it is in regard to anger, iniquity, or in remembrance of something. Why is anger such a crippling disease of the heart?

"The Lord God hath commanded that men should not contend one with another" (2 Nephi 26:32). King Benjamin taught, "Ye will not suffer your children that they . . . fight and quarrel one with another" (Mosiah 4:14). The moment we yield to anger in our hearts, we have withdrawn from the Holy Spirit and Satan gains power over us.

How can we resist the temptation of allowing our hearts to be stirred up to anger? Mormon described the state of the Nephites' hearts in AD 100. He said, "There was no contention in the land, because of the love of God which did dwell in the hearts of the people" (4 Nephi 1:15). Anger must be supplanted with love. When anger boils up within us toward a family member, we would do well to remember how much we truly love them and how any act of anger would hurt them. When our hearts are at war with another, we see people very differently than they are seen through the eyes of our Savior. He sees the spark of divinity in all of us. He loves us in the face of even our most ugly weaknesses.

We will never build up and strengthen a relationship by seeing and expecting the worst in another. At times when our hearts are stirred up to anger, we would do well to remember President Gordon B. Hinckley's counsel: "I am asking that we look a little deeper for the good, that we still voices of insult and sarcasm, that we more generously compliment virtue and effort . . . [That we] look for the remarkable good among those with whom we associate, that we speak of one another's virtues more than we speak of one another's faults."[7] The antithesis of being stirred up to anger is being stirred up in a remembrance of all that is good and to repentance within ourselves. Those are the thoughts that must work within us.

When our hearts are at war with another, we would do well to not only accentuate all that is good and worthy in the other person, but also to perform an honest assessment of our own shortcomings and weaknesses. When we recognize any measure of ugly pride or vain ambition within ourselves, we will be more forgiving of others. We will come to grasp our own dependence on our Savior's mercy. When we cease covering our own sins by unfairly "horribilizing" others, we will be led by our Savior's hand to repent of that which is amiss in our own lives (see D&C 121:37).

The apostle Paul asked, "Can ye be angry, and not sin?" (Ephesians 4:26, footnote a; from Joseph Smith Translation). The answer is no! Anger is never justified as taught by the Savior. The Savior appears to have left some wiggle room for us to justify our anger when He gave the Sermon on the Mount. He supposedly taught, "But I say unto you, That whosoever is angry with his brother without a cause shall be in danger of the judgment" (Matthew 5:22). It is worth noting that this phrase "without a cause" is not found in the Savior's sermon to the Nephites in 3 Nephi 12:22 or in the Joseph Smith Translation of Matthew 5:22. There is no acceptable reason for us to use anger as a release of our emotions.

Elder Lynn G. Robbins said plainly, "Anger is a yielding to Satan's influence by surrendering our self-control."[8] What a remarkably humbling and sobering appraisal of anger! It is spiritually perilous and destructive to lose control of our emotions. If we are living in a way that invites the Spirit, any moments of anger will quickly and inevitably produce regret and remorse. One of our greatest tests in life is to learn self-control—to learn to master our thoughts, passions, and appetites within heavenly bounds.

EXPOSING SATAN'S GAME PLAN

The Book of Mormon provides a more concise description of Satan's strategies than any other book of scripture. Nephi prophesied of our day:

> For the kingdom of the devil must shake, and they which belong to it must needs be stirred up unto repentance, or the devil will grasp them with his everlasting chains, and they be stirred up to anger, and perish;
>
> For behold, at that day shall he rage in the hearts of the children of men, and stir them up to anger against that which is good.
>
> And others will he pacify, and lull them away into carnal security, that they will say: All is well in Zion; yea, Zion prospereth, all is well—and thus the devil cheateth their souls, and leadeth them away carefully down to hell.
>
> And behold, others he flattereth away, and telleth them there is no hell; and he saith unto them: I am no devil, for there is none—and thus he whispereth in their ears, until he grasps them with his awful chains, from whence there is no deliverance. (2 Nephi 28:19–22)

This passage makes it very clear that Satan is real. He is a fallen spirit that does indeed exist and is actively trying to influence us and take control of our hearts. Nephi uses some very powerful imagery in this passage to demonstrate how Satan goes about his work. He can rage in our hearts. He can stir us up to anger. He can pacify us and lull us away into security. He can flatter us. He can also whisper cunning lies to us and then forcefully grasp us with his chains. Nephi uses the word *stir* in two different ways in these verses. He mentions how Satan can rage in our hearts and stir us up to anger. But he also teaches that we need to be stirred up to repentance if we are denizens of the kingdom of the devil.

We are living in that prophesied time when Satan is raging in the hearts of the children of men. He wants to make all men miserable like unto himself. He wants us to dig pits for our neighbors and then bury us in those same pits that we ourselves dug (see 1 Nephi 14:3). Satan's allegiance to us is a fraud. His loyalty to us is counterfeit. He wants us to follow him, but in the great day of harvest, he will not be there to console or support us. Instead, he will be laughing at us for the despair and misery that we experience because of him. Satan desires to have us that he may sift us as wheat (see Luke 22:31). He seeks the misery of all mankind (see 2 Nephi 2:18).

President Ezra Taft Benson declared, "The Book of Mormon exposes the enemies of Christ. God, with His infinite foreknowledge, so molded the Book of Mormon that we might see the error and know how to combat false educational, political, religious, and philosophical concepts of our time."[9] We definitely live in a time where false concepts are proliferating at an astonishing rate. Social media, as well as the media at large, are flooded with the poisonous philosophies of men and women masquerading as truth. Are we effectively using the Book of Mormon to recognize false teachings and learn how to ward off such offenses?

SAMUEL THE LAMANITE

One of the great stories in the Book of Mormon that illustrates how Satan tries to get hold of our hearts centers on the night of Jesus's birth and the signs that the people saw in the Americas to celebrate that blessed day.

Samuel the Lamanite came to the Nephites in 6 BC to prophesy about the coming birth of our Savior and to call the people to repentance. Approximately one or two years before the Savior's birth, "great signs were given unto the people, and wonders; and the words of the prophets began to be fulfilled. And angels did appear unto men" (Helaman 16:13–14).

Satan quickly went to work to discount these spectacular signs and wonders in the people's eyes. He planted some ideas in their hearts such as this: "Some things they may have guessed right, among so many" (Helaman 16:16); "It is not reasonable that such a being as a Christ shall come" (verse 18); "This is a wicked tradition, which has been handed down to us by our fathers" (verse 20); "They can keep us in ignorance, for we cannot witness with our eyes that they are true" (verse 20); "They will, by the cunning and the mysterious arts of the evil one, work some great mystery which we cannot understand" (verse 21).

The similarity in technique and method between these arguments and those that are rampant today is striking and not coincidental. These descriptions are included in the Book of Mormon to help us recognize Satan's methods and combat them in our day. Samuel the Lamanite faced not-so-subtle variations of today's frequent criticisms of the Church and Christian principles in general.

Satan may even work on us by occasionally presenting some truths in order for us to believe a larger lie (see Alma 1:4; Genesis 3:4–5). He plays on our senses in numerous ways. He may entice us with the beautiful concepts of love, unity, and acceptance of others before cunningly convincing us to abandon our adherence to ethical and moral absolutes. He asks us, "If we cannot see something, how can we know that it is true?" He also plants seeds of doubt in our minds by saying that anyone could guess right on some things. He tries to confuse us in regard to the promptings we receive from the Holy Ghost. He is quick to discount personal revelation and say we conjure up all of our own thoughts. He would have us completely disregard this member of the Godhead, even the Holy Ghost!

Mormon summarized Satan's work at this time. He wrote:

And many more things did the people imagine up in their hearts, which were foolish and vain; and they were much disturbed, for Satan did stir them up to do iniquity continually; yea, he did go about spreading rumors and contentions upon all the face of the land, that he might harden the hearts of the people against that which was good and against that which should come.

And notwithstanding the signs and the wonders which were wrought among the people of the Lord, and the many miracles which they did, Satan did get great hold upon the hearts of the people upon all the face of the land. (Helaman 16:22–23)

Despite the miraculous signs and wonders the Nephites experienced, Satan was successful in getting hold over their hearts, and in short manner! We should never discount Satan's devices or efforts. They are extremely effective and we must ever be on guard against them. The venom he spews against the truth should also never surprise us. He will spread rumors and contentions and work continually to try to make us miserable as he is.

SATAN'S PATTERN OF CONFUSING, CHEAPENING, AND DISMISSING

From the story of Samuel the Lamanite, we learn that mocking faith and testimony solely as foolish and vain imaginations in people's hearts is another tool in Satan's arsenal. This reference to the vain imaginations of the heart is mentioned on four different occasions in the Book of Mormon. Twice, it is used by Satan to explain away the signs and wonders the people had seen marking Christ's birth. The other two mentions are of Laman and Lemuel's description of their father, Lehi. Laman and Lemuel thought Lehi had foolish and vain imaginations in his heart to up and leave Jerusalem and depart into the wilderness for a promised land they did not think they would ever see.

Today's world is also quick to dismiss personal revelation, visions, and signs as foolish and vain imaginations. The world teaches that revelation is something that was given to prophets in Biblical, ancient times, and if by chance it still exists today, surely it is only received by a select few. Satan thus makes a mockery of the notion that regular people can receive revelation for themselves. The adversary works hard to delegitimize revelation as he knows what a powerful tool for righteousness it is. He continually attempts to cheapen, confuse, and muddle even very clear feelings of the Spirit. He will attack the process of revelation every step of the way, in any way possible.

Today, some people are quick to say that certain doctrines of the Church are foolish and vain. Some declare that the leaders of the Church are outdated and need to "get with the times" on certain issues. Thus, people's testimonies become weaker and weaker and Satan's control over their hearts grows stronger and stronger. This tactic has worked for Satan for thousands of years, so why would he stop using it today?

Satan continued his diabolical work on the Nephites' hearts at the time of Jesus's birth and shortly thereafter. "There began to be *greater* signs and *greater* miracles wrought among the people" than had been shown a year or two earlier (3 Nephi 1:4, emphasis added). Despite all the incredible signs and wonders that occurred in the Americas when Jesus was born, it only took Satan a short time to convince people to disbelieve what they had seen.

And the people began to forget those signs and wonders which they had heard, and began to be less and less astonished at a sign or a wonder from heaven, insomuch that they began to be hard in their hearts, and blind in their minds, and began to disbelieve all which they had heard and seen—Imagining up some vain thing in their hearts, that it was wrought by men and by the power of the devil, to lead away and deceive the hearts of the people; and thus did Satan get possession of the hearts of the people again, insomuch that he did blind their eyes and lead them away to believe that the doctrine of Christ was a foolish and a vain thing. (3 Nephi 2:1–2)

Within four years of the Savior's birth, people were already forgetting the miraculous signs and wonders they were given to commemorate this event.

These two verses, which mention the word *heart* four times, show how hard Satan worked upon people's hearts. He worked on the people's minds and eyes simultaneously, but his focus was concentrated on their hearts. Can you imagine seeing what the people saw when Jesus was born? A night without any darkness? A brilliant new star appearing in the sky? Prophets had prophesied of these events for hundreds and hundreds of years, and here they were being fulfilled with exactness. The night had come, proving the prophecies were true, and still the people began to forget. Some of Satan's best work occurred at this time, to get people to dismiss these miraculous signs that had been given. He applies these same techniques to create doubt in our lives today.

THE GREAT DISCOURAGER

President James E. Faust called Satan the "Great Imitator, the Master Deceiver, the Arch Counterfeiter, and the Great Forger."[10] We would like to add that Satan is also the Great Discourager. As 3 Nephi 2:1–2 illustrates, Satan wants nothing more than to deceive and eventually take possession of our hearts. He will do whatever it takes to fulfill his mission. We must ever be on guard against his methods and rebuke him. We cannot afford to lose our hearts to the darkness.

Elder Jörg Klebingat said of Satan, "He will seek access to your heart to tell you lies—lies that Heavenly Father is disappointed in you, that the Atonement is beyond your reach, that there is no point in even trying . . . and a thousand variations of that same evil theme."[11] We have all felt Satan's influence as he has attempted to spread these lies in our hearts.

The harder we try to purify our hearts, the harder Satan will work to introduce spiritual disease into our hearts. A familiarity with the specific devices Satan employs can be a powerful support when we get discouraged about our efforts to sanctify our hearts.

Discouragement runs rampant among Church members today. Frequently, Church members are too hard on themselves and believe perfection is to be achieved in this life. We will inevitably fall short and quickly become discouraged if we think this is what is expected of us today. While we are commanded to be perfect, Heavenly Father and our Savior knew that we would not achieve perfection here in mortality. We will continue on our journey to perfection after we die. The fact that we are not yet perfect does not mean that our Heavenly Father is disappointed in us.

We'd like to briefly relate Derek's experience with Satan's efforts to discourage him. While we don't want this experience to take away from the book's main focus, what follows illustrates Satan's efforts to discourage us. Our hope in sharing this is to increase awareness of Satan's desires to dishearten and depress us while on our journey. In Derek's words:

> I have struggled with general anxiety disorder and depression for about six years now. I have always been a somewhat anxious person, but after a particularly challenging and traumatic experience at work, I developed anxiety and depression with such force that I couldn't properly function on my own. These illnesses have stayed with me ever since that time.
>
> I know there are many Church members that struggle with mental illness. The number of people battling anxiety and depression has risen dramatically in recent years. Discouragement is one of the most prominent fruits of these illnesses. President Ezra Taft Benson said, "Many are giving up heart for the battle of life. Suicide ranks as a major cause of the deaths of college students. As the showdown between good and evil approaches with its accompanying trials and tribulations, Satan is increasingly striving to overcome the Saints with despair, discouragement, despondency, and depression."[12]
>
> I am very familiar with each of the "4 Ds" President Benson referenced. I feel despair, discouragement, despondency, and depression more often than most people as a result of my illness. If you struggle with mental illness, you have undoubtedly experienced similar feelings on a frequent basis. If so, you are uniquely qualified to know how Satan is trying to inflict men, women, and children's hearts

with despair and discouragement. You know the destructive impact such feelings can bring upon people.

If there is anything I've learned from my personal battle with these feelings, it is that we must fight on. Don't give up heart in this battle of life! That is exactly what Satan would want us to do. We should strive to become better Saints, but we cannot afford to be too hard on ourselves. At particularly difficult times, the victory of our hearts is achieved by simply getting through the day. Above all other heart conditions that we will study in this book, we cannot afford to give up heart along the way.

We need to develop faith in the ability of the Atonement of Christ to bless our own lives. It is a lot easier to have faith that the Savior's Atonement will bless someone else's life instead of our own. As we repent, we need to remember to forgive ourselves as well. Heavenly Father forgives us and remembers our sins no more when we repent (see D&C 58:42). Can we do the same and forgive ourselves and move forward?

There is a pattern most of us will experience as we try to sanctify and purify our hearts. We might work and labor and toil on breaking a habit, and momentarily think we are making great progress, only to slip back to what we have always done. This is one of Satan's favorite times to exploit any feelings of discouragement or lack of worth we might have. He will tell us we cannot do it. He will try to discourage us from continuing on. He will say it is pointless to try to change because no one is perfect on earth, and surely we never will be. He will make us feel like the course we are taking is being graded on a pass-fail scale—and that we are failing. Though we experience both successes and failures, progress and direction along the journey while here on earth is what defines success.

If we turn to the Savior at this moment of truth, after we have slipped up while trying to improve, He will lovingly work with us and grant us greater resolve and power to change. His might, His omnipotence, will overwhelm Satan's force. His merciful, open, ever-extended arms will lift us up. His ability to cleanse us will make whole any destruction the devil can inflict. If we pray for assistance to overcome Satan's foolish and vain imaginations, we will become more Christlike and be given added strength to build upon positive changes in our lives.

LESSONS FROM THE GADIANTON ROBBERS

Using other people to influence and sway us to do evil is another very effective tool Satan uses to get power over our hearts. His work becomes much easier when others are doing it for him. The Book of Mormon is filled with stories of wicked individuals trying to get others to join in their wickedness. Many of these stories will be fleshed out in subsequent chapters, but some names are worth mentioning here. Nehor, Amlici, Korihor, Zoram, and Amalickiah all worked relentlessly to convince people to turn their hearts to Satan (see Alma 1; Alma 2; Alma 30; Alma 31; and Alma 48, respectively).

The Gadianton robbers did more to turn the hearts of the people over to Satan than any other group or person in the Book of Mormon. The Gadianton robbers are an interesting case study in swaying people's hearts. There were three main eras for the Gadianton robbers' influence in the land that we learn about in the Book of Mormon.

We learn about the first iteration of the Gadianton robbers in Helaman 1. In this period, the Gadianton robbers flourished from about 52–17 BC. Kishkumen led this band that was initially formed during a heated election among three brothers to determine the chief judge. Kishkumen was a follower of Paanchi, who lost the election and was sentenced to death for treason. This only enraged Paanchi's supporters further, and Kishkumen ended up murdering the rightfully elected chief judge, Pahoran.

After Pahoran's successor was killed by a Lamanite leader in battle, Helaman, the son of Helaman, became chief judge. Kishkumen wanted to kill him as well. Helaman's servant agreed to take Kishkumen to see Helaman and learned more about "the heart of Kishkumen" along the way (Helaman 2:8). Consider the way Kishkumen's heart is described. "It was his object to murder, and also that it was the object of all those who belonged to his band to murder, and to rob, and to gain power" (Helaman 2:8). Helaman's servant fittingly stabbed Kishkumen's wicked heart and killed him before Kishkumen could murder the chief judge. Gadianton then took over as the leader of these robbers, and they were known by this name ever after.

It is important to understand that the Gadianton robbers could never have prospered without the support and backing of the people. These robbers were to be executed according to the laws of the land for their treason (see Helaman 2:10). However, the Nephites allowed the robbers to even live in the more settled parts of the land and did not identify these robbers to the government (see Helaman 3:23). Gradually, those that upheld the robbers surrendered their hearts to the darkness this group offered. Hate, murder, and a thirst for power eventually filled the hearts of those who supported the robbers.

The Lamanites "destroyed" the first iteration of the robbers from their midst by preaching the word of God unto them (see Helaman 6:37). In stark contrast, the Nephites continued to support the robbers at this time. They even mourned the murder of their chief judge, himself a Gadianton robber, who was killed by another Gadianton robber! Eventually, Nephi, the son of Helaman, asked for a famine to come upon the land wherein thousands of these robbers perished. The rest of the people repented and "swept away the band of Gadianton from amongst them insomuch that they have become extinct" (Helaman 11:10).

A second iteration of the Gadianton robbers was formed in 12 BC, only five years after the first band was swept from the earth. This band became stronger than the armies of both the Nephites and the Lamanites in less than two years' time! Again, Mormon says they were stirred up to anger, which led to murder and plunder (see Helaman 11:24–25). This group of robbers was destroyed when Gidgiddoni, the Nephite commander, led those who opposed the robbers to gather food and supplies and come together as one. They essentially waited the weakened robbers out until the robbers were forced to come down to battle the Nephites in their strength. The Nephites prayed for deliverance from the robbers, and the Lord delivered them.

Mormon marveled at how quickly the Nephites went from destroying the original band of Gadianton robbers to allowing them to regenerate just five short years later. This second band of robbers had become extremely formidable in a very small window of time.

Mormon lamented, "Yea, and we see *at the very time* when he doth prosper his people, yea, in the increase of their fields, their flocks and their herds, and in gold, and in silver, and in all manner of precious things of every kind and art; sparing their lives, and delivering them out of the hands of their enemies; softening the hearts of their enemies that they should not declare wars against them; yea, and in fine, doing all things for the welfare and happiness of his people; yea, then is the time *that they do harden their hearts,* and do forget the Lord their God, and do trample under their feet the Holy One—yea, and this *because of their ease, and their exceedingly great prosperity*" (Helaman 12:2, emphasis added).

Mormon had personally witnessed the entire destruction of his people. As a compiler and abridger, he had read and studied about the devastation among the Nephites and Lamanites in earlier times. He was quick to point out what he saw from this unique vantage point in speaking about the past. He had read about the Nephites' prosperity at this time after they destroyed the first band of Gadianton robbers. He read how the Lord had blessed them, prospered them, and delivered them. How frustrating it must have been for Mormon to then read about the return of the Gadianton robbers five short years later! He knew how wicked and powerful these secret combinations were because the land was filled with robbers during his day (see Mormon 2:8). He saw firsthand the destruction they caused.

With Mormon's background in mind, it would be foolish to simply dismiss his solemn warning and feel secure and confident that we will not experience the same fate. He was shown our day and was intimately familiar with the battles we would fight. Mormon saw prosperity and ease as an enormous danger and challenge for members of the Church in the latter days. Mormon desperately wanted to warn us and help us not fall into the same trap that led to the Nephites' destruction. Mormon warned us that we cannot afford to forget the Lord our God. We cannot afford to trample Him under our feet. We cannot afford to harden our hearts and think that we are able to do it all on our own.

Lastly, the book of 4 Nephi describes a third generation of Gadianton robbers that was formed around AD 260. And why was this group formed at this time? "And this church did multiply exceedingly because of iniquity, and because of the power of Satan who did get hold upon their hearts" (4 Nephi 1:28). An evil and destructive disease was again planted in the people's hearts by the devil.

The people became more and more hardened in their hearts and were taught to hate the people of God until finally they "began to build up the secret oaths and combinations of Gadianton" (see 4 Nephi 1:31, 34, 42). Murder, plunder, and seeking for power quickly followed. Mormon credits the followers of Gadianton as an instrument that destroyed the Nephite civilization. Said he, "And behold, in the end of this book ye shall see that this Gadianton did prove the overthrow, yea, almost the entire destruction of the people of Nephi" (Helaman 2:13).

With each iteration of the Gadianton robbers, they were able to gain great power over the hearts of the people and in rapid order. It is vital to be extremely wary and vigilant of groups that may lead us away to do wickedly, no matter how well they conceal their true aims. We should never embrace or even casually support groups that want to lead us astray from the safety of the gospel fold.

THE SURE FOUNDATION

In order to ward off Satan's attempts to access our hearts, we need to build our foundation upon our Redeemer, Jesus Christ. Only through His power can we "cast out devils, or the evil spirits which dwell in the hearts of the children of men" (Mosiah 3:6). Only through Him can we access grace sufficient to cleanse and heal our hearts.

Grace is described in the Bible Dictionary this way: "It is likewise through the grace of the Lord that individuals, through faith in the Atonement of Jesus Christ and repentance of their sins, receive strength and assistance to do good works that they otherwise would not be able to maintain if left to their own means."[13] It is only through the grace of our Savior that we are given the strength to move on from these diseases of the heart and make permanent, positive changes in our lives as we repent.

Have you noticed this grace working in your life? Bad habits and patterns, even those that may seem simple to master, cannot be overcome without divine grace operating in our lives. For example, at the time of this writing, the Sabbath Day has become a specific central focus of the prophet and apostles in the last couple of years. We have been taught on many occasions about how we can make the Sabbath a more sacred and spiritual day. Both of us have each felt the Spirit's witness to heed the counsel of our leaders and keep the Sabbath Day holy.

Although there are many weaknesses and bad habits yet to break, we look back over the last few months and years and can see small areas of progress in keeping the Sabbath Day holy. Many habits and shortcomings, such as watching sports on TV or surfing the internet for worldly distractions, were initially difficult to change in keeping the Sabbath Day holy, and there have certainly been times when we have not used our time for better Sabbath Day pursuits. Improvement can be a lengthy process at times; however, through the Lord's grace, changes happen and eventually stick. With diligent effort, time spent watching sports and being distracted on the internet can be replaced with time spent focusing on the Lord and making efforts to better keep His day holy. Throughout the process of change and repentance, the Atonement of Christ provides us with strength to rid ourselves of bad habits and patterns and replace them with virtues and good habits. Weaknesses become strengths, and what was once hard can be made easy.

Helaman said, "And now, my sons, remember, remember that it is upon the rock of our Redeemer, who is Christ, the Son of God, that ye must build your foundation; that when the devil shall send forth his mighty winds, yea, his shafts in the whirlwind, yea, when all his hail and his mighty storm shall beat upon you, it shall have no power over you to drag you down to the gulf of misery and endless wo, because of the rock upon which ye are built, which is a sure foundation, a foundation whereon if men build they cannot fall" (Helaman 5:12). As we repent and strive to better live the gospel every day, not only can we be forgiven of our sins and have them remitted, but we can also be given additional power in our hearts to resist evil through the Atonement of our Savior.

Chapter 2

HARDHEARTEDNESS

Hardheartedness is by far the most frequently mentioned type or condition of the heart in the Book of Mormon. Having a hard heart is mentioned 97 times in the Book of Mormon, comprising over one-fifth of the total mentions of the heart in the Book of Mormon, and in none of these references can we find it esteemed as something desirable!

Scientifically speaking, what exactly is a hard heart? The most common physical condition associated with a hard heart occurs in the heart's arteries. These arteries carry blood from the heart to other parts of the body. Fat gets deposited on the inside walls of the arteries and then can calcify or harden. It becomes more difficult for blood to pass through the arteries to other organs as this plaque grows. This hardening can lead to heart attacks, stroke, congestive heart failure, and even death.[1]

The medical aspects of such heart disease help us understand how hardheartedness, as it is used in the Book of Mormon, is symbolically and spiritually similar to a physically diseased heart. Our spiritual health can be severely damaged by hardheartedness.

Spiritual hardheartedness is quite broadly defined in the scriptures. However, each unique definition or example of hardheartedness found in the Book of Mormon provides additional insight and meaning. Some of the more applicable definitions include being unfeeling, insensitive, or indifferent (see Mormon 4:11). Hardheartedness is likewise defined as being cold, pitiless, unmerciful, and having no concern for the welfare of others (see Jacob 1:15; Alma 21:3). Hardheartedness is lacking in understanding, having a resistance to instruction and the truth, complaining about life's circumstances, and being unteachable (see 1 Nephi 16:22; 2 Nephi 33:2; Mosiah 13:32; 26:3; 3 Nephi 2:1).

SAM TSUYA

Ryan had a remarkable experience on his mission in Brazil with someone who had once suffered from a hard heart and all that accompanies one. In Ryan's words:

> I served in the São Paulo Brazil East Mission. During my first months in the mission, I met an elderly Japanese-American missionary couple that served in various capacities within the mission home. Elder and Sister Tsuya were well known for two things. The first was the haircuts Elder Tsuya gave the missionaries on transfer days—haircuts of such unusual method and result that the mission president gently asked him to retire his clippers shortly after I arrived.
>
> The other thing that the Tsuyas were known for was their incredible love for others and sharing the gospel. Everything they did was infused with a fiery spirit of missionary work. Their presence in Brazil was quite unusual because they spoke no Portuguese and only spoke English with a thick accent, though the lack of Portuguese didn't seem to slow them down. Each week they went to the fruit market, taking with them a box of Books of Mormon they had purchased with their own money. They always returned home empty-handed. They invited anyone and everyone they encountered to come unto Christ, regardless of their inability to speak the language. They carried the

Spirit with them, and you couldn't help but feel the Spirit when you were around them.

One transfer day, I had the chance to visit with Elder Tsuya. While listening to his story, I discovered that he had joined the Church in Hawaii. I found that interesting and told him that my grandfather had served a mission in Hawaii and was on Oahu during the attack on Pearl Harbor. Elder Tsuya was very surprised at this and said he had joined the Church during that time on Oahu, but didn't remember an Elder Squire. I told him that it was my mom's father, Elder Thurgood, who had served in Hawaii.

Elder Tsuya almost fell out of his chair. He stood up and yelled out, "Elder Thurgood is your grandpa?!?" By this time, many missionaries had gathered around to listen to the conversation. Elder Tsuya then related the story of meeting my grandpa. He said one night he was eating a meal with a large group of people in his community. Elder Tsuya was being inappropriate and was taking the Lord's name in vain, among other things. A man with a nametag of some sort, my grandfather, had spoken up and asked him to stop. Elder Tsuya, being a thoughtless teenager, didn't think much of the interruption and once again took the name of the Lord in vain.

When Elder Tsuya did that, he said my grandpa jumped up from his seat, came over to him, and hit him hard on the shoulder. My grandpa lectured him about how little he knew about life, how he wasn't as smart as he thought, how he needed to quit smoking and do a bunch of things differently, and come unto Christ, or he wouldn't ever amount to anything in this life. Elder Tsuya said that he would always remember that moment and found the experience extremely embarrassing and humiliating.

Elder Tsuya described himself at that time in his life as being tremendously insensitive and indifferent to things of religion and to God. He was entirely unconcerned for the welfare of others and lacked any understanding of spiritual things. He wasn't looking to be taught by any-body and felt like he had all the answers he needed in life. In short, he could have been described as a poster boy of hardheartedness.

Elder Tsuya told me that when he went home that night, the words directed at him sunk deep into his soul. He thought and thought about things that had been said, and he concluded he needed to make some changes in his life. He ran into two similarly dressed missionaries a couple of weeks later and stopped them to ask their purpose on the islands. He quickly agreed to listen to the discussions with a sincere desire to change and was baptized very shortly thereafter. Elder Tsuya gave much of the credit for his deci-sion to listen to the missionaries to that experience with my grandpa. He even had a journal entry of sorts from that night (which he later kindly provided me a copy) that recorded the events of the night, the desire he had to change, and included the name on the nametag of the man that had hit him: Elder Thurgood.

I quickly wrote home telling my family I had *huge* news and that Grandpa Thurgood needed to be in the room when I made my telephone call at Christmas, which was a couple of months away. I felt like this story was worth shar-ing over the phone, and I spent several letters getting the family excited about the news I would share.

When I called home, the first item of business was to get to the bottom of what I wanted to share. With everyone listening, I finally told my grandfather I had met somebody who came into the Church because of him. I will always remember how quiet the phone call became, with all the background chatter coming to an abrupt stop. Finally, Grandpa Thurgood spoke softly and said, "Ryan, you are mistaken. I never baptized anybody on my mission."

I then asked him if he remembered hitting a Japanese-American kid, who was a real smart aleck, at dinner on Oahu one night and then lecturing him on how much he needed to change his life. He became confused, then flustered, and said that he did remember the incident well as it was the only time he had ever done anything like that. He wanted to know what this had to do with anything and how I knew about that experience.

I told my grandfather that a couple weeks later that boy had stopped similar-looking missionaries and decided to listen to the discussions because of what he had said to him that night. That boy later married in the temple in Hawaii. That boy grew to serve in various callings in the Church and blessed many, many lives. That boy later served as a mission president in Tokyo, Japan, for three years. That boy also served as president of the Tokyo MTC in Japan. That boy also served several other missions with his wife. He was now in Brazil because they never placed any limitations of where they would serve or what language they would be willing to learn to speak. That boy had many children and grandchildren that were faithful in the Church.

My Grandpa Thurgood was in tears and unable to talk for the remainder of the phone call. He had spent 54 years thinking his mission hadn't made a difference to anybody other than himself. My grandparents were later able to attend the temple with the Tsuyas and had a tearful and very joyous reunion when the Tsuyas completed their mission service in Brazil.

How reassuring it is to know that hardheartedness does not have to be a permanently soul-destroying condition! We are all not only invited to overcome hardheartedness, but we are also assisted in our battles to overcome its effects.

Those who are spiritually hardhearted reject the Savior, reject the Spirit, reject the Lord's servants, and do not look to the Lord (see 1 Nephi 15:3; 17:30; 2 Nephi 25:12, Mosiah 11:29, Ether 8:25). The hardhearted refuse to ask in faith and depend upon their own strength and wisdom (see 1 Nephi 15:10–11, Helaman 16:15).

They resist the Spirit of truth and are offended by the strictness of the word of the Lord (see Alma 30:46; 35:15). The hardhearted are unrepentant (see Mosiah 12:1, Alma 15:15; 34:31). These were all aspects of hardheartedness that Elder Tsuya was able to overcome in his life.

With the many variations of hardheartedness, this disease also produces many different consequences and outcomes. The fruits of hardheartedness are indeed destructive to the soul. We are taught that the hardhearted will disbelieve signs and wonders from God and will decrease in faith and righteousness (see 3 Nephi 1:22, 30). It is amazing to think that hardheartedness kept the disciples from understanding the miracle of the loaves in the feeding of the five thousand (see Mark 6:52).

The hardhearted will receive the lesser portion of the word (see Alma 12:10–11). On many occasions, a hard heart is coupled with a blind mind in the Book of Mormon (see 1 Nephi 7:8; 14:7; Jarom 1:3; Alma 13:4; 3 Nephi 2:1; 7:16; Ether 4:15; 15:19). The hardhearted are unable to see spiritually what is being taught. Great and marvelous things will be withheld from them (see Ether 4:15). The hardhearted will moreover miss out on the great privilege of priesthood blessings (see Alma 13:4). The Spirit withdraws from those who harden their hearts and has no place in those who are already hardhearted (see 2 Nephi 33:2; Helaman 6:35). Sins, iniquities, wicked practices, and abominations likewise result from hardheartedness (see Jacob 1:15; Alma 21:3; 37:10). Perhaps most damning of all, the hardhearted forget the Lord their God and trample Him under their feet (see Helaman 12:2).

We will not be able to deliver essential spiritual nutrients to the rest of our body if we have a hard heart spiritually. Spiritual fitness and well-being are impossible if our hearts are hard. We may show glimpses of other spiritual strengths and partially develop them, but deep and balanced spiritual growth will be prevented as our hard hearts keep our spirits from functioning properly.

LAMAN AND LEMUEL—THEY MIGHT HAVE BEEN HAPPY

One of the Book of Mormon's greatest examples of hardheartedness is found in observing the lives of Laman and Lemuel. Nephi describes Laman and Lemuel as being hardhearted eleven times in the book of 1 Nephi. If Nephi wrote this down eleven times in limited space on hard-to-engrave plates of ore, we are sure he felt that way about his brothers even more often than that.

The first signs of hardheartedness for Laman and Lemuel seemed to surface as their father pulled them away from Jerusalem. In their minds, it was Lehi's "foolish imaginations" that forced them from their lives of comfort and ease into the wilderness. Laman and Lemuel "murmured in many things against their father" because they "knew not the dealings" of God (see 1 Nephi 2:11, 12). It was at this critical time that Nephi did a very smart thing. When he and his family were in the valley of Lemuel, Nephi said, "I did cry unto the Lord; and behold He did visit me, and did soften my heart" (verse 16).

Nephi received a personal witness that the Lord would be leading their journey and his father was the Lord's mouthpiece. Their journey did not result merely from foolish imaginations. This blessing came to Nephi from a gracious, merciful Father because Nephi desired it and asked for it. After receiving his witness, Nephi pleaded for his brothers Laman and Lemuel to obtain a similar witness for themselves.

Laman and Lemuel stubbornly would not do this! Their hearts were already so completely hardened that they refused the invitation to call upon the Lord. Their inability to humble themselves enough to seek an answer from the Lord was a morally destructive symptom of their hardheartedness.

The blessings and answers that prayer yields were shut off from Laman and Lemuel as a result of this disease in their hearts. These two never received their own spiritual witness that the Lord would lead the expedition. As a result, their hearts were continually hardened, particularly at key moments of the journey. Their hardheartedness continued to frustrate their spiritual development throughout the remainder of their lives.

Laman and Lemuel considered going back to Jerusalem to get the brass plates "a hard thing" (1 Nephi 3:5). Such commands and doctrine are hard for the hardhearted to understand (see 1 Nephi 15:3). After failing twice to get the plates, Laman and Lemuel spoke "many hard words" unto Nephi and Sam and blamed them for their failings (1 Nephi 3:28). Only the appearance of an angel unto Laman and Lemuel caused them to cease beating their younger brothers with an undoubtedly hard rod. To summarize, the command was considered a *hard* thing and was *hard* for them to understand, many *hard* words were spoken, and a *hard* rod was used against their younger brothers. This experience demonstrates the destructive depths of spiritual desensitization a hard heart can bring about.

Laman and Lemuel again began to murmur almost before the glow of the angel's visitation had dimmed, questioning moments later how it would be possible for the Lord to best Laban (see 1 Nephi 3:31). Laman and Lemuel's hard hearts resulted in spiritual ignorance, caused them to murmur, drove them to darkness, allowed violence to be introduced in their hearts, and eventually resulted in filling their hearts with murder.

There are many examples where the hardness of Laman and Lemuel's hearts resulted in spiritual decay where there might have been growth. When they returned to Jerusalem to get Ishmael and his family, Laman and Lemuel were brought painfully close to the comfort and ease they had enjoyed while living at home. With a renewed proximity to the luxuries of the world, they did not want to return to the wilderness because of the hardness of their hearts and rebelled against Nephi (see 1 Nephi 7:6–7). They bound Nephi with cords and sought to kill him. Nephi was given strength to loosen the bands, and again, they sought to lay hands on Nephi. It took the pleading of members of Ishmael's family and Nephi's wife to soften Laman and Lemuel's hearts (see 1 Nephi 7:16–19).

After listening to the tree of life vision received by their father, and then listening to Nephi's own inspired vision, Laman and

Lemuel still did not understand the meaning of the vision because of the hardness of their hearts. They told Nephi that he had declared "hard things" unto them (1 Nephi 16:1). In reality, "the guilty taketh the truth to be hard" and are actually the ones hardening the message (1 Nephi 16:2).

When Nephi broke his bow in the wilderness, Laman and Lemuel again hardened their hearts and were found "complaining against the Lord their God" (1 Nephi 16:22). When Nephi later asked them to help build a ship, they again hardened their hearts and were reluctant to labor. They could not imagine their humble family accomplishing so mighty a task (see 1 Nephi 17:17–19). Hardheartedness prevented them from gaining the invaluable testimony that the Lord will always prepare a way for his commandments to be accomplished. They had lost sight and understanding that not only building this ship, but the entire journey, was a commandment of the Lord. They bemoaned the life they left behind in Jerusalem where they "might have been happy" (1 Nephi 17:21). There can truly be no vision where there is hardness of heart.

Laman, Lemuel, and others made themselves merry and spoke with much rudeness while sailing on the ship to the promised land. They forgot by what power they were crossing the ocean. Laman and Lemuel bound up Nephi with cords when Nephi's righteous desires became a killjoy to the party. A terrible tempest ensued, and after four long days, Laman and Lemuel finally loosed the bands from Nephi. They were driven by nothing more than self-preservation at this point. Their hearts had become so hardened that only the threat of destruction could soften them (see 1 Nephi 18:19–20).

Finally, once they arrived in the promised land, Laman and Lemuel again sought to kill Nephi. The Lord warned Nephi to depart from them and flee into the wilderness with his family and anyone else that would go with him (see 2 Nephi 5:5). Nephi described Laman and Lemuel's hearts again using the hardest substance he could imagine. He said, "For behold, they had hardened their hearts against him, that they had become like unto a flint" (2 Nephi 5:21). He thought they were as hard as the substance that was used to make weapons. When broken up, flint results in many sharp edges as well. Unfortunately, this was an apt description of Laman and Lemuel's hearts.

LIKENING THE SCRIPTURES UNTO OURSELVES

Laman and Lemuel's hardheartedness is mentioned in each of the above situations. We think it might be overlooked, or in the least understated at times, how demanding this journey would have been. It is easy to read about each scenario in this journey and identify what course of action they should have taken with the benefit of hindsight and the companionship of the Spirit. It is not hard to pick apart the anemic spiritual performance of Laman and Lemuel. However, would we really act much differently given similar circumstances?

Imagine your family traveling many weeks into the wilderness and being at the mercy of the land for your food and subsistence. You are living on raw meat, unable to even build fires in order to stay below the radar of robbers for your own safety. It may have been a change in climate that had rendered your wooden bows from Jerusalem useless, causing their springs to be lost some time earlier. Your family finds itself dependent on your brother's fine steel bow, it being your lone source of harvesting food. Then, the unthinkable happens and the steel bow breaks too. Your family's living conditions demanded great faith even before the use of bows was lost, and now you are living in your extremity unsure of your next meal.

Who wouldn't be complaining and murmuring at a time like this? Not only would you be hungry, but you would also have a deep sense of longing for the security and comfort you enjoyed in Jerusalem. It was in these circumstances that even the prophet Lehi began to murmur. We must remember that softening our hearts is a lifelong process. There will be times when we will all be tested to our limits.

Imagine being commanded to help build a ship, one that would possibly take two years of colossal effort and hard work to build. Would you really jump right into the project and say, "Great! Let's make some tools and get behind this younger brother of ours, the one that appears to want to be our leader?" Before you consider your response to this circumstance, maybe consider the level of enthusiasm you exhibited the last time a picture needed to be hung on the wall.

Do we assess the condition of our own heart and seek help in cultivating a softer heart when reading these stories in the scriptures? Do we take the time to try to visualize ourselves in similar circumstances? Do we earnestly seek to discern and internalize the principles that are being taught? Or do we read through the story as simply that, a story about something abstract, in a faraway land and from a time long ago?

If we try to recognize the difficulty of his situation and circumstance, Nephi's example during such trying times becomes amazing and awe-inspiring! Nephi was not perfect, but he did some key things that allowed the Lord to soften his heart and mold him into the pioneer, prophet, and king he became.

THE ADVERSARY'S USE OF HARDHEARTEDNESS

We gain some valuable insights into hardheartedness from carefully studying the visions Lehi and Nephi received about the tree of life. The angel taught Nephi, "And the mists of darkness are the temptations of the devil, which blindeth the eyes, and hardeneth the hearts of the children of men, and leadeth them away into broad roads, that they perish and are lost" (1 Nephi 12:17). Temptations led to three different conditions in this verse, namely blind eyes, hard hearts, and being led away into broad roads.

While serving as a member of the Seventy, Elder Rulon G. Craven said, "To blind the eyes is to not see or acknowledge the consequences of our actions. To harden the heart is to ignore or not be willing to accept counsel. To be led into the broad roads is to give in to worldly enticements and lose the influence of the Holy Spirit in our lives. Temptation is like a magnetic force which holds a metal object in its power. It loses its magnetic force and power when you turn away from it."[2]

We are walking closer to that pull and may get so close that we cannot back away if we are entertaining a temptation placed before us. We have to spurn the temptation and turn completely away from it for that magnetic draw to have no effect. One of the most effective ways we can turn away from temptation is to turn to something else, namely the word of God. How did people in Lehi's dream get through the mists of darkness? "They did press their way forward, continually holding fast to the rod of iron, until they came forth and fell down and partook of the fruit of the tree" (1 Nephi 8:30).

People with hard hearts do the polar opposite when it comes to their treatment of the word of God. "But behold, there are many that harden their hearts against the Holy Spirit, that it hath no place in them; wherefore, they cast things away which are written and esteem them as things of naught" (2 Nephi 33:2). Hardheartedness prevents people from looking to the scriptures for any guidance at all, and the still and steady voice of the prophets and Holy Ghost go unheard over the din of the world. Elder Michael John U. Teh said, "Neglecting to study the scriptures on a regular basis is a form of hardening our hearts."[3] The hardhearted reject the Savior, the Spirit, prophets, and the word of God.

Were Laman and Lemuel willing to accept counsel from Lehi, from Nephi, or from angels? No! This led to their downfall. They were staggeringly, jaw-droppingly unteachable!

Nephi further saw in his vision that the Bible had "many parts which are plain and most precious" taken away with the intent that it would blind our eyes and harden our hearts (1 Nephi 13:27). In 1 Nephi 14, the Gentiles were warned three times to not harden their hearts against the Lamb of God and His word, lest they be brought down into captivity and be destroyed (see 1 Nephi 14:2, 6, 7). As we diligently study the Book of Mormon, it will act as an elixir against the adversary's attempts to harden our hearts. The Book of Mormon will open our eyes to the effects of our actions, open our hearts to receive counsel, and empower us against the temptations of the enticements of the world.

ZEEZROM

Another enlightening example of hardheartedness is that of Zeezrom, a lawyer in the city of Ammonihah who contended against Alma and Amulek as they preached to the people. In Alma 11, Zeezrom tried to bribe Amulek with silver to deny the existence of God (see Alma 11:22). From Zeezrom's point of view, nothing was more valuable than money. Not understanding Amulek's spiritual depth, Zeezrom tried to bribe him with silver, the only currency Zeezrom seemed to understand.

How appropriate it is that *Ze-ezrom* has a unit of silver in the Nephite monetary system in his name preceded with the common prefix "ze-," possibly translating to "he of the silver!" (see Alma 11:6). As a side note, it is also interesting that the chief ruler of Ammonihah, Antionah, has a unit of gold as a part of his name coupled with the common suffix "-ah" (see Alma 11:19). Clearly, earthly riches were at the forefront of this people's hearts and minds.

In Alma 12, Alma begins speaking to Zeezrom and delivers the most comprehensive sermon on hardheartedness in the Book of Mormon. In the span of 33 verses (see Alma 12:10–37; 13:1–5), Alma mentions hardheartedness twelve times. Ten of these references are part of a more cohesive grouping in Alma 12. The numbers 10 and 12 are very significant numbers in the scriptures. The number 10 represents perfection or completeness. The number 12 represents divine government, God's authority, and the priesthood.[4]

There is rich symbolism in scripture, and we should always have our hearts open and our minds in tune with the Spirit to learn more of the mysteries of God as we are reading. John, in the Book of Revelation, uses the symbolism of certain numbers repeatedly in his prophecies. It is clear that he was intentionally using the symbolism behind these numbers to provide deeper meaning to his teachings. Likewise, it is clear to us that Jacob specifically used ten woes in 2 Nephi 9 to bring the Ten Commandments to people's remembrance. We will study more about those woes in a later chapter.

Although we want to be cautious about overemphasizing numerology, its tenets add an extra layer of emphasis and meaning to Alma's sermon. Did Alma want us to think about the number ten and some sort of completeness when we see these references grouped together in Alma 12? Did he want us to think about the number twelve and the priesthood when we total all references mentioned? It could very well be surmised that Alma intended such additional meaning.

Alma groups five references together in Alma 12:10–13 and then another five references in Alma 12:33–37, three of which come directly from Heavenly Father. Like the ten commandments or Jacob's ten woes, perhaps Alma wanted us to more easily recall the consequences of being hardhearted in our pursuit of spiritual knowledge and how this condition relates to our ability to obtain mercy and be exalted. Alma describes a completeness or finality of our soul's fate based on whether we are hardhearted or not. He finishes each grouping by speaking of the judgment we all must face and proclaiming what will happen to the state of our souls based on the malleability of our hearts.

Alma does a masterful job describing to Zeezrom and the people of Ammonihah the striking contrast in the spiritual health of those with hard hearts versus those who have soft hearts. Alma makes a natural progression in his argument as he goes from point to point, showing that those with hard hearts are not favored of God and miss out on tremendous blessings of the gospel promised to those with soft hearts. These points escalate in importance and consequence as he speaks with Zeezrom.

Alma begins by teaching about the relationship between hardheartedness and spiritual knowledge. Alma taught, "And therefore, he that will harden his heart, the same receiveth the lesser portion of the word; and he that will not harden his heart, to him is given the greater portion of the word, until it is given unto him to know the mysteries of God until he know them in full" (Alma 12:10). Here, Alma makes the effect very clear that a hard heart impedes a person's ability to gain spiritual knowledge. Alma's first five references to a hard heart concern our capacity to know and understand God's word.

Alma continues to raise the stakes to show how serious this disease of the heart can be: "And they that will harden their hearts, to them is given the lesser portion of the word until they know nothing concerning his mysteries" (verse 11). Consequently, not only do the hardhearted receive the lesser portion of the word, but they also end up knowing nothing of God's word if they continue on in this state! Alma then goes one step further, "Then if our hearts have been hardened, yea, if we have hardened our hearts against the word, insomuch that it has not been found in us, then will our state be awful, for then we shall be condemned" (verse 13). Thus, the hardhearted have lost all knowledge of the gospel and find themselves in an awful state and condemned of God.

Alma says that eventually the hardhearted will know nothing of God's mysteries. This is consistent with the Lord's teachings when He says, "For unto him that receiveth I will give more, and from them that shall say, We have enough, from them shall be taken away even that which they have" (2 Nephi 28:30). As far as our gospel knowledge is concerned, we are either acquiring more knowledge or losing that which we once had. Our knowledge cannot simply be set aside and then drawn upon whenever we want if we stop studying. It can only be drawn upon if we continue to study. Therefore, daily scripture study is vital to our spiritual health, not just to acquire more knowledge, but also to not lose what we have already been given.

Alma then focuses on the relationship between hardheartedness and repentance, mercy, and the Lord's rest in his next grouping of five references on the subject. At this point, his sermon escalates in its consequences of hardheartedness to the very salvation of our souls. The Father Himself uses this term three times in Alma 12:33–35 as He lays out the plan of redemption to all of us. He states, "Therefore, whosoever repenteth, and hardeneth not his heart, he shall have claim on mercy through mine Only Begotten Son, unto a remission of his sins; and these shall enter into my rest" (Alma 12:34). This reassuring promise of having a claim on the Savior's mercy is a comfort to all of us. People with hard hearts have a very difficult time admitting to sins or mistakes they have made. By softening our hearts sufficiently, we are able to humbly reach out to our Heavenly Father in prayer, confess our wrongs, and ask for forgiveness. Only then do we obtain such mercy through the Atonement of Christ.

Alma continues to show the contrast between those with hard hearts and those with soft hearts. People with hard hearts commit sin and do not repent (see verse 35). Hence, they do not have a claim on the Savior's mercy and ultimately experience the Lord's wrath and the everlasting destruction of their souls (see verse 36). On the other hand, people with soft hearts will have mercy granted unto them and will enter into the Lord's rest (see Alma 12:33, 34, 37). Alma emphasizes that the stakes are extremely high with this disease of the heart. We need to soften our hearts sufficiently to be able to draw upon the power of the Savior's Atonement.

Alma finishes speaking about hardheartedness by highlighting the impact hardheartedness has on our ability to serve within the priesthood, bringing the final tally to twelve mentions in this sermon. This aligns perfectly with the symbolism associated with the number twelve and the priesthood. By remembering that there are twelve total references to hardheartedness in Alma's sermon, we more readily recall his teachings about the effect a hard heart has on our ability to enjoy the great privileges the priesthood affords (see Alma 13:4).

Alma says that this holy calling, this great privilege and blessing, was available to everyone from the beginning, when we were all on equal footing. Alma again explains the difference between those with hard hearts and soft hearts in regard to the priesthood. Those with hard hearts miss out on the blessings of the priesthood while those with soft hearts are called to this holy calling (see Alma 13:4–5). What a beautiful and inspired sermon on this disease of the heart!

OTHER EXAMPLES OF HARDHEARTEDNESS

There are numerous other examples in the Book of Mormon of individuals and groups with hard hearts. Korihor, Amalickiah, and the Jaredites were all described as hardhearted. Many other descriptions could be given of all these people, and some were, but Mormon and Moroni continually chose to focus on the description of their hard hearts. This condition sadly led to the destruction of each of the aforementioned people, some in heartbreaking and horrific ways.

While in prison in Ammonihah, Alma and Amulek were stripped of their clothes, beaten by all that came forth to see them, and suffered hunger, thirst, and fatigue. Eventually, "the Lord granted unto them power and they straightway came forth out of prison; and they were loosed from their bands; and the prison had fallen to the earth, and every soul within the walls thereof, save it were Alma and Amulek, was slain" (Alma 14:28).

Even after witnessing Alma and Amulek coming forth from the prison, the surviving population still were not convinced. Unfortunately, the people of Ammonihah were described as remaining "hardhearted and stiffnecked . . . ascribing all the power of Alma and Amulek to the devil" (Alma 15:15). The people of Ammonihah, even "every living soul," were all destroyed by the Lamanites a short time later (Alma 16:9).

Korihor, an anti-Christ, suffered a gruesome fate because of his hardheartedness as well. Korihor began to preach unto the people in Zarahemla that there would be no Christ. After having found success there, he went to the land of Jershon and was thrown out by Ammon. He did not have much success in his next stop in the land of Gideon either. He was brought before the high priest, Giddonah, as well as the chief judge over that land while there.

Giddonah asked Korihor why he was doing what he was doing. He described Korihor's hardheartedness and did not feel it was worthwhile to even respond to his false teachings (see Alma 30:29). Korihor was bound and sent back to the land of Zarahemla to be judged by Alma, the high priest and chief judge over all the land. Alma was also grieved because of the hardness of Korihor's heart (see Alma 30:46). Eventually, Korihor was struck dumb by Alma. He went from house to house begging for food and was trampled to death.

Amalickiah was extremely hardhearted. In his efforts to become king over the dissenters from the Nephites and eventually over the Lamanites, "he led away the hearts of many people to do wickedly" (Alma 46:10). Amalickiah's design included arranging the murder of the king of the Lamanites, plotting for him to be stabbed in the heart. Having accomplished this, Amalickiah, as next in line to be king, took over the throne. Once his strategy had worked to become king of the Lamanites, he is described as "having gained the hearts of the people" (Alma 47:30). What did he do with these hearts he had gained? "He had hardened the hearts of the Lamanites, and blinded their minds, and stirred them up to anger" (Alma 48:3). Amalickiah stirred them up to anger, to fight against the Nephites.

Amalickiah's grisly fate played out in similar fashion to that of others with hardened hearts mentioned previously. Teancum, a mighty Nephite warrior, "stole privily into the tent of the king, and put a javelin to his heart" (Alma 51:34). The symbolism of Amalickiah being stabbed in the heart is not lost on us. It was perhaps fitting that Teancum would cast his fateful javelin through Amalickiah's heart—a heart that had led him to do so much evil and caused him to lead away so many others' hearts.

We will not shed too much detail on the Jaredites' story at this point, but much of their story is the result of having hard hearts and rejecting the prophets while in the Americas. Moroni aptly described the adversary's strategy, "The devil, who is the father of all lies; even that same liar who beguiled our first parents, yea, even that same liar who hath caused man to commit murder from the beginning; *who hath hardened the hearts of men* that they have murdered the prophets, and stoned them, and cast them out from the beginning" (Ether 8:25, emphasis added).

Truly, it is Satan himself who works tirelessly to harden our hearts. He was successful with the Jaredites in this regard. When prophets came to call the Jaredites to repentance, they met a hardened and resistant people. "And it came to pass that the people hardened their hearts, and would not hearken unto their words" (Ether 11:13). This hardheartedness led to rejection and even murder of the prophets, which led to the entire civilization being destroyed.

HE WHO LOOKETH SHALL LIVE

One of our favorite Book of Mormon stories on hardheartedness is actually a Bible story. In Numbers we read the following:

> And the Lord sent fiery serpents among the people, and they bit the people; and much people of Israel died.
>
> Therefore the people came to Moses, and said, We have sinned, for we have spoken against the Lord, and against thee; pray unto the Lord, that he take away the serpents from us. And Moses prayed for the people.
>
> And the Lord said unto Moses, Make thee a fiery serpent, and set it upon a pole: and it shall come to pass, that every one that is bitten, when he looketh upon it, shall live.
>
> And Moses made a serpent of brass, and put it upon a pole, and it came to pass, that if a serpent had bitten any man, when he beheld the serpent of brass, he lived. (Numbers 21:6–9)

This is all that is said of this miraculous event in the Old Testament. We are not told how the story ends. We are left to wonder how many people were willing to look to the serpent. From the Bible account, we can glean the teaching that we should follow the prophet of God and do what he says. We could also look for symbolism that might be present. Truly, "all things which have been given of God from the beginning of the world, unto man, are the typifying of him" (2 Nephi 11:4).

Jesus actually explains the symbolism of the serpent to us while He ministered on the earth. He declared, "And as Moses lifted up the serpent in the wilderness, even so must the Son of man be lifted up: That whosoever believeth in him should not perish, but have eternal life" (John 3:14–15).

Three different Book of Mormon prophets also reference this event to teach the people. They provide us with additional information, details, and valuable insight that we otherwise would not have. The Book of Mormon is a remarkable complement and companion to the Bible in such situations!

Much of the additional meaning that the Book of Mormon provides is focused on the people who actually refused to look to the serpent and live. This story provides an astonishingly clear example of how the hard-hearted are stubborn and unteachable. When facing the doom of a poisonous snakebite that was killing people all around, to *not* look seems like it would have required very real effort and resolve, perhaps even more effort than it would have taken to look. It must have taken an extremely determined and conscientious effort to *not* follow the counsel that was given. The deliberate disregard to Moses's counsel would almost have been comical to witness had it not been so tragic.

Nephi, Alma, and Nephi, the son of Helaman, all taught the people different things about this episode and how we can apply it in our lives. Hardheartedness was at the forefront of all their teachings about this story. Book of Mormon insights into this experience are a sobering warning that we need to be aware of times when we are deliberate in our disobedience to God's law. There are likely examples in our own lives of premeditated rebellion if we are honest with ourselves.

Nephi observed, "And he [Moses] did straiten them in the wilderness with his rod; for they hardened their hearts, even as ye have; and the Lord straitened them because of their iniquity. He sent fiery flying serpents among them; and after they were bitten he prepared a way that they might be healed; and the labor which they had to perform was to look; and because of the simpleness of the way, or the easiness of it, there were many who perished. And they did harden their hearts from time to time, and they did revile against Moses, and also against God" (1 Nephi 17:41–42).

Nephi also noted, "And as the Lord God liveth that brought Israel up out of the land of Egypt, and gave unto Moses power that he should heal the nations after they had been bitten by the poisonous serpents, if they would cast their eyes unto the serpent which he did raise before them . . . yea, behold I say unto you, that as these things are true, and as the Lord God liveth, there is none other name given under heaven save it be this Jesus Christ, of which I have spoken, whereby man can be saved" (2 Nephi 25:20).

There is so much to ponder in these verses. The act of casting our eyes unto the Lord, the power to heal the nations, being bitten by poisonous serpents—the symbolism is very powerful and can be very instructive to us as we ponder each element.

Alma taught:

Behold, [the Son of God] was spoken of by Moses; yea, and behold a type was raised up in the wilderness, that whosoever would look upon it might live. And many did look and live.

But few understood the meaning of those things, and this because of the hardness of their hearts. But there were many who were so hardened that they would not look, therefore they perished. Now the reason they would not look is because they did not believe that it would heal them.

O my brethren, if ye could be healed by merely casting about your eyes that ye might be healed, would ye not behold quickly, or would ye rather harden your hearts in unbelief, and be slothful, that ye would not cast about your eyes, that ye might perish? (Alma 33:19–21)

Alma also taught his son Helaman to look and live that he may live forever (see Alma 37:46).

Finally, Nephi, the son of Helaman, concluded:

Yea, did [Moses] not bear record that the Son of God should come? And as he lifted up the brazen serpent in the wilderness, even so shall he be lifted up who should come.

And as many as should look upon that serpent should live, even so as many as should look upon the Son of God with faith, having a contrite spirit, might live, even unto that life which is eternal. (Helaman 8:14–15)

Many people would not look to the serpent to be healed because of their hard hearts. Hardheartedness led to their lack of belief. It led the people to completely miss the touching symbolism of the serpent raised up on the pole. It filled them with determination to not be influenced by very basic and easy-to-understand counsel.

What serpents do we refuse to look upon in our lives? Do we refuse to quickly return to our spouses and admit wrongdoing after an argument? Do we refuse to forgive someone that has offended us? Do we refuse to fulfill a calling or assignment from our Church leaders? We are refusing to look upon the serpent, refusing to look to Christ and live, if we do such things. We are refusing His most precious gift to us, His Atonement. His grace and mercy are sufficient for us (see Ether 12:27). We just need to look!

THE NEED FOR DISCOMFORT

It is very natural for us to appreciate and relish physical comfort, to want to be healthy and strong, to crave food in our stomachs, to not want to feel hot or cold, and to long for safety in our environment. It is also natural for us to want to feel emotional comfort, to feel successful and secure, to be loved and admired, to feel confident and self-assured, to not overextend ourselves, and to not dwell on our weaknesses or shortcomings. These desires for comfort can lead to, or be a symptom of, hardheartedness, and can become the enemy of personal growth when they are overemphasized.

We cannot come to value comfort and security above that which the Lord would have us experience to expand ourselves. It is often precisely discomfort that leads to growth and development beyond our current capacity. We become less fearful of, and more open to, discomfort as we soften our hearts. We become more willing to follow the promptings of the Spirit to do things that may be hard for us. It can be a test of faith to approach Heavenly Father in prayer to ask for help to be better, knowing that the answer to such a prayer sometimes involves a great degree of effort and uneasiness. Are we willing to soften our hearts and pray for the opportunity to grow, knowing full well that things may get particularly arduous and demanding?

The Jaredites were pushed by what is described as a "furious wind" that blew on the face of the waters when they journeyed to the promised land (Ether 6:5). They were "tossed upon the waves" and "buried in the depths of the sea" (verses 5–6). There were "mountain waves" that broke upon them and "great and terrible tempests" (verse 6). In fact, "the wind did never cease to blow" (verse 8)! Calm weather would have made for far more enjoyable travel conditions, but in calm weather they would not have traveled at all. The very assistance they needed from the Lord to reach the promised land, the furious wind, was the very reason for their discomfort. As we look at life, it is precisely the times when we are exhausted, overwhelmed, stretched way too thin, working long hours, or in hard situations that produce the most substantial bursts of needed personal growth.

A SOFT HEART IS A SPIRITUAL GIFT

It is interesting to note that the Holy Ghost can carry messages *unto* our hearts, but not *into* our hearts (see 2 Nephi 33:1). Indeed, "there are many that harden their hearts against the Holy Spirit that it hath no place in them" (2 Nephi 33:2). We need soft hearts to allow the Spirit's message to be received into our hearts. Messages delivered unto a hard heart will not be given audience. We have to open up our soft hearts to receive the truths and mysteries of the gospel that are available to us.

How many of us harden our hearts when we hear someone begin a talk or lesson in Church by stating the topic is faith or tithing or family history? If we consider the topic too elementary and feel like we have heard it all before and know everything about it already, the word of God and the Spirit can have no place in our hearts at that point. We miss out on the opportunity to learn by the Spirit what He would have us know at that particular time.

After examining some of these examples of hardheartedness, how can we soften our hearts? Where do we start? Going back to Nephi, "And also having great desires to know of the mysteries of God, wherefore, I did cry unto the Lord; and behold he did visit me, and did soften my heart that I did believe all the words which had been spoken by my father" (1 Nephi 2:16). A softened heart is a spiritual gift, bestowed through the Spirit by a loving Heavenly Father.

The Lord promised, "A new heart also will I give you, and a new spirit will I put within you: and I will take away the stony heart out of your flesh, and I will give you an heart of flesh" (Ezekiel 36:26). This verse encapsulates how we can change our hearts from being hardened, prideful, and set upon riches. We must approach our Heavenly Father in prayer, continually petitioning for a new heart. As we pray, we will begin to notice our hearts changing. We will begin to partake of the fruits of the Atonement and the Spirit. We will be more loving, peaceful, patient, kind, and gentle, among many other positive changes (see Galatians 5:22–23).

King Anti-Nephi-Lehi told his people, "And behold, I thank my great God that he has given us a portion of his Spirit to soften our hearts" (Alma 24:8). The Holy Ghost softens our hearts as we live worthy of His influence. Thus, anything we can do to have a greater measure of the Spirit in our lives will help to soften our hearts.

We all have sins from which we struggle to break free. Repetitive and habitual sins harden our hearts and stunt our progression. As we pull away from such sins, our hearts will begin to shed layers of hardness, one by one. We then will be able to make other necessary changes in our lives and become what the Lord would have us be.

The Savior warned, "And even so will I cause the wicked to be kept, that will not hear my voice but harden their hearts, and wo, wo, wo is their doom" (D&C 38:6). Here the Lord gives us the "triple wo"! Only three other times in the standard works does this "triple wo" occur (see Revelation 8:13; 2 Nephi 28:15; 3 Nephi 9:2). As bad as one wo is, or even two woes, three woes is very serious indeed! And it is used here to warn those with hard hearts.

Satan wants nothing more than to afflict us with this disease of the heart. He knows that hardheartedness can lead to spiritual death if left untreated. The adversary's job becomes much easier if he doesn't have to worry about us pouring out our hearts unto the Lord asking for help. He knows he has us right where he wants us if we will not even open our scriptures to study them or listen to our Church leaders. This signifies we are not willing to look up to our Savior to be healed spiritually. We will walk aimlessly on broad roads and will be lost if we reject guidance from the Spirit of God due to hard hearts, even until we are grasped with Satan's awful chains (see 1 Nephi 12:17; 2 Nephi 28:22). We cannot allow this to happen!

The Savior stated, "For mine elect hear my voice and harden not their hearts" (D&C 29:7). Amulek instructed us, "Yea, I would that ye come forth and harden not your hearts any longer; and therefore, if ye will repent and harden not your hearts, *immediately* shall the great plan of redemption be brought about unto you" (Alma 34:31, emphasis added). The great privileges of having the priesthood be effective in our lives and receiving the promised blessing of entering into the Lord's rest also come to those with soft hearts (see Alma 13:4–13).

What powerful promises can be ours! We will be among the elect of God, immediately have the plan of redemption brought about unto us, and receive cherished priesthood blessings if we harden not our hearts. Mercy will be bestowed upon us as we continually strive to soften our hearts. We will also be allowed to enter into covenants with the Lord leading us to admittance into the Lord's rest and exaltation.

We must plead unto Heavenly Father for a softened heart. We can focus on our "favorite sins" and rid ourselves of them. We must plead unto the Father for the companionship of the Holy Ghost to be with us and carefully examine how we may be causing the Spirit to withdraw from us by our actions. As the Spirit sends messages unto our hearts, we will be blessed if we listen to these promptings and follow them with exactness. The more the Holy Ghost is with us, the more softened our hearts will become. What a miracle this is! Our Savior will take away our stony hearts and give us new hearts of flesh if we will but invite Him.

Chapter 3

PRIDE IN OUR HEARTS

Much has been written about the pride cycle in the Book of Mormon. President Ezra Taft Benson delivered an authoritative and timeless sermon on the subject entitled "Beware of Pride" in April 1989 that drew heavily from the Book of Mormon.[1] We will study some of President Benson's teachings on this subject, but we will focus more specifically on the pride in our hearts. By concentrating on the heart in regard to pride, additional insights can be gained about pride's effects on our hearts, the pervasiveness of this disease in our society and individually, and some methods and means we can employ to heal our hearts of pride.

Pride is obviously a frequently addressed topic and overarching theme in the Book of Mormon. This is likely due to pride's extraordinary impact on the Nephites and their civilization, as well as the need we have in our day for these same lessons. Pride is mentioned almost 100 times in the Book of Mormon and is described in many different and distinct ways. There is mention of "pride in our hearts," "pride in our eyes," "being puffed up in pride," "being lifted up in pride," "being swallowed up in pride," "walking after or in pride," "growing in pride," and even "waxing in pride" (see Jacob 2:20; 2 Nephi 26:20; 2 Nephi 28:15; Jacob 2:13; Alma 31:27; Helaman 13:27; Helaman 3:36; Alma 4:6, respectively). Pride is also coupled with many other vices, including arrogance, boasting, and having stiff necks and high heads. Each subtle variance in how pride is described is worth critical examination. Questions such as "Why did this prophet choose to describe pride in this way?" and "What can I deduce about pride from this description?" can lead to invaluable personal revelation and instruction.

PRIDE AS THE GREAT DESTROYER

Pride in people's hearts is specifically mentioned twenty-nine times and will be the focus of our study. Pride in people's hearts is mentioned as a destroying force in the Book of Mormon more often than all other diseases of the heart combined. Pride is indeed the great destroyer. In the Book of Mormon, it is shown to be the destroyer of both individual souls as well as entire civilizations. There are also illuminating references to pride's destructive power in the Bible. We learn in Proverbs, "The Lord will destroy the house of the proud," and "Pride goeth before destruction" (Proverbs 15:25, 16:18).

Nephi declared the reason behind the fate of the great and spacious building and gives little room for interpretation. "And it came to pass that I saw and bear record, that the great and spacious building was the pride of the world; and it fell, and the fall thereof was exceedingly great. And the angel of the Lord spake unto me again, saying: Thus shall be the destruction of all nations, kindreds, tongues, and people, that shall fight against the twelve apostles of the Lamb" (1 Nephi 11:36).

Many other prophets have warned of pride's great destroying power. Jacob warned, "Let not this pride of your hearts destroy your souls!" (Jacob 2:16). Nephi quoted Zenos or Isaiah in admonishing his own people, "The time cometh speedily that Satan shall have no more power over the hearts of the children of men; for the day soon cometh that all the proud and they who do wickedly shall be as stubble; and the day cometh that they must be burned," a prophecy he later repeated as a warning to us as well as to his own people (see 1 Nephi 22:15; 2 Nephi 26:4). Jesus Christ warned the people using these same words in 3 Nephi 25:1. Nephi quoted Isaiah, "Every one that is proud shall be thrust through; yea, and every one that is joined to the wicked shall fall by the sword" (2 Nephi 23:15). Such is the fate of the proud as has been testified again and again by Christ and many prophets alike.

In Helaman 4, Mormon succinctly summed up why the Nephites suffered catastrophic losses at that particular period of time around 30 BC. He writes, "Now this great loss of the Nephites, and the great slaughter which was among them, would not have happened had it not been for their wickedness and their abomination which was among them. . . . *And it was because of the pride of their hearts*, because of their exceeding riches, yea, it was because of their oppression to the poor, withholding their food from the hungry, withholding their clothing from the naked" (Helaman 4:11–12, emphasis added).

Later, Mormon taught that pride was again leading the people to destruction. He said, "And it came to pass in the eighty and fifth year (about 6 BC) they did wax stronger and stronger in their pride, and in their wickedness; and thus they were ripening again for destruction" (Helaman 11:37).

Pride is declared to be the reason for the final destruction of the Nephites. Mormon tersely summarized his people's fate when he said, "Behold, the pride of this nation, or the people of the Nephites, hath proven their destruction except they should repent" (Moroni 8:27).

So how exactly is pride in our hearts such a destructive force? Why does such pride more hastily and assuredly lead us to destruction than other offenses might? While serving as an Assistant to the Twelve, Elder Theodore M. Burton said, "Such pride, haughtiness, and willful disobedience bring people into desperate conditions where repentance is almost impossible. When repentance becomes impossible and people refuse to change their ways from evil, then destruction by the Lord is the only alternative left."[2]

"Destruction by the Lord" is an interesting way to describe this unfortunate state. When people have pride in their hearts, they tend to fight amongst themselves and destroy each other quite proficiently without any need for the Lord's intervention. And the Lord's intervention is exactly what is missing! At such times, the Lord's promises of mighty deliverance from all types of bondage are not available to people who continue to walk along in their prideful manner.

Elder Richard G Scott said, "For the proud and haughty, it is as though there never were an Atonement made."[3] What a damning indictment! Making the Atonement of our Savior ineffective in our lives is surely the most destructive consequence of pride. Without the Atonement of Christ in our lives, we have no hope for change in our hearts and justice will rule over us without mercy's tender sway. For those without access to the Savior's mercy and grace through His atoning sacrifice, destruction becomes the only possible end.

We will not repent of our wickedness if we have pride in our hearts (see Alma 6:3). We will not be receptive to the instructive whisperings and promptings of the Spirit. We will be less teachable and won't give heed to the direction and guidance of the prophet as well as other church leaders. We will boast in our own strength (see Mosiah 11:19). Those with pride in their hearts seek to counsel the Lord and follow their own path, driven by selfish motives. Anger and resentment fill prideful hearts, much like what Laman and Lemuel experienced toward their brother Nephi. Those with pride in their hearts will seek to acquire riches and honors, placing them above their fellow man (see Jacob 2:13). Those with pride in their hearts will persecute and afflict their neighbors and others because of their perceived superiority (see Jacob 2:20; Helaman 3:34). This is not the Lord's program. These feelings and prideful ambitions will surely lead to destruction.

Pride in our hearts can destroy marriages and other close relationships if we allow it. Those who are prideful do not listen intently, do not seek to counsel with their spouse, nor do they value the feelings, thoughts, and opinions of their spouse. Pride will only allow for its own predetermined course regardless of the input another might have.

While oblivious to ugly flaws and defects within themselves, those with pride in their hearts will see the worst in others and exaggerate their mistakes. This fabricated and false comparison with others is often the fuel that feeds pride. The proud will never give another the benefit of the doubt for a perceived misstep; rather, they will judge others harshly for any fault that is revealed or error they commit.

THE PERILS OF PRIDE IN THE ISAIAH CHAPTERS

Nephi includes thirteen chapters from Isaiah in 2 Nephi 12–24 in which the dangers of pride are a dominant theme. In these chapters, cities and empires are added to the Book of Mormon's somber list of destructions in pride's aftermath. Isaiah described the destruction of Judah/Jerusalem and blamed their destruction on pride. He warned:

> And it shall come to pass that the lofty looks of man shall be humbled, and the haughtiness of men shall be bowed down, and the Lord alone shall be exalted in that day.
>
> For the day of the Lord of Hosts soon cometh upon all nations, yea, upon every one; yea, upon the proud and lofty, and upon every one who is lifted up, and he shall be brought low. (2 Nephi 12:11–12)

Isaiah further described the destruction of Ephraim. He prophesied:

> And all the people shall know, even Ephraim and the inhabitants of Samaria, that say in the pride and stoutness of heart:
>
> The bricks are fallen down, but we will build with hewn stones; the sycamores are cut down, but we will change them into cedars. (2 Nephi 19:9–10)

Isaiah similarly described the destruction of Assyria. He stated:

For [Assyria] saith: By the strength of my hand and by my wisdom I have done these things…and my hand hath found as a nest the riches of the people. . . . Shall the ax boast itself against him that heweth therewith? Shall the saw magnify itself against him that shaketh it? As if the rod should shake itself against them that lift it up, or as if the staff should lift up itself as if it were no wood! Behold, the Lord, the Lord of Hosts shall lop the bough with terror; and the high ones of stature shall be hewn down; and the haughty shall be humbled. (2 Nephi 20:13–15, 33)

The people of Assyria suffered a fate similar to that of Syria and Ephraim. Their great pride and boasting in their own strength and wisdom led to their destruction.

Isaiah likewise prophesied the destruction of Babylon. "And I will punish the world for evil, and the wicked for their iniquity; I will cause the arrogance of the proud to cease, and will lay down the haughtiness of the terrible" (2 Nephi 23:11). Babylon was destroyed according to the prophecy of Isaiah because of the pride of the nation. The symbolic Babylon—the world and all of the evil thereof—will also suffer a similar destruction because of pride at the Second Coming.

And finally, Isaiah described Satan's ultimate destruction and ascribed it to pride in his heart.

For thou hast said in thy heart: I will ascend into heaven, I will exalt my throne above the stars of God; I will sit also upon the mount of the congregation, in the sides of the north;

I will ascend above the heights of the clouds; I will be like the Most High.

Yet thou shalt be brought down to hell, to the sides of the pit. (2 Nephi 24:13–15)

Elder Neal A. Maxwell liked to call all of these "I's" that Satan uses "vertical pronouns [that] are usually accompanied by unbending knees."[4] We know that Satan wanted all of the glory unto himself. His insatiable ambition, powered by a heart filled with pride, led to his destruction.

We realize the peoples mentioned in these prophecies from Isaiah are quite extensive. Greater depth of study can and should be given to each of the examples that he mentions. However, we find it very noteworthy that Isaiah described the destruction of so many different nations and peoples as a consequence of pride: Judah, Syria/Ephraim, Assyria, Babylon, the world, and even Satan himself. And how significant it is that Book of Mormon prophets repeatedly attributed the destruction of the Nephites to the pride of its people.

PRIDE IN OUR EYES VERSUS PRIDE IN OUR HEARTS

While we will discuss some of Jacob's teachings on hearts being set upon riches in greater depth in the next chapter, there is significant doctrinal overlap between the dangers of wealth and pride in the heart. Jacob helped us distinguish the difference between the two. He observed, "And the hand of providence hath smiled upon you most pleasingly, that you have obtained many riches; *and because some of you have obtained more abundantly* than that of your brethren *ye are lifted up in the pride of your hearts*, and wear stiff necks and high heads *because of the costliness of your apparel*, and persecute your brethren because *ye suppose that ye are better than they*" (Jacob 2:13, emphasis added).

Pride in our hearts often goes hand in hand with our hearts being set upon riches. C. S. Lewis said, "Pride gets no pleasure out of having something, only out of having more of it than the next man."[5] Pride in our hearts is more concerned with comparing our riches to those of our brothers and sisters than in merely acquiring wealth. We then lift ourselves up thinking we are better than others because we have more. Jacob pleaded with us to overcome the pride in our hearts. He said, "Think of your brethren like unto yourselves" (Jacob 2:17). He wanted to root the tendency to compare ourselves with others out of us. We will further distinguish between these two distinct but related diseases of the heart in the next chapter.

Costly or fine apparel is mentioned eleven times in the Book of Mormon as something we need to avoid. Though the exact words of the warning vary, the counsel remains clear and constant. Why is costly apparel so significantly emphasized in the Book of Mormon? Why did the prophets of the Book of Mormon, who had seen our day and were writing to us, worry so considerably about what we are wearing? Costly apparel has a unique ability to lift up the wearer above others. Those of the world often wrongly equate fashionable apparel and what one wears with the intrinsic value or worth of the individual wearing it. Book of Mormon prophets understood very well the effect costly apparel has on our hearts today!

Those who wore costly apparel in the Book of Mormon are said to have had both pride in their eyes and pride in their hearts. What is the difference between pride in our hearts and pride in our eyes? The description of pride in our eyes is only found in the Book of Mormon among the standard works. Why would Mormon and other prophets deliberately use one of these sayings over the other at times?

Prideful eyes are constantly looking at what others are wearing, what cars people are driving, and the size and condition of people's houses. Prideful eyes are worldly, always on the lookout for the next trendy, must-have thing. Prideful eyes are always longingly gazing at material possessions, be it their own or the possessions of others. Prideful eyes are drawn to the superficial, the artificial, and the phony—that which is on the outside, that which has no real value. Prideful eyes do not have the ability to see past the façade to the intrinsic value and worth of an individual. Prideful eyes are one of the symptoms of being spiritually blind.

A prideful heart, on the other hand, is an even more serious and destructive condition than prideful eyes. A prideful heart takes into account what prideful eyes see, processes this information, and then takes the sin one perilous step further. A prideful heart *compares* what prideful eyes see between two individuals and then *determines* or *judges* that because of one person's lack and another's abundance, the person with the abundance is superior to the other. The prideful heart always makes this comparison and judgment.

People in the Book of Mormon such as Nehor, the apostate Zoramites, and the Nephites in Alma and Samuel the Lamanite's days all wore costly apparel and did not make an effort to care for the poor and the needy. They were too consumed in the pride of their hearts to worry about others in less fortunate circumstances. They instead worried about having more or better possessions than those to whom they were comparing themselves. Thus, they did not have any excess resources to give to the poor and the needy because they desperately needed all they possessed to keep up with others' acquisition of wealth. They lusted after riches, and regardless of what they had, it was never enough. There was always somebody that had more, and always somebody with whom to compare.

What can we do to overcome this disease of the heart? One solution is found in Mormon's description of members of the Church who were not proud of heart: "And they did impart of their substance, every man according to that which he had, to the poor, and the needy, and the sick, and the afflicted; and they did not wear costly apparel, yet they were neat and comely" (Alma 1:27). An added measure of humility comes to those who generously give to the poor and the needy.

While this verse does not directly come out and say so, it infers that if we are buying costly apparel, we are in effect robbing the poor and the needy. We are making the choice to clothe ourselves in extravagant things instead of using our surplus resources to care for the poor. The more frequently we refuse to give to the poor and needy or show reluctance in doing so, the more prideful we become.

Imagine living for an entire day in an impoverished place where people go without fundamental necessities every day—a place with no access to clean water, a place where children and their parents regularly go hungry, a place where people do not have access to basic treatment of their diseases or life-changing medicines, a place where the people have no access to immunizations; in short, a place where a modest amount of resources could make a world of difference.

Then, imagine leaving that place and on your way home spending money on expensive designer apparel. Maybe you feel like you can afford it, but that money may have made an enormous and lasting difference in the life of another for a year or more! Maybe it is from such situations that the inference is made that we rob the poor when we use our resources selfishly in this manner. The situation just described is not a fictional or imagined place. There are people suffering for want of resources in all corners of the world and ours is the responsibility to alleviate their suffering if we are able.

Maybe it was thoughts such as these that led Moroni to share the following: "Why do you adorn yourselves with that which hath no life, and yet suffer the hungry, and the needy, and the naked, and the sick and the afflicted to pass by you, and notice them not?" (Mormon 8:39). The Lord is particularly concerned about this sin because He has declared that "the earth is full, and there is enough and to spare" (D&C 104:17).

Nephi went further to make it perfectly clear that we are, in fact, robbing the poor because of dressing ourselves in fine clothing. He taught:

> Because of pride, and because of false teachers, and false doctrine, their churches have become corrupted, and their churches are lifted up; because of pride they are puffed up.
>
> They rob the poor because of their fine sanctuaries; they rob the poor because of their fine clothing; and they persecute the meek and the poor in heart, because in their pride they are puffed up. (2 Nephi 28:12–13)

Sanctuaries are defined as places of refuge or rest. Though we may tend to think of sanctuaries only as religious structures, our homes can also be considered sanctuaries. It may be worth asking, are we robbing the poor because of the excessive size and quality of our homes? Is our appetite for material consumption depriving those in need? If we have riches, have they corrupted us to the point we persecute those around us that are less fortunate? Do we persecute others because of our pride? Has the disease of pride spread from our eyes to our hearts?

Book of Mormon prophets considered this a critical area of doctrine worthy of our attention. The question of whether we are doing enough with our resources to bless others will likely always rest in the minds of those seeking to follow Christ. The Book of Mormon reminds us of our great responsibility to use our abundance of resources to care for those less fortunate.

It is important to remember that Nephi is not describing his own people in these verses. In his vision, he was shown our day, and he prophesied and taught based on the needs he saw. He was shown a people that were dripping in selfishness and pride. President Spencer W. Kimball said that selfishness "snares the soul, shrinks the heart, and darkens the mind."[6] How ironic and sad it is that as we are puffed up in pride and attempt to lift our hearts above others, our hearts are actually shrinking!

Nephi gives us a higher standard of stewardship for caring for the poor and the needy than what people tend to think would be required. If we are buying a bunch of expensive clothing or building fine sanctuaries unto ourselves, we are, by Nephi's definition, robbing the poor. What a humbling and sobering thought! Do we sufficiently consider the impact our personal purchases and consumption patterns have on the poor and needy around us? If we can get ourselves to even ask this question, our hearts are already a little less prideful than they were before.

Mormon gave us very simple counsel on how we should dress. He said we should have clothing that is "neat and comely" (Alma 1:27). We do not, however, need to go crazy and buy the most exclusive designer shoes and clothing, the most lavish and luxurious cars, or any other such wasteful extravagances. That money would be far better used by helping the poor. If an active concern for the poor and needy were never far from our thoughts, we would be that much closer to living the law of consecration. Such giving would result in great blessings being showered down upon our hearts. It is a humbling opportunity to possibly be an instrument of deliverance for those around us.

Lehi described the great and spacious building in his vision of the tree of life. He said, "And it was filled with people, both old and young, both male and female; and their manner of dress was exceedingly fine; and they were in the attitude of mocking and pointing their fingers towards those who had come at and were partaking of the fruit" (1 Nephi 8:27). It is significant that even in Lehi's dream, the fine apparel of the world is a focus.

Nephi also commented on the significance of precious clothing when he had his similar vision.

> And it came to pass that I beheld this great and abominable church; and I saw the devil that he was the founder of it.
>
> And I saw also gold, and silver, and silks, and scarlets, and fine-twined linen, and all manner of precious clothing; and I saw many harlots.
>
> And the angel spake unto me, saying: Behold the gold, and the silver, and the silks, and the scarlets, and the fine-twined linen, and the precious clothing, and the harlots, are the desires of this great and abominable church. (1 Nephi 13:6–8)

"Behold the gold," the angel said. This catchy rhyme helps us remember how this abominable church is defined. The angel explained to Nephi that these worldly riches, which included silks and scarlets, fine-twined linen, and precious clothing, were the desires of the great and abominable church. Herein lies a key for us to consider. When our eyes see such worldly riches, if we allow our desires to gravitate toward them, our hearts will become corrupt and prideful. Once again, it starts with our eyes, which leads to our thoughts and desires, and eventually to our hearts.

We need to be cognizant of our fixation on things of the world and the excessive amount of time we waste thinking about such things. Any time we find ourselves desiring such things, we need to check ourselves and understand our motivations for wanting them. The glitter and glamor of fine and costly apparel attracts the eye's gaze, which can quickly lead to pride in our hearts if we are not careful. These distractions can fill our eyes and hearts with vanity and a love of the world.

THE "DOCTRINAL DIAMOND" OF THE DAY TO DAY

There are certain phrases and teaching moments in the Book of Mormon to be loved and treasured. Many of them are repeated frequently over the pulpit and during lessons, while others are more subtle and uncommon. We often call these phrases and teaching moments "scriptural gems" that provide strength, comfort, and insight to those searching for them. Such nuggets of wisdom deserve our time and focus to find deeper meaning and application in our lives.

Elder Neal A. Maxwell calls these gems "doctrinal diamonds. And when the light of the Spirit plays upon their several facets, they sparkle with celestial sense and illuminate the path we are to follow."[7] We love the fact that these gems have several facets upon which the light can play. One day, the Spirit might teach us one thing about a particular verse in scripture. The next day, the light might shine on a different facet of the same verse and increase our understanding further.

Our scripture study can be likened to the Liahona, upon which new writing "was written and changed from time to time, according to the faith and diligence we gave unto it" (1 Nephi 16:29). While the writing does not actually change in the scriptures, our understanding of, and the impact we place on, certain passages can change from time to time. Such is the beauty and miracle of the scriptures!

One of our favorite gems in the Book of Mormon is offered by Mormon as he observed the Nephites' pride. He noted, "And it came to pass that the fifty and second year ended in peace also, save it were the exceedingly great pride which had gotten into the hearts of the people; and it was because of their exceedingly great riches and their prosperity in the land; *and it did grow upon them from day to day*" (Helaman 3:36, emphasis added).

We are taught again and again to do certain things daily, weekly, and monthly to keep our hearts humble and our testimonies strong and bright. We are taught to study the scriptures daily, to pray daily, and to take care of the poor and needy daily, among other things (see Mosiah 4:26). We are taught to attend our church meetings weekly, to partake of the sacrament and renew our covenants weekly, and to have family home evening weekly. We are taught to fast and give a generous fast offering at least monthly. We are instructed to minister to others and attend the temple on a regular basis as well. These are the very activities that will prevent pride from growing upon our hearts from day to day!

The subtlety of pride in our hearts and other sins growing upon us from day to day, week to week, and month to month is a significant doctrine that is worth our time studying and pondering. Helaman 3 provides one of the most recognizable synopses of the pride cycle in the Book of Mormon. It provides a sobering description of pride growing upon the people from day to day. This chapter illustrates the impact of pride over a period of ten years. We will focus on the ten-year period from the forty-third to the fifty-second year of the reign of the judges.

We are told that in the forty-third year there "was no contention among the people of Nephi save it were a little pride which was in the church, which did cause some little dissensions among the people" (Helaman 3:1). This doesn't sound so bad, does it? Overall, the church seemed to be prospering notwithstanding some "little" hiccups along the way. We see that the forty-fourth year had "no contention" and the forty-fifth year did not have much contention either (verse 2). The forty-sixth year, however, "had much contention and many dissensions" (verse 3).

The forty-seventh and forty-eighth years had "great contention," which sounds like even more than "much" used earlier (verse 19). Then, in the forty-ninth year, "continual peace [was] established in the land" and the people enjoyed "exceedingly great prosperity" except for some secret combinations that were not known to the government yet (verses 23, 24). The fiftieth year also had "continual peace and great joy" (verse 32).

The fifty-first year had "peace also, save it were the pride which began to enter into the church—not into the church of God, but into the hearts of the people who professed to belong to the church of God" (verse 33). The fifty-second year had "peace also, save it were the exceedingly great pride which had gotten into the hearts of the people" (verse 36). We have provided a summary below that gives a better picture of these changes from year to year.

YEAR	MORMON'S SYNOPSIS OF YEARS 43–52 OF THE REIGN OF THE JUDGES
43	No contention save it were a little pride in the church, some little dissensions
44	No contention among the people
45	Not much contention among the people
46	Much contention and many dissensions
47	Great contention in the land
48	Great contention in the land
49	Continual peace established in the land, exceedingly great prosperity in the Church
50	Continual peace and great joy in the land
51	Peace in the land, but also pride began to enter into the Church members' hearts; humble people suffered great persecutions
52	Peace in the land, but also exceedingly great pride in the hearts of the people

Mormon was truly inspired by the Holy Ghost to add these descriptions to the record we have today. He prayerfully considered what to include in his abridgement. So, why does Mormon take us on this ten-year journey from the forty-third year to the fifty-second year and describe things in this way? He undoubtedly reviewed many more records from Helaman, the son of Helaman, and could have included much more about these years if he wished. Mormon repeatedly told us he could not write even a hundredth part of what was on the large plates and in fact did so in this very chapter (see Helaman 3:14). Instead, he succinctly and powerfully shows us that the people went from no contention and a little pride to great contention, then back to continual peace, and then back to exceedingly great pride, all in the span of ten years.

Mormon summarized the desolate state of the Nephites' condition. He said, "They had fallen into a state of unbelief and awful wickedness . . . *in the space of not many years*" (Helaman 4:25–26, emphasis added). One of the messages we glean from these verses is that if we are not doing the day-to-day, week-to-week, and month-to-month things we should be doing, it won't take too long, even "not many years," before we completely lose our way.

Mormon provided a similar insight into the actions that resulted in the apostate Zoramites' condition. He noted, "But they had fallen into great errors, for they would not observe to keep the commandments of God. . . . Neither would they . . . continue in prayer and supplication to God daily, that they might not enter into temptation" (Alma 31:9–10).

If we are not doing things that enlarge and expand our testimony and spirituality daily, we are not merely standing still. We are, in fact, losing ground, and our spirituality and testimony diminish. How sad that day will be if we look back over our lives and realize that our day-to-day shortcomings resulted in so many empty years void of spiritual growth!

MORONI'S SERMON IN MORMON 8

One of the most powerful sermons on pride in our hearts is given by Moroni in Mormon 8. Moroni has witnessed the entire destruction of the Nephite civilization including the death of his father, Mormon, at this point. He stops talking about the destruction of his people and changes direction in verse 13. He writes what, at the time, he thinks are his final words, and he directs them to us in the latter days. In the middle of his impassioned sermon, he reminds us that he sees us and knows our doing. "Behold, I speak unto you as if ye were present, and yet ye are not. But behold, Jesus Christ hath shown you unto me, and I know your doing" (Mormon 8:35). With a vision somewhat similar to what Nephi experienced, Moroni describes our day and the pride of people's hearts that is prevalent among us.

Moroni writes of churches, and the leaders and teachers of these churches, rising up in the pride of their hearts (see Mormon 8:28). He then continues, "And I know that ye do walk in the pride of your hearts; and there are none save a few only who do not lift themselves up in the pride of their hearts, unto the wearing of very fine apparel, unto envying, and strifes, and malice, and persecutions, and all manner of iniquities; and your churches, yea, even every one, have become polluted because of the pride of your hearts" (verse 36).

The admonitions in these two verses alone reference prideful hearts five times! Moroni then continues to describe the condition of our world today: "For behold, ye do love money, and your substance, and your fine apparel, and the adorning of your churches, more than ye love the poor and the needy, the sick and the afflicted" (Mormon 8:37). This is Moroni's second mention of fine apparel in the last two verses as well. He writes of secret combinations built up to get gain and all because of the pride in people's hearts. Having a prophet of ancient times tell us that Jesus Christ has shown us to him and that he knows our doing should cause us to take very serious notice of this message.

There are other compelling teachings that stand out to us from Moroni's cautionary prophecy. With a striking resemblance we find significant, both Moroni and Nephi mentioned that only a few would not be lifted up in pride. Moroni said there were none "*save a few only* who did not lift themselves up in the pride of their hearts" (Mormon 8:36). Nephi said, "Because of pride . . . they have all gone astray *save it be a few*" (2 Nephi 28:14). Pride in people's hearts is truly a pandemic today! To be one of the few who will be spared from this widespread outbreak, we must be vigilant and alert to even the smallest dose of pride that creeps into our lives. Both Nephi and Moroni pleaded for us to come unto Christ, knowing the damning consequences that come from having prideful hearts. Thankfully, the Book of Mormon teaches us not only about the bitter repercussions of this disease, but also how to overcome the affliction of a prideful heart.

We would do well to remember who does the actual lifting in our lives instead of having our hearts lifted up in pride. The Savior told Moroni, "And blessed is he that is found faithful unto my name at the last day, for he shall be lifted up to dwell in the kingdom prepared for him from the foundation of the world" (Ether 4:19).

Both Moroni and Nephi cautioned us to not walk in a prideful manner. Moroni saw people walking in the pride of their hearts (see Mormon 8:36). Nephi quoted Isaiah when he warned, "The daughters of Zion are haughty, and walk with stretched-forth necks and wanton eyes, walking and mincing as they go, and making a tinkling with their feet" (2 Nephi 13:16). Samuel the Lamanite also described those who walked in the pride of their hearts and in the pride of their eyes (see Helaman 13:27). These warnings are given to us specifically as Church members. We must learn to walk differently. We are to walk uprightly before God and in the paths of righteousness (see 1 Nephi 16:3, 5). We should walk circumspectly and humbly before the Lord (see Mosiah 26:37, Ether 6:17).

BE NOT ASHAMED

We would like to highlight one other point that Moroni makes in Mormon 8. Moroni writes of people in the last days being ashamed to take upon them the name of Christ, a possible reference to Lehi's vision of the tree of life (see Mormon 8:38). One of the four groups that Lehi saw came and partook of the fruit of the tree of life. "And after they had tasted of the fruit they were ashamed, because of those that were scoffing at them; and they fell away into forbidden paths and were lost" (1 Nephi 8:28).

We read in the Bible, "When pride cometh, then cometh shame" (Proverbs 11:2). Shame is thus related to pride and works with it hand in hand. Not only do the prideful shun and mock others, bringing them to shame, but they also will grow ashamed of the Savior and things related to His gospel and Church.

It is one thing to be ashamed of your favorite sports team after a bad game or during a dreadful season and not wanting to wear their team gear as a result. However, we should *never* be ashamed of the gospel of Christ! What a blessing it is to have a Heavenly Father and a Savior who love us perfectly, in spite of our sins and weaknesses. We should all feel deep gratitude for the doctrines of the gospel and that for which the Church stands. We should never cower in front of others because of our faith and beliefs. Rather, we are to be a light unto the world (3 Nephi 18:24). We are to wait for the Lord's coming without shame (2 Nephi 6:7, 13). We should find honor and happiness in being enlisted in this conflict as disciples of Christ.

The apostle Paul provides a very humbling thought: "Wherefore God is not ashamed to be called [our] God" (Hebrews 11:16). God is not ashamed of us with all of our faults, weaknesses, and sins, and chooses to call Himself our God. If God is not ashamed to be our God despite our wildly imperfect lives, how much worse is it for us to think so highly of ourselves that we are ashamed of our Creator, our God, and our Redeemer, and of being called His people?

The apostle Paul was not ashamed of the gospel of Christ once he became converted. In our estimation, Paul declared the gospel message as boldly and confidently as anyone ever has. Paul testified, "For I am not ashamed of the gospel of Christ: for it is the power of God unto salvation to every one that believeth" (Romans 1:16). Paul, in speaking with many different peoples, regularly taught them not to be ashamed of the Church. He mentioned this subject well over a dozen times in his epistles. Imagine seeing Paul loudly and courageously declare the truths of the gospel, having no shame in doing so. What a great example to all of us!

There are many in the Book of Mormon that boldly testified of Christ and were not ashamed of His gospel, including Abinadi, Nephi while on his garden tower, Abish, Samuel the Lamanite, and many, many others. The most touching example in all of holy writ may be the group of men, women, and children who believed in Alma and Amulek's words. They were cast into the fire along with their scriptures because they were not ashamed to be called followers of Christ. A part of becoming more humble is learning to gracefully receive persecutions from others instead of being the one to dole out persecutions to others. Do we have the courage to be called a disciple of Christ if persecutions arise? Do we humbly and gratefully remember our Savior's Atonement and pledge to follow Him through good times and bad? Are we delighted in and grateful for our membership in the Church?

HOW CAN WE OVERCOME PRIDE IN OUR HEARTS?

If the natural man or woman in us has a strong tendency to be prideful in our hearts, how can we overcome it and instead be humble before others and the Lord? President Ezra Taft Benson, in his talk titled "Beware of Pride," told us we can choose to be humble. Choosing to be humble eliminates pride from our hearts.

We love the prophetic counsel that President Benson gave us. Even though this list is somewhat long, it is well worth studying and pondering. He taught the following:

> Let us choose to be humble. We can choose to humble ourselves by conquering enmity toward our brothers and sisters, esteeming them as ourselves, and lifting them as high or higher than we are. We can choose to humble ourselves by receiving counsel and chastisement. We can choose to humble ourselves by forgiving those who have offended us. We can choose to humble ourselves by rendering selfless service. We can choose to humble ourselves by going on missions and preaching the word that

can humble others. We can choose to humble ourselves by getting to the temple more frequently. We can choose to humble ourselves by confessing and forsaking our sins and being born of God. We can choose to humble ourselves by loving God, submitting our will to His, and putting Him first in our lives.

Let us choose to be humble. We can do it. I know we can.[8]

Studying the Book of Mormon is the best way to learn how to be humble in the ways President Benson mentioned. The Book of Mormon is the elixir for overcoming enmity toward our brothers and sisters. This precious book of scripture teaches us how to receive counsel from the Lord and others in a number of different places. It teaches us to understand that the Lord will even chastise us from time to time out of love. It powerfully teaches the importance of forgiving others. It teaches us masterfully about service through King Benjamin's address to his people and from the resurrected Savior's acts of service to the Nephites.

Through studying the Book of Mormon, we learn of faith-promoting stories of people serving missions and preaching the gospel. The Book of Mormon teaches us about the importance of temples in a more comprehensive way than anywhere else in scripture. It teaches us clearly about repentance and the proper steps we must take to have repentance change our hearts. Through the Book of Mormon's teachings on the Atonement of the Savior, we learn about submitting our will to God and the importance of putting Him first in our lives. If we study and ponder the Book of Mormon and do our best to follow its teachings, we will become a more humble people.

The battle to extirpate pride from our lives will likely be a continual one. Alma poses a question to the members of the Church in Zarahemla:"Behold, are ye stripped of pride? I say unto you, if ye are not ye are not prepared to meet God" (Alma 5:28). The imagery of being "stripped" of pride is powerful. We are commanded to strip away each layer of pride that is a part of us, like paint is stripped from a wall or like layers of skin are stripped from an onion. Stripping ourselves of pride is a lengthy and involved process and will take great effort on our part. We cannot expect it to happen all at once.

More importantly, it is only through the Atonement of Christ that we can become more humble and see lasting change. We must do our part and focus on President Benson's list of ways to become more humble. However, every item on his list relies on the same thing—the Atonement of Christ. Elder Patrick Kearon said, "Our Savior is the Prince of Peace, the Great Healer, the only One who can truly cleanse us from the sting of sin and the poison of pride and change our rebellious hearts into converted, covenant hearts. His Atonement is infinite and embraces us all."[9]

As we look over President Benson's counsel on how we can choose to be humble, the Holy Spirit will guide us to know the best direction to aim our efforts. We can gain further knowledge on each of these actions by studying teachings in the Book of Mormon. If we earnestly strive to become more humble and prayerfully work through the process, the Holy Ghost will work in us through the Savior's Atonement and we will be given the power necessary to change. Not only will we be able to repent of our prideful nature, but we will also find ourselves with a greater ability to resist pride from taking root in us. We will build stronger defenses to prevent this poison from creeping into our hearts.

There is great power to be gained in reviewing President Benson's counsel frequently. Continually working on one or two of these items at a time will make us "stronger and stronger in [our] humility, and firmer and firmer in the faith of Christ" (Helaman 3:35). A prophet of the Lord has promised us we will become a more humble people by doing the above things. As we work to develop more humility, the Lord can and will sanctify our hearts through the power of the Holy Ghost, and the destroying angel will pass over us.

Chapter 4

HEARTS SET UPON RICHES

A heart set upon riches, treasure, or the vain things of the world is a very pervasive and common disease of the heart and a consistent theme throughout the Book of Mormon. Nowhere in scripture is a heart set upon riches emphasized so frequently as it is in the Book of Mormon. Such a phrase is mentioned eighteen times in the Book of Mormon, and it is indirectly mentioned another seven times as having pride in our hearts due to riches. Despite their similarities, there is an important distinction to be made between prideful hearts and hearts set upon riches. We will carefully examine this critical difference in this chapter.

Much of the pride that entered and affected the Nephites' hearts at various times throughout their history was due to the riches they acquired and *how they saw themselves in comparison to others* as a result of these riches. Pride in our hearts is based largely on this comparison mentality. A heart set upon riches focuses more acutely on *the heart's desire to acquire such riches, and on the focus, time, and effort given to this pursuit* instead of more worthy endeavors. If left untreated, this disease leads to a love of riches that is greater than a love of God.

JACOB'S EARNEST AND HEARTFELT COUNSEL

Riches and how they affected the Nephites' hearts were of particular concern to Nephi's brother Jacob. After Nephi's death, Jacob went up to the temple and addressed the Nephites. We are certain his brother's death added greatly to the emotion of the moment for Jacob. Jacob mentioned that he was "weighed down with desire and anxiety for the welfare of their souls" (Jacob 2:3). He declared that the people were "beginning to labor in sin" (verse 5). He said that it grieved his soul and caused him to shrink with shame before the presence of his Maker that he had to come testify against the wickedness of the people's hearts (see verse 6).

What a vivid portrayal of Jacob's feelings on that solemn occasion! Not only had his beloved older brother, prophet, and king died, but now Jacob had the task to call his people to repentance and talk about the wickedness of their hearts. The people should have been hearing "the pleasing word of God . . . which healeth the wounded soul," but instead of consoling and healing their wounds, Jacob was sent "to enlarge the wounds of those who [were] already wounded" (verses 8–9).

So what did Jacob first talk about with the Nephites on this special occasion in relation to their hearts? He described how the people had begun to search for gold and silver and other precious ores. Some had been quite successful in this endeavor (see verses 12–13). The Psalmist warned, "If riches increase, set not your heart upon them" (Psalm 62:10). Unfortunately, the people's hearts were already beginning to be set upon their riches.

Adding to the spiritual peril, those who obtained more riches than others had begun to be proud in their hearts because they had more. "And *because some of you have obtained more abundantly than that of your brethren* ye are lifted up in the pride of your hearts, and wear stiff necks and high heads because of the costliness of your apparel, and persecute your brethren *because ye suppose that ye are better than they*" (verse 13, emphasis added).

In Jacob's discourse, we see the comparison facet of pride in our hearts mentioned earlier in this chapter. We studied costly apparel in the previous chapter on pride in our hearts, but it just as easily fits into this chapter for a different reason. Costly apparel led the Nephites to compare themselves to their peers, and pride inevitably followed as they saw that they were better dressed and had more riches. The acquisition of costly apparel became a top priority of the Nephites and took their hearts' focus and attention away from higher, more righteous pursuits. The Nephites found themselves seeking for gold and silver and precious ores and were very successful in finding such things. But why were they seeking for such riches? What was their motivation?

Jacob gave his people prophetic counsel that applies as much today as at any other time. He taught:

> Think of your brethren like unto yourselves, and be familiar with all and free with your substance, that they may be rich like unto you.
>
> But before ye seek for riches, seek ye for the kingdom of God.
>
> And after ye have obtained a hope in Christ ye shall obtain riches if ye seek them; and ye will seek them for the intent to do good—to clothe the naked, and to feed the hungry, and to liberate the captive, and administer relief to the sick and the afflicted. (Jacob 2:17–19)

This is one of the greatest and most powerful recorded teachings that we have from Jacob. These verses are to be loved and cherished. Do we read and interpret Jacob's counsel literally, or do we gloss over it and just determine that we need to try to give some money to the poor when it is convenient for us? If we are seeking for riches, are we really seeking them for the intent to do good? Are our motives pure and righteous in regard to acquiring riches?

Jacob declared ten woes that the people needed to avoid in 2 Nephi 9:27–38. We like to call these ten woes the "Be-not-attitudes." We are taught not to be spiritually deaf, spiritually blind, liars, uncircumcised of heart, or murderers, among other woes. The second of Jacob's ten woes reads, "But wo unto the rich, who are rich as to the things of this world. For because they are rich they despise the poor, and they persecute the meek, *and their hearts are upon their treasures; wherefore, their treasure is their god*. And behold, their treasure shall perish with them also" (2 Nephi 9:30, emphasis added). Jacob pronounced this wo on the rich who have their hearts set upon their treasures, not on those who are simply rich. The Savior taught this same principle to the Jews and the Nephites. He said, "For where your treasure is, there will your heart be also" (3 Nephi 13:21, Matthew 6:21). The danger of setting our hearts upon treasures is that they become our god. Jesus taught that we cannot serve God and mammon (see 3 Nephi 13:24).

SACRIFICE SHOULD PINCH

C. S. Lewis gave his thoughts on charitable giving. He said, "I am afraid the only safe rule is to give more than we can spare. If our charities do not at all pinch or hamper us, they are too small. There ought to be things we should like to do and cannot do because our charitable expenditure excludes them."[1] What a thought! We would be so much closer to living the law of consecration and so much closer to our Savior if we thought and acted even a little along these lines. Our hearts would become more set upon the kingdom of God than upon any earthly riches.

Although merely giving financial resources can pinch, it will serve us well to be open to the Spirit on how to best allow the pinch of charitable giving into our lives. Ryan got creative in an experiment on C. S. Lewis's teachings on this subject. In Ryan's words:

> While I felt that my family's fast offering was adequate and generous, I also felt very little to no "pinch" in what was being given. Money was being given to help the poor and needy, but it was difficult to feel any discomfort or see any impact in our day-to-day finances. I didn't feel any real connection to the act other than the daily fast once a month. I wanted to make the experience more personal,

something I felt regularly throughout the month. I wanted to feel an impact in giving to others in need.

To this end, I decided in addition to fasting for the month, I would give up a less-than-optimal habit of soda pop consumption and donate the money that would have been spent on that, in addition to our regular fast offering. Each time I realistically would have purchased soda—be it with a meal, or by the can for home, or grabbing a drink from a convenience store—I recorded the exact amount I would have spent. It was surprising to see just how much soda I was really consuming. It was also very rewarding to feel the "pinch" of giving to those less fortunate.

By creating an impact in my own life and tying it to helping others in need, I felt closer to the Spirit and closer to those I was trying to help. I am sure one result was a bishopric member and financial clerk that were also likely curious and amused as to such an uneven amount of dollars and cents for our family's monthly fast offering check. More importantly, by giving up a common and somewhat poor habit for the month, my thoughts were turned toward giving to those less fortunate almost daily.

OUR STEWARDSHIP TO REALLOCATE RESOURCES

When we are blessed with resources, we become answerable for the allocation of those resources, whether that be for our own use or for the service of others. This earth has more than enough resources for all mankind. According to the Food and Agriculture Organization of the United Nations, the world produces more than 1½ times enough food to feed everyone on the planet.[2] And yet, approximately 821 million people go to bed hungry across the globe, almost one out of nine according to the World Food Programme.[3] This catastrophic failure to distribute food to those in need is an incredibly disheartening situation. How often do we think about the hungry? We often think of the pioneers' trek across the plains and remember stories of some of them eating rawhide to avoid starvation. Many suffered with hunger as they came to the Salt Lake Valley. These stories and scriptural doctrines should make us want to be more aware of helping the hungry and not wasting what we have been given.

What a sacred stewardship it is for those who have more than they need to try to make a difference with those who hunger and go without! We all play a small role in this fight. One of the enduring messages of the Book of Mormon is to take care of the poor and the needy. This is also one of the four pillars of the four-fold mission of the Church today. We all need to play a more active role in this effort. This does not mean that we simply give our money to the poor and the needy and check this commandment off the list. There is far more to it than that.

There are so many ways that we can take care of the poor and the needy that do not require grandiose monetary contributions. We can offer dinner to the less fortunate. We can volunteer our time and serve at a food bank. We can serve at Church mills or canneries if we have them in our area. We know of someone that goes around to people's houses and asks if he can pick fruit from their trees that would otherwise go to waste and donate it to the food bank. In the Lord's eyes, our time and sacrifice is just as valuable, if not more valuable, in serving the poor and needy than our monetary resources.

President Thomas S. Monson said, "At baptism, we covenanted to 'bear one another's burdens, that they may be light.' How many times has your heart been touched as you have witnessed the need of another? How often have you intended to be the one to help? And yet how often has day-to-day living interfered and you've left it for others to help, feeling that 'Oh, surely someone will take care of that need.'"⁴ As our hearts are touched by the promptings of the Holy Ghost, we would do well to quickly follow these promptings to lighten others' burdens. After we follow a prompting in this fashion, additional promptings will assuredly come. Our eyes will be opened to the needs around us, and we will be lifted up as we lift up others.

One way we can all impart of our substance to the poor today is by paying a generous fast offering. In a 1971 Church Welfare Meeting, President Marion G. Romney said, "If the members of the Church would double their fast offering contributions, the spirituality in the Church would double. We need to keep that in mind and be liberal in our contributions."[5]

On another occasion, President Romney promised, "Pay an honest tithe and a generous fast offering if you want the blessings of heaven. I promise every one of you who will do it that you will increase your own prosperity, both spiritually and temporally. The Lord will reward you according to your deeds."[6]

When the Savior visited the Nephites, he quoted Malachi's prophecy regarding tithes and offerings and offered this promise, "And I will rebuke the devourer for your sakes, and he shall not destroy the fruits of your ground; neither shall your vine cast her fruit before the time in the field" (3 Nephi 24:11, Malachi 3:11). Don't we all want these abundant blessings associated with our obedience to the law of the fast and the law of tithing? We cannot afford to pay less than a full tithe in an attempt to hide up such treasure unto ourselves!

President Russell M. Nelson said, "At least once a month, fast and pray and contribute generous fast offerings. We will all be blessed and protected from apostasy by so doing."[7] Amulek teaches us that the efficacy of our prayers is dependent upon how we take care of the needy, the naked, the sick, and the afflicted. He said, "For after ye have done all these things, if ye turn away the needy, and the naked, and visit not the sick and afflicted, and impart of your substance, if ye have, to those who stand in need—I say unto you, if ye do not any of these things, behold, your prayer is vain, and availeth you nothing" (Alma 34:28).

The aforementioned teachings have had a tremendous impact on both of our lives. When Derek first found and read President Romney's promise of increased spirituality if we double our fast offering, his family decided then and there to be more generous, to give more, and to pray for these blessings to be given to his family. In Derek's words:

> I understand that my family's humble offerings are a small pittance in both amount and/or proportion sacrificed in comparison to the offerings of so many faithful members of the Church. However, when we heard President Romney's promises of temporal and spiritual prosperity, we chose to increase our fast offerings and saw immediate blessings. I share this experience because I know that President Romney's blessings promised are not only real, but are still applicable today.
>
> Our family has seen this blessing of increased spirituality in our lives. I have personally had some poignant experiences with prayer and feel closer to my Heavenly Father. I know that He hears our prayers. Our prayers are not offered in vain if we do our part to take care of the poor and the needy. If we do not have money to give to the poor and the needy, we can still qualify for the promised blessings of this commandment if in our hearts we say, "I give not because I have not, but if I had I would give" (Mosiah 4:24).

King Benjamin's Counsel

Do we look to the beggar on the street and wonder if that person brought his or her position upon himself or herself? King Benjamin does a masterful job of making the point that we are all beggars on this earth and should not withhold our substance from, or rain judgment upon, any beggars around us. He pleads with us, "And now, if God, who has created you, on whom you are dependent for your lives and for all that you have and are, doth grant unto you whatsoever ye ask that is right, in faith, believing that ye shall receive, O then, how ye ought to impart of the substance that ye have one to another" (Mosiah 4:21).

King Benjamin continues, "And now, for the sake of these things which I have spoken unto you—that is, for the sake of retaining a remission of your sins from day to day, that ye may walk guiltless before God—I would that ye should impart of your substance to the poor, every man according to that which he hath, such as feeding the hungry, clothing the naked, visiting the sick and administering to their relief, both spiritually and temporally, according to their wants" (verse 26).

King Benjamin suggests to us that caring for the poor and needy needs to be a daily duty as we are seeking to retain a remission of our sins from day to day. Although donating money every day to the poor might be impractical, our stewardship for the poor and needy should be at the forefront of our minds each day. We should be actively engaged in the pursuit of opportunities to serve and care for those less fortunate.

This verse also mentions non-monetary substances with which we can help. It is easy to wrongly narrow the definition of imparting of our substance to the poor and needy as strictly pertaining to monetary donations. However, this verse as well as Amulek's use of this phrase in Alma 34:28 suggest that imparting of our substance is so much more than simply donating money to the poor. So often, *time* is the substance we have to give! Imparting of our substance can mean imparting of our time. It includes visiting the sick and afflicted and administering to their relief, spiritually as well as temporally. It includes helping the needy through the gift of service in addition to helping with monetary needs. Heartfelt prayer followed up with diligence in heeding the promptings of the Spirit will lead us to those in need. Everyone is in need from time to time in some way, and we are all called to minister to those around us. We all have resources that we can impart to the poor and the needy when time is deemed substance. In the final reckoning, time and attention may be the most valuable substance we have to impart to others.

King Benjamin warns that none of us have the right to feel that we are better than someone else, or even that we are so much "as the dust of the earth" (Mosiah 2:25). People often fall into the enticing trap of believing they have acquired their wealth on their own merits. It might be heard, "Why should others deserve any of my money when it was I who worked so hard to earn it in the first place?" If we have been given stewardship over money and resources, we have a mighty responsibility to use those resources in the care of those around us.

The Savior said, "And the rich have I made" (D&C 38:16). How beneficial it would be for us to remember this thought if we are fortunate enough to prosper temporally! Our riches all come from the same source. We have felt this in our own lives in deeply personal ways. We owned a business together for several years and saw the hand of the Lord in it many times. Tender mercies very literally saved our business from going bankrupt in one or two instances. It can be a very humbling thing to own a business upon which the livelihood of others depends. We were driven to our knees in prayer and fasting many times.

We often felt that the business was prospering better than our best efforts warranted. To this day, we frequently remark to each other about the utter reliance we had on the Lord in that period of our careers. We cannot honestly look at ourselves now and say that *we* earned that money or that *we* made the business prosper. Often, the very merits people reference in speaking about how they succeeded in life or business are nothing more than gifts from God: health and strength; physical, mental, or emotional abilities; opportunities; chances for learning and education; kind and helping mentors and supporters; and everything else in the environment in which we work and live. Every mite of our substance represents a blessing from above and was not created or made through our merits.

HEARTS SET UPON TREASURE

As we indicated earlier, caring for the poor and the needy is a huge focus of the Church and one of its four missions. This parallels the Book of Mormon's pervasive focus on this subject. How much thought have we put into this stewardship? Can we do more? If we sacrifice a little more, our hearts will focus less and less upon earthly possessions and more and more upon our Savior and our fellow man.

King Noah did exactly the opposite of this in his life. "He did walk after the desires of his own heart" (Mosiah 11:2). He put a twenty percent tax on the people to support his riotous and prodigal living. So, not only did he not help the poor, he burdened the poor and all of his people with increased taxes to further indulge himself. He built a spacious palace made of gold and all sorts of other expensive metals and woods in which he and his high priests spoke "lying and vain words to his people" (verse 11). He had other great towers and buildings built with these taxes as well. Mormon describes King Noah thus, "And it came to pass that he placed his heart upon his riches. And he spent his time in riotous living with his wives and concubines" (verse 14).

The prophet Abinadi arrived on the scene in Mosiah 12 and posed several stinging questions to King Noah in his luxurious palace. One of the most forthright of these questions he posed was, "Why do ye set your hearts upon riches?" (Mosiah 12:29). Abinadi could clearly discern how corrupt King Noah's heart was as a result of his focus on riches. This disease of the heart destroyed King Noah. His life had a miserable ending. He was burned to death by some of his followers. His wealth and riotous living led to his destruction.

The prophet Nephi, as he prayed upon his garden tower, expressed grave concern about his people setting their hearts upon riches and the vain things of the world (see Helaman 7:21). He felt this condition of the heart went hand in hand with forgetting God. The effort to accumulate wealth can distract and consume to the point that God and His kingdom are forgotten. Accumulating wealth can come to take priority over living the gospel. Hugh Nibley said, "The more important wealth is, the less important it is how one gets it."[8] Compromising one's integrity for the sake of obtaining additional riches is even worse than aggressively or foolishly investing in high-risk assets.

Mormon focused on the topic of hearts being set upon riches as he described the early years of the Church under Alma the

Younger. Mormon noted that members of the Church did not send away the hungry, sick, or afflicted. "They did not set their hearts upon riches; therefore they were liberal to all . . . having no respect to persons as to those who stood in need" (Alma 1:30).

Five short years later, they had begun to wear costly apparel and "set their hearts upon riches and the vain things of the world" (Alma 4:8). Such behavior became a great stumbling-block to the church. Alma decided to give up his position as the chief judge and began to travel from city to city to preach to the members of the Church and bring them to repentance.

While preaching to those in Zarahemla, Alma asked, "Yea, will ye still persist in the wearing of costly apparel and setting your hearts upon the vain things of the world, upon your riches? Yea, and will you persist in turning your backs upon the poor, and the needy, and in withholding your substance from them?" (Alma 5:53, 55). When Alma went to the land of Gideon, he was still focused on the people's hearts being set upon riches and the vain things of the world, but he trusted that people in this land were not in as alarming a condition as the people of Zarahemla (see Alma 7:6).

Samuel the Lamanite warned the Nephites of having their hearts set upon worldly treasures and riches as well. In a beautiful chiasmus, he taught, "And he that hideth not up his treasures unto me, cursed is he, and also the treasure, and none shall redeem it because of the curse of the land. And the day shall come that they shall hide up their treasures, because they have set their hearts upon riches; and because they have set their hearts upon their riches, and will hide up their treasures when they shall flee before their enemies; because they will not hide them up unto me, cursed be they and also their treasures" (Helaman 13:19–20).

For those unfamiliar with chiasmus, it is a literary form that is succinctly described as inverted parallelism. Chiasmus is in the form of A-B-C-D-C-B-A, where "D" is the central focus of the chiasmus.

We believe that one of the reasons this style of writing was used so frequently in the Book of Mormon was because of the difficulty for everyone to have access to the scriptures and other writings in their day. We believe prophets were able to use chiasmus to impress their message upon listeners' minds in a way that they could more easily remember it and retain it.

The central phrase of the chiasmus in Helaman 13:19–20 is the people having their hearts set upon riches. Samuel the Lamanite saw what this condition was doing to the people and wanted to impress upon them the curse that would follow as a result.

SLIPPERY TREASURES IN ANCIENT TIMES

Samuel the Lamanite prophesied, "And behold, the time cometh that he curseth your riches, that they become slippery, that ye cannot hold them; and in the days of your poverty ye cannot retain them" (Helaman 13:31). This phrase *slippery treasures* has always fascinated us.

The Nephites' treasures became slippery because they set their hearts upon them and brought on this curse. So, what exactly does "slippery treasures" mean? How can we avoid having our treasures become slippery unto us or have our "riches make themselves wings and fly away?" (Proverbs 23:5).

There was an ancient practice with the Saints to hide up their treasures unto the Lord at certain times while living the law of consecration. If everyone had what was necessary for their needs and a surplus still remained, then Saints would hide up their treasures for future Saints' needs. If they hid up these treasures in such a way, in the name of consecration, then the Lord would not curse these treasures. Samuel the Lamanite exempted such people from the curse when he said, "Whoso shall hide up treasures in the earth shall find them again no more, save he be a righteous man and shall hide it up unto the Lord" (Helaman 13:18). However, these Saints would be cursed if they hid treasures up for personal use.

Another reason people hid up their treasures was out of fear that someone would steal them. This was the case with the Nephites during Samuel the Lamanite's day.

The curse of slippery treasures had a literal fulfillment for the Nephites. When Samuel's prophecy was fulfilled over three hundred years later, the Gadianton robbers overran the land and stole that which was hid up in the earth. Mormon observed, "And these Gadianton robbers, who were among the Lamanites, did infest the land, insomuch that the inhabitants thereof began to hide up their treasures in the earth; and they became slippery, because the Lord had cursed the land, that they could not hold them, nor retain them again" (Mormon 1:18).

Mormon continued, "For behold no man could keep that which was his own, for the thieves, and the robbers, and the murderers, and the magic art, and the witchcraft which was in the land" (Mormon 2:10).

Such a plight had actually occurred hundreds of years before with the Jaredites as well. Moroni wrote:

> And now there began to be a great curse upon all the land because of the iniquity of the people, in which, if a man should lay his tool or his sword upon his shelf, or upon the place whither he would keep it, behold, upon the morrow, he could not find it, so great was the curse upon the land.
>
> Wherefore, every man did cleave unto that which was his own, with his hands, and would not borrow neither would he lend; and every man kept the hilt of his sword in his right hand, in the defense of his property and his own life and of his wives and children. (Ether 14:1–2)

These verses have such striking imagery! Can you imagine holding your riches in one hand and holding your sword in your other hand to try to protect them? What an awful scenario!

SLIPPERY TREASURES TODAY

How does the idea of slippery treasures apply to us today? Do we see examples of slippery treasures around us? How can we avoid this curse coming upon ourselves?

It would stand to reason that we are under this same condemnation as those who have gone before us if we do not hide up our treasures unto the Lord. Our treasures may not be as slippery as they were around 6 BC or AD 325, but we are getting closer and closer to the same state. We need to be wary of this curse in our day.

At first glance, we may think we are decidedly different than the Nephites, but we actually do very similar things to what they did. We save our money in banks for security and to accumulate interest. We invest in the stock market with surplus income and via retirement accounts and pensions to try to increase such wealth. We purchase real estate and rental properties in the hopes of getting a return on our investment. All of these activities can be responsible ways to save or accumulate wealth. Prudently investing our resources for the right reasons can allow us opportunities such as family vacations, missionary service, and the freedom to serve others and build the kingdom of God in retirement.

However, greed can overtake the heart and become the primary financial motivation. Greed can cause one to become loose with one's ethics, steal from a neighbor, or gamble with one's treasures in the form of perilous and risky financial speculation. Insatiable greed can cause treasures to become slippery as we lose focus on the Lord. Some of us may pay less than a full tithe and so hide up treasures unto ourselves in this way.

Using such good and bad scenarios, it is easy to see how treasures can become slippery to us. Banks can and do fail. Inflation or even hyperinflation could lead to our money being worth much less than it is today. The stock market has crashed on numerous occasions and most likely will have significant drops or crashes in the future. Real estate can sharply decrease in value depending on the overall market, as it has in the past. Fortunes can be lost when speculating in the name of investing. We can close the windows of heaven and lose out on temple blessings if we fail to pay a full tithe.

How can we avoid this curse coming upon ourselves? Do we simply need to give away our surplus in everything we have to the poor and the needy? If we were fully living the law of consecration, that would be the right action to take. We are not fully living that law today, so such an action is not technically required of us at this time. However, the prophets have provided a great deal of both counsel and warning on how to handle our finances.

President Thomas S. Monson said, "Avoid the philosophy and excuse that yesterday's luxuries have become today's necessities. They aren't necessities unless we ourselves make them such. It is essential for us to live within our means."[9] What a simple yet profound piece of counsel. Falling into the trap of redefining more and more of our luxuries as necessities can be both temporally and spiritually perilous. Taking a closer look at assessing how we choose to distinguish between luxuries and necessities in our lives with an honest heart may yield striking results. This practice, if undertaken, will help us follow the prophet's counsel to live more fully within our means.

President Gordon B. Hinckley said, "I am suggesting the time has come to get our houses in order. So many of our people are living on the very edge of their incomes. In fact, some are living on borrowings. We have witnessed wide and fearsome swings in the markets of the world. The economy is a fragile thing. It can eventually reach down to each of us as individuals. There is a portent of stormy weather ahead to which we had better give heed."[10]

This stormy weather that President Hinckley warned about hit not too long after he first gave this address to us in 1998. The dot-com crash went from 2000–2002. More stormy weather hit with the Great Recession of 2007–2009. Additional turbulent weather will inevitably hit us again in the future. Following the prophet's counsel to get our houses in order and to live within our incomes will help us weather these storms.

Do we keep a family budget with individual categories for things like gas, groceries, and clothing? Do we separate categories into wants and needs? Do we make sure to set aside some money each month for the storms that lie ahead? Budgets are great tools to use for our financial planning and can shed light on trends and spending habits. They can help target areas in which improvement needs to be made.

We have seen the reality and impact of slippery treasures in our own lives. We have experienced times when treasures have been laid up righteously, times where money was set aside for the poor and needy, and great blessings have flowed into our lives. We have also experienced more selfish times, times when perhaps too much focus was spent on personal consumption. We have felt enormous blessings rain down in our lives as tithes and fast offerings have been faithfully given. We have experienced seasons of abundance and plenty in which we were showered with temporal blessings from above. We have also experienced many times of much less, seasons of scarcity when temporal wealth was rare and illusive. We have seen conservative and disciplined investing strategies yield positive results, and we have seen times when those same strategies have created loss and reduced resources. It is not uncommon to pass through both seasons of abundance and saving as well as seasons of slipperiness and loss when it comes to management of our resources. Some slipperiness comes as a natural part of our mortality; other seasons of slipperiness are the consequence of our own poor decisions and judgment.

HEARTS THAT BECOME COLD

From observing the members of the Church during Nephi's time, we learn that having hearts set upon riches and the vain things of the world leads to personal apostasy. President Brigham Young said, "The Latter-day Saints who turn their attention to money-making soon become cold in their feelings toward the ordinances of the house of God. They neglect their prayers, become unwilling to pay any donations; the law of tithing gets too great a task for them; and they finally forsake their God, and the providences of heaven seem to be shut from them—all in consequence of this lust after the things of this world, which will certainly perish in handling, and in their use they will fade away and go from us."[11]

What an unsettling statement! Setting our hearts upon riches makes us cold in our feelings toward the temple and the ordinances received there. As one feels more and more distant from the temple, an assessment of the heart in regard to the love of riches should be honestly undertaken. On the other hand, going to the temple and serving there more frequently will warm our hearts toward the gospel while cooling our hearts from the love of material possessions.

Another consequence of having hearts set upon riches is given by the Savior in the parable of the sower. He taught, "And the care of this world, and the deceitfulness of riches, choke the word" (Matthew 13:22). We choke the word of God out of our lives as we worry more and more about acquiring riches. Riches can truly be deceitful and damaging to our spiritual welfare in this regard. They are so attractive and so desirous, yet they are completely worthless and will not even exist in the eternal realm. Rather than treasure up riches, we are told to treasure up in our minds the words of life (see D&C 84:85).

At this point it is worth noting a quote from President Dallin H. Oaks. He said, "Those who believe in what has been called the theology of prosperity are suffering from the deceitfulness of riches. The possession of wealth or significant income is not a mark of heavenly favor, and their absence is not evidence of heavenly disfavor."[12] Although such thinking continues to be prevalent in society and sometimes within members of the Church, such thinking is an absolute falsehood. We cannot afford to confuse our individual net worth with our individual worth. The riches of this world are certainly not how God measures our value as His children.

Elder Franklin D. Richards said, "We are living . . . in an age . . . when many men's hearts are set upon worldly treasures, pleasures, and influence. One of the great challenges facing us today is to develop sufficient wisdom, understanding, and inner strength so that we can live happily and successfully in our complex and difficult world and not be caught up in the mad scramble for the material things and pleasures."[13] He said this in 1976. Over forty years later, the mad scramble has only become more and more mad and more and more of a scramble. It is astonishingly easy to get caught up in the pursuit of material things. There are mad scrambles for cars, houses, and other possessions. Every Christmas season, there is a mad scramble for the popular gifts of the year. Happiness should not be attached to the accumulation of things.

OVERCOMING THE APPETITE FOR RICHES

How do we combat this worldly desire from taking over our hearts? How do we keep from being caught up in this "mad scramble" to acquire riches? The Savior taught, "But lay up for yourselves treasures in heaven, where neither moth nor rust doth corrupt, and where thieves do not break through nor steal" (3 Nephi 13:20). The most effective way to keep our hearts from being set upon riches is to focus on laying up treasures for ourselves in heaven.

As we cannot take our earthly riches with us to the other side, what treasures can we lay up in heaven while here on earth? The scriptures offer us many examples of things we can take with us. Joseph Smith taught, "Whatever principle of intelligence we attain unto in this life, it will rise with us in the resurrection" (D&C 130:18). Our pursuit of learning, especially of things of God, is a worthy pursuit and will result in treasures being laid up in heaven for us.

Mormon teaches us that charity endureth forever (see Moroni 7:47). Any effort and progress we make to cultivate charity in our lives will be laid up as a treasure unto us in heaven. The development of any spiritual gifts will be a treasure that can be taken with us into the eternities. These spiritual gifts and virtues come only to us through the grace of Jesus Christ and the enabling power of His Atonement.

Joseph Smith also taught that "the same sociality which exists among us here will exist among us [in heaven]" (D&C 130:2). Building and developing relationships with others is a heavenly pursuit, especially with our families and those to whom we are entrusted to minister. The treasures of these relationships will accompany us into the eternities.

Jacob counseled, "Wherefore, do not spend money for that which is of no worth, nor your labor for that which cannot satisfy" (2 Nephi 9:51). Do we spend our labor magnifying our Church callings? Do we minister to our neighbors and loved ones? Do we actively seek out opportunities to bless those that are in need? These are examples of labors that can satisfy, labors that provide heavenly wages!

President Henry B. Eyring taught us an additional way that the Atonement works on hearts set upon riches. He said, "The companionship of the Holy Ghost makes what is good more attractive and temptation less compelling. That alone should be enough to make us determined to qualify for the Spirit to be with us always."[14] There is much to learn about the Holy Ghost and how He works directly through the Atonement. This is one of the beautiful ways the Holy Ghost works through us. If we are worthy of having the Spirit in our lives, He will bless us by making temptations appear less attractive. Riches and treasures of the world will not be as appealing to us the more we have the Spirit with us. Riches will take lower priority on our demands and in our thoughts.

Keeping our hearts from being set upon riches and treasures is a lifelong pursuit. Money and material wealth are often at the forefront of what we see and what we hear in conversation. The pursuit of wealth can easily dominate our thoughts. It is easy to see the riches of others and covet what they have. Responsibility will require the analysis of our own financial position frequently in life while determining ways to improve it. At such times, motivations and desires should be checked to ensure they align with the Lord's. There is no room for greed when working with the management of resources. Needs must be met and taken care of, a process that must be accompanied by a wariness of luxuries and desires that may dominate our thoughts.

If we are blessed with worldly riches, may we use them "for the intent to do good—to clothe the naked, and to feed the hungry, and to liberate the captive, and administer relief to the sick and the afflicted" (Jacob 2:19). May we be a tender mercy to others in their time of need. May we focus on the riches of the gospel and set our hearts more fully upon them, for they are plentiful and endless.

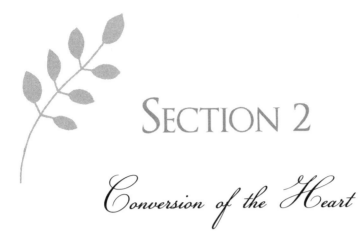

SECTION 2

Conversion of the Heart

Elder David A. Bednar said, "The journey of mortality is to progress from bad to good to better and to experience the mighty change of heart—to have our fallen natures changed. The Book of Mormon is our handbook of instructions as we travel the pathway from bad to good to better and strive to have our hearts changed."[1]

Much of what we have studied up to this point involves changing our hearts from bad to good by eradicating certain diseases from our hearts. We can work on changing our hearts to be less prideful, to be less set upon riches, or to be softer than they are currently. The Book of Mormon provides a detailed look at the mighty change that needs to occur within each of our hearts to be truly converted unto the Lord. It also explains how we can actually make lasting changes to our hearts. This initiates our journey to progress from good to better.

The following three chapters will discuss conditions or actions of the heart that are identifiable with our personal conversion to the gospel and our Savior. Elder Bednar related this part of our journey to becoming more like a Saint. These conditions of the heart will help us become more saint-like.

Our conversion of the heart begins with experiencing a mighty change of heart. This is also frequently described in scripture as spiritually being born again. When we experience a mighty change of heart, we have "no more disposition to do evil" (Mosiah 5:2). Not only that, but we focus more on doing the right things for the right reasons.

After we have experienced a mighty change of heart and are baptized and receive the gift of the Holy Ghost, we are blessed with the opportunity to receive personal revelation and inspiration from Him on a daily basis. President Russell M. Nelson said, "In coming days, it will not be possible to survive spiritually without the guiding, directing, comforting, and constant influence of the Holy Ghost. I plead with you to increase your spiritual capacity to receive revelation."[2]

Pondering the gospel in our hearts is the key that unlocks the door to personal revelation. The Church is built upon the rock of revelation. We need to learn the language of the Spirit and understand how to access this incredible gift. We will study how we can more effectively ponder the scriptures and doctrines of the gospel in our hearts to get answers to our questions and to receive needed guidance along our journey.

We will then study the virtue of lowliness of heart that is most often coupled with meekness. This attribute is key to our personal development and our ability to gain knowledge and understanding of the gospel. If we are not lowly in heart, we will not be teachable or humble enough to be instructed by the Spirit or by our prophets and apostles. We will also study the law of gaining knowledge as it relates to being lowly in heart.

We invite you to assess the condition of your heart as you read the following chapters. Have you experienced a mighty change of heart? If not, what can you do to bring about this change? Has your heart truly been converted to Christ and His Church? Do you ponder upon the word of God, or do you simply read or only read and study His word? Do you know how to ponder? How teachable are you? Are you humble enough to be taught by the Spirit? Are you meek in your interactions with your fellow man?

As you measure your heart and prayerfully work on these things, the Savior has promised to give you a new heart. Great blessings will flow into your lives. You will receive personal revelation on a more frequent basis that will benefit not only yourselves but also your families and those to whom you minister. You will have the Holy Ghost's companionship more frequently in your life. You will receive instruction and gain knowledge from on high. You will receive specific, personalized guidance and ensure that you learn what you should from certain experiences as you seek to know Heavenly Father's will.

Chapter 5

A Mighty Change
of Heart

A mighty change of heart or simply a change of heart is mentioned nine times in the Book of Mormon. The phrases *change of heart* and *mighty change* are both unique to the Book of Mormon among the standard works. The eloquent and descriptive language in the Book of Mormon adds so much beauty to our knowledge of the gospel! Alma, the son of Alma, mentions a change of heart five times, and King Benjamin mentions a change of heart twice.

The distinct descriptor *mighty* is found in four of these nine mentions. This mighty change of heart is usually accompanied with the principle of being spiritually born again, which is more widely recognized in religious circles. There are many accounts in the Book of Mormon of people that experienced a mighty change of heart, and profound insights can be gleaned from their careful study.

It Began under a Tree

Ryan had the privilege of witnessing a mighty change of heart several times while serving a mission in Brazil. Perhaps his most memorable example of this change of heart was with a young man named Beto. In Ryan's words:

> We met Beto one day while making a visit to a recent convert. He was a friend that happened to be visiting when we arrived. He was very rough in appearance, language, and manner. In short, we weren't thrilled he was associating with our ward's newest member. He mocked our appearance and condescendingly asked what we did as missionaries. When we told him that we shared a message of hope about the Savior, Jesus Christ, he asked to hear it. We set a meeting with him under a tree in the neighborhood for the next day and were frankly surprised when he showed up.
>
> His manner was more polite, and he seemed receptive that day. When we shared Joseph Smith's experience, his already softened defenses and attitude crumbled. He openly wept and was astonished and confused at what he was feeling. The Spirit attended that meeting under a tree in unmistakable fashion that Friday afternoon. We took advantage of the moment and explained to him what these feelings meant. We challenged him to be baptized, and he accepted without hesitation. We then challenged him to give up smoking, drugs, and alcohol, all of which he regularly participated in. He readily accepted. We spoke of the law of chastity and told him he would need to live it. We went so far as to explain that his appearance, manner, and speech needed to change. He committed to every invite we threw at him, and we told him we would see him at church in two days.
>
> When Sunday came, Beto showed up in a beautiful three-piece suit with a clean white shirt. He even sported a gold tie clip and pocket watch with a chain. He had not only cleaned up well, but his haircut was noticeably and drastically different. It was a fast Sunday, and as soon as the Bishop finished his testimony, Beto was the first one up to the pulpit. As missionaries, we were a little concerned and

alarmed, since we had told him nothing about fast meeting and how it works. Beto stood up, greeted everyone, and introduced himself. He then bore a humble testimony that everything he had been taught by the missionaries felt true, that he had felt the Spirit testify to him, that he knew Jesus was his Savior, and that the Book of Mormon was true. He concluded his humble testimony by inviting everybody to his baptism in a week or two.

I will always remember the bishop making eye contact with me from the stand and mouthing the words, "Who is this guy?" Beto kept his commitments and changed so many things in his life to align with the gospel of Jesus Christ. But the next time he came to Church, he was in blue jeans and a clean but casual shirt. He continued attending meetings in that dress, including on the day of his baptism. I finally asked him on the day of his baptism why he wasn't wearing his beautiful suit. He replied that the member we brought to that first discussion had stayed and told him about Church and about the fast and testimony meeting that would be held that Sunday. He said that he had taken pretty much all the money he had and rented a suit in the city for that Sunday. He said that he wanted to look the part when he bore testimony of the true Church for the first time. He felt a little sheepish about the casual clothing he had been wearing since that first Sunday, but he had spent all his money and couldn't do anything about it yet.

In the next three months, Beto was kicked out of the home he was living in because of the gospel, and then a month later he was kicked out of the friend's house into which he had moved because of the gospel. He lost all of his friends and closest family relationships because of his choice to join the Church. He ended up moving in with the bishop's family, but left for the north of Brazil after a few months because he felt like an imposition. The last we heard while in Brazil was that there was not a ward in the city to which he moved. He had to save money and took a two-hour bus ride to church on Sundays as often as he could.

That was the last I heard from him until years later I received a letter in the mail from Manaus. It was from Beto. He was a zone leader in the Brazil Manaus Mission and had just run into an old ward member that was able to track down my address. We stayed in touch after that, and I count his friendship a great privilege. After finishing his mission, he was later married in the temple and served faithfully in his ward.

Beto's entire life changed because of what happened in the span of a few quick weeks, or it could even be said his entire life changed during a discussion under a tree. Some changes of heart come in quick and overwhelming fashion; others are a slow and steady process of growing and cultivating greater and greater light. So, what does it mean to have a mighty change of heart?

Four Characteristics of a Mighty Change of Heart

President Ezra Taft Benson said, "When we have undergone this mighty change, which is brought about only through faith in Jesus Christ and through the operation of the Spirit upon us, it is as though we have become a new person. Thus, the change is likened to a new birth. Thousands of you have experienced this change. You have forsaken lives of sin, sometimes deep and offensive sin, and through applying the blood of Christ in your lives, have become clean. You have no more disposition to return to your old ways. You are in reality a new person. This is what is meant by a change of heart."[1]

After King Benjamin taught his people at the temple, he asked them if they believed his teachings. His people responded, "Yea, we believe all the words which thou hast spoken unto us; and also, we know of their surety and truth, because of the Spirit of the Lord Omnipotent, which has wrought a mighty change in us, or in our hearts, that we have no more disposition to do evil, but to do good continually" (Mosiah 5:2).

This is the first time this mighty change of heart is recorded in scripture. The people wanted to emphasize that they thought much differently than they had before and that they no longer resembled their old selves. This was indeed a significant and mighty change that they experienced in their hearts, and it seems to have come as the result of a great and powerful spiritual experience. It was the Holy Ghost that wrought this change within them.

There are four distinct characteristics of a mighty change of heart that are consistently mentioned in the examples found in the Book of Mormon. First of all, a mighty change of heart is brought about through studying or hearing the word of God. Second, it involves repentance and an overwhelming desire to do good continually and to abandon all evil practices. Third, a mighty change of heart is always coupled with making covenants with Heavenly Father. Fourth, it has a long-lasting impact on the individual's life.

King Benjamin's people fit this narrative perfectly. They heard the word of God as it was preached by King Benjamin. We are told that they had "no more disposition to do evil, but to do good continually" (Mosiah 5:2). They made a covenant with God "to do his will, and to be obedient to his commandments in all things" (verse 5). And this change was long-lasting. We read later on that the rising generation did not believe King Benjamin's words like their parents did (see Mosiah 26:1–5). It is implied that the people who entered into covenants to keep the commandments after King Benjamin's address were still faithful to these covenants.

King Benjamin provides additional insight of what a mighty change of heart entails. We are to become "as a child, submissive, meek, humble, patient, full of love, willing to submit to all things which the Lord seeth fit to inflict upon [us], even as a child doth submit to his father" (Mosiah 3:19). This is in contrast to being carnal, sensual, and devilish if we yield ourselves to Satan's influence (see Mosiah 16:3, Alma 42:10). The conversion of our heart is our journey to become Saints and followers of our Savior, Jesus Christ. To become a Saint is to change our hearts to be more like the Savior's. We are to progress from bad to good to better, as Elder David A. Bednar stated.[2]

ALMA THE YOUNGER'S MIGHTY CHANGE

Alma the Younger focused on this doctrine of experiencing a change of heart more than anyone else in the Book of Mormon. Perhaps he did so because of the mighty change that happened both to his own heart as well as to the heart of his father. He had intimate experience with undergoing a mighty change of heart. As Alma the Younger spoke to the members of the Church in Zarahemla in Alma 5, he mentioned this subject five times.

Alma the Younger said of his father, Alma the Elder:

And according to his [Alma the Elder's] faith there was a *mighty change* wrought in his heart. . . . And behold, he preached the word unto your fathers, and a *mighty change* was also wrought in their hearts, and they humbled themselves and put their trust in the true and living God. And behold, they were faithful until the end; therefore they were saved.

And now behold, I ask of you, my brethren of the church, have ye spiritually been born of God? Have ye received his image in your countenances: Have ye experienced this *mighty change* in your hearts? (Alma 5:12–14, emphasis added)

This mighty change experienced by Alma and his followers has similar characteristics to King Benjamin's people. It fits the four criteria that we mentioned previously. Alma the Elder was taught the word of God by Abinadi and then subsequently taught others the word of God. The desire of this people's hearts was to keep the commandments and serve God until they died (see Mosiah 18:10–11). Alma's followers all entered into a covenant to keep the commandments and follow the Savior as they were baptized in the waters of Mormon (see Mosiah 18:8–10, 15–16). Finally, Alma the Younger related that these people "were faithful until the end" (Alma 5:13).

Alma does a masterful job of teaching his people in Alma 5 by asking them fifty introspective questions. Alma wanted the people of Zarahemla to look inside themselves and assess their own spirituality and the condition of their hearts. He wanted them to consider their personal standing with the Lord. His questions motivate and inspire us to want to better understand what a change of heart is, and to grow within us a desire to experience this change of heart.

The questions that Alma poses encourage spiritual introspection and an honest measurement of the condition of our own heart. Not only does Alma speak of a mighty change of heart in this sermon, but he also asks questions about the purity of our hearts. He asks whether we continue to have pride in our hearts. He asks if we have our hearts set on riches and the vain things of the world. These questions are not merely a checklist of actions we need to perform to qualify for heaven; rather they examine the very motives and desires for doing what we do. In the end, Alma says it comes down to a choice of hearkening to the voice of the Good Shepherd or not. Will we follow Him and leave wickedness behind? Will we allow Him to change our hearts and give us a new heart like unto His?

Alma the Younger provided some great descriptions of what it was like for his father's followers to experience a mighty change of heart. Their souls were "illuminated by the light of the everlasting word" (Alma 5:7). They humbled themselves and put their trust in the true and living God (see Alma 5:13). They received Christ's image in their countenances and were spiritually born of God (see Alma 5:14, 19). They also "felt to sing the song of redeeming love" (Alma 5:26).

President Dallin H. Oaks taught that a change of heart includes new attitudes, priorities, and desires.[3] Elder L. Whitney Clayton said this change causes people to treat others with meekness.[4] Indeed, this is a *mighty* change of heart we must all experience, not just some small tweak or slight adjustment. This change of heart, with its accompanying character traits and attributes, is made possible only through the sanctifying power of the atoning blood of Christ. The presence of the Holy Ghost empowers us to access the enabling power of Jesus Christ.

CHANGE CAN HAPPEN IN A HEARTBEAT OR OVER A LIFETIME

Change is one of those words that strikes fear into most people. In our professional lives, we have changed enough systems and business practices to know that resisting change comes quite naturally. Most team members would shudder at even the prospect or possibility of change, even when it would benefit them greatly. Generally speaking, people are creatures of habit. We like to eat the same thing for breakfast. We like to exercise at a certain time of day. We like to shower and brush our teeth in a certain way. Many specific actions and ways of doing things become ingrained in us at work as well as in our lives at home. If any of our routines are disrupted, we often make it more chaotic and disconcerting than it should be. If you don't think this is true, think of the last time someone was sitting where you usually do at Church. Did it give you pause? Is it even possible to change something as complex and multifaceted as our hearts?

One of our favorite quotes on the subject is from author Andy Andrews. He said, "Most people think it takes a long time to change. It doesn't. Change is immediate! Instantaneous! It may take a long time to decide to change . . . but change happens in a heartbeat."[5] We are firm believers in this concept of change—the concept that it only takes one heartbeat to change.

Elder Jeffrey R. Holland taught of a similar speed to making changes. He said, "You can change anything you want to change and you can do it very fast. It is another Satanic falsehood to believe that it takes years and years and eons of eternity to repent. It takes exactly as long to repent as it takes you to say, 'I'll change'—and mean it. Of course there will be problems to work out and res-titutions to make. You may well spend—indeed, you had better spend—the rest of your life proving your repentance by its permanence. But change, growth, renewal, and repentance can come for you as instantaneously as it did for Alma and the sons of Mosiah."[6]

We've seen positive changes come to fruition in our own lives as quickly as described above. Often, it's the time it takes for us *to decide to change* that can take so long, even years.

It may be illuminating to consider the patterns and choices that so many make with regard to their personal health. Many people spend significant time considering the state of their health. There are many, ourselves included, that spend an inordinate amount of time deliberating on the present situation of their physical health. We will wish we had the body and energy of a teenager. We will think about the various forms of exercise that would help us get to where we want to be. We will also consider the cost of giving up certain favorite foods and quantities of those foods that would enable us to be in a different situation. We will fret and dread the possible changes, and agonize about the effort that the process will require. We will plan around certain times of the year during which we think we will lack the will power to execute change. We will plot and strategize what times of the year are best to make the needed changes. We will read books and scheme about the best approach for this change of diet. Sometimes, hundreds of hours of mental exertion take place in considering all of the facets of this change.

It is our guess that these thoughts and considerations are not unique to us. But even with all the planning and maneuvering, if you asked the vast majority of people that have made the transition from an unhealthy lifestyle to a healthy one, most can point to a very short period in their life, a day, or even a moment, that they just changed. They can point to a moment in time from whence they changed the way they ate and the way they exercised. We personally know people that have completely changed the nature of their health, and that change can be traced to a single day and moment in which they changed.

The buildup to change can take months or even years depending on our mental process, preparation, and deliberation. However, once we truly decide to do something, change can come instantaneously. In the end, we may end up asking ourselves, "Why didn't I do this earlier?" To effect change, our thoughts must be focused on the positives that will come from changes we are trying to make rather than what we think we may be losing or missing. If the benefit of change outweighs the cost in our minds, we will more likely move forward and change. The blessings and benefits of living the gospel always outweigh any carnal practice that we enjoy or feel we cannot live without.

While some changes of the heart are sudden and instantaneous, many changes happen slowly and methodically over time. Most will experience changes in their hearts over time as habits are formed to follow our Savior and keep His commandments. The momentum of these positive habits must be great enough to overcome occasional relapses that can take us off our course. During such relapses, if we will quickly return to our course after slipping up, the Holy Ghost will strengthen us even more in adopting a new way of life.

President Henry B. Eyring said, "Not only is your feeling the influence of the Holy Ghost a sign that the Atonement, the cure for sin, is working in your life, but you will also know that a preventative against sin is working."[7] Our hearts will change here a little and there a little as the Spirit works upon us. The Holy Ghost will give us greater resolve and power to maintain the changes we have made. He will help guard us from further sin and will make these new actions easier for us to repeat. This is the grace available to all of us because of the Atonement of our Savior, and it is only through His grace that we can improve.

SAMUEL THE LAMANITE'S ROADMAP TO CHANGE

How can we experience a mighty change of heart? And how can we ensure that our newly changed heart gets the proper care it needs to not only survive, but to thrive in the gospel for the rest of our mortal lives?

Samuel the Lamanite provided the pattern to follow to experience a mighty change of heart. He offered a key insight as to how we can begin this process. He taught, "And behold, ye do know of yourselves, for ye have witnessed it, that as many of them as are brought to the knowledge of the truth, and to know of the wicked and abominable traditions of their fathers, and are led to believe the holy scriptures, yea, the prophecies of the holy prophets, which are written, which leadeth them to faith on the Lord, and unto repentance, which faith and repentance bringeth a change of heart unto them" (Helaman 15:7).

Samuel's teaching is truly profound! We need to have faith and exercise repentance to bring about a change of heart, but what leads us to have this faith? What leads us to want to repent in our lives? Samuel testifies to us that we must believe the holy scriptures and the prophecies of holy prophets which are written. The action of *studying* the word of God leads to *faith*, which leads to *repentance*, which then brings about a *change of heart*. This is the pattern! A mighty change of heart is preceded by scripture study about the truths and prophecies contained therein. When we consider a mighty change of heart, it is often forgotten that scripture study and hearing the word of God is where it all begins. That is why we include this as the first step to experiencing a mighty change of heart.

Prophets, priests, and teachers were laboring throughout the land during Jarom's time. They were actively engaged in teaching the people the word of God. Jarom observed, "And it came to pass that by so doing they kept them from being destroyed upon the face of the land; *for they did prick their hearts with the word,* continually stirring them up unto repentance" (Jarom 1:12). The word of God has the power to prick our hearts and remind us of the divine potential within us. The scriptures can motivate us to change. Again, the word of God leads to faith, which leads to repentance, which leads to this mighty change of heart.

Samuel the Lamanite continued to explain the three other characteristics of a mighty change of heart. Samuel spoke of the people of Ammon and other Lamanites that had come unto Christ. They came to fear sin. They buried their weapons of war in covenant with God to keep His commandments. Finally, Samuel reminded us that those who had experienced a change of heart were "firm and steadfast in the faith" (see Alma 24:17–18; Helaman 15:8–10).

Enos had a similar experience. He said that the words that his father had taught concerning eternal life and the joy of the saints sunk deep into his heart. He asked for forgiveness from his sins and was granted this desire because of his faith (see Enos 1:3–8).

President Henry B. Eyring said, "That mighty change is reported time after time in the Book of Mormon. The way it is wrought and what the person becomes is always the same. The words of God in pure doctrine go down deep into the heart by the power of the Holy Ghost. The person pleads with God in faith. The repentant heart is broken and the spirit contrite. Sacred covenants have been made. Then God keeps His covenant to grant a new heart and a new life, in His time."[8]

President Eyring teaches that it starts with the word of God and follows the pattern outlined by Samuel the Lamanite. Studying the scriptures and the words of our prophets and apostles today is one of the most effective ways we can invite the Holy Ghost into our lives. Are we continually holding fast to the rod of iron and studying the scriptures daily? Do we frequently study the words of living prophets and apostles when they address us in general conference? We must be diligent students of the word of God to experience a mighty change of heart in our lives. This will lead to increased faith and the desire to repent. What an effective and unambiguous roadmap we have been given!

The missionary stories in the book of Alma share powerful examples and teachings that beautifully lay forth the doctrine of a change of heart. In that book, we learn about the remarkable missionary efforts of Alma and the sons of Mosiah. The sons of Mosiah performed many miracles, with the Lord's help, as they preached to the Lamanites. One of these sons of Mosiah, Ammon, first journeyed to the land of Ishmael and became a servant to King Lamoni. Ammon defended the king's flocks, and due to his astonishing example of obedience, loyalty, and strength, he was eventually given the opportunity to teach the king about the Savior and His gospel.

King Lamoni and his people followed the same pattern taught by Samuel the Lamanite to experience a mighty change of heart. After Ammon taught King Lamoni the plan of redemption from the beginning, King Lamoni fell unto the earth as if he were dead. He had faith, and his heart recognized the truth of Ammon's teachings. He knew then that he had done many things that were contrary to the commandments of the Lord, and he cried for mercy upon his soul. A great scene unfolded in which the Spirit was manifest so powerfully that eventually the king, the queen, the king's servants, and Ammon all fell to the earth with joy.

Abish, an existing Lamanite convert, saw this as an opportunity for others to come and believe in the power of God. She ran from house to house, calling the people to come and see what was happening. A crowd gathered and as the king, queen, and those that had fallen to the earth arose, they testified of Jesus and of the gospel that Ammon had taught unto them. Many believed their words and were converted also (see Alma 17–19).

Alma recorded, "And it came to pass that when Ammon arose he also administered unto them, and also did all the servants of Lamoni; and they did all declare unto the people the selfsame thing—*that their hearts had been changed; that they had no more desire to do evil*" (Alma 19:33, emphasis added).

These people had been touched from listening to the word of God that Ammon delivered to them. They had faith in what they were hearing, which led to them desiring to repent of their sins. President Ezra Taft Benson said, "Repentance involves not just a change of action, but a change of heart."[9] Again, the Lord is as concerned or even more concerned with our hearts and motives than the actual actions we perform.

Lamoni's people, along with Lamanites that were converted in other lands, gave themselves a new name to be known by—the people of Anti-Nephi-Lehi or the people of Ammon. This group went to extraordinary lengths to show the Savior that their hearts had been changed.

Alma testified, "Yea, I say unto you, as the Lord liveth, as many of the Lamanites as believed in their preaching, and were converted unto the Lord, never did fall away. For they became a righteous people; they did lay down the weapons of their rebellion, that they did not fight against God any more, neither against any of their brethren" (Alma 23:6–7). These people buried their weapons of war deep within the earth and refused to fight ever again. Alma concluded, "And this they did, vouching and covenanting with God, that rather than shed the blood of their brethren they would give up their own lives" (Alma 24:18).

Lamoni and his people aptly demonstrated the four main characteristics of a change of heart. They were taught the word of God by Ammon. They had no more desire to do evil. They made a sacred covenant to bury their weapons of war and not shed anyone's blood. They never did fall away after their hearts had been changed.

One of the questions Alma posed earlier was, "If ye have experienced a change of heart, and if ye have felt to sing the song of redeeming love, I would ask, can ye feel so now?" (Alma 5:26). Alma was asking if we still feel the burning in our hearts from having experienced a change of heart the first time. Sister Bonnie D. Parkin, the fourteenth general president of the Relief Society, said, "If your heart is not singing the song of redeeming love, return to your covenants. Celebrate them."[10] What inspired doctrine! Returning to and keeping covenants is how we can properly care for our changed hearts.

Elder Dale G. Renlund gave us further instruction on maintaining a changed heart. He stated:

A mighty change of heart is just the beginning. Indeed, equal, if not greater care, must be taken with a spiritually changed heart than with a physically transplanted heart if we are to endure to the end.

We must identify temptations that easily beset us and put them out of reach—way out of reach. Finally, we need to frequently biopsy our mightily changed hearts and reverse any signs of early rejection.

Please consider the state of your changed heart. Do you detect any rejection setting in as a result of the tendency of the natural man to become casual? If so, find a place where you can kneel. Remember, more than mortal years on this earth are at stake. Do not risk forfeiting the fruits of the ultimate operation: eternal salvation and exaltation.[11]

As Elder Renlund taught, we must consider the state of our hearts frequently. As we do so, we will identify where our hearts might be wandering and be able to make quick course corrections. A changed heart has no room for casual complacency! We must also recognize temptations that come into our lives and distance ourselves from them. We will always be tempted, but we can choose to distance ourselves from certain temptations that continually afflict us.

"AND THUS WE SEE"

Going back to the people of Ammon, these converted Lamanites suffered greatly on this earth for their sacrifice to join the Church. On more than one occasion, hundreds and even thousands of Ammonites were killed while not ever wielding a weapon in their own defense as they kept their covenants. Others were kicked out of their homeland and had to begin life anew in the land of Jershon.

A tremendous battle ensued not long after they moved to Jershon between the Nephites and the Lamanites, "such an one as never had been known among all the people in the land" (Alma 28:2). Many thousands of Nephites and Lamanites were slaughtered. Mormon interjected, "And thus we see how great the inequality of man is because of sin and transgression, and the power of the devil, which comes by the cunning plans which he hath devised to ensnare the hearts of men" (Alma 28:13).

What a wonderfully enlightening verse! Mormon described the people of Ammon being converted to the Lord and then having numerous, challenging struggles. They were all kicked out of their homeland and many were murdered by their fellow man.

Someone without any spiritual insight might look at this situation and conclude, "I agree. This is definitely an inequality! People became converted to the gospel and then experienced all sorts of difficulties, tragedies, and challenges. They were forced to leave their homeland. They were even put in positions in which many of them were murdered while defenseless. Obviously, life was much harder on those that became converted than it was for those who chose not to be converted."

And yet, Mormon was highlighting the eternal perspective and the contrast between the rewards reserved for the righteous and the hopeless state of the wicked. Mormon knew that those who died willingly without wielding their weapons after conversion had gone on to a glorious eternal life. And those Lamanites who were killed in battle that had not been converted were unprepared to meet their God.

We should not ever expect life to be fair or we will dwell on frequent feelings of injustice and be regularly disappointed. However, unlike the mortal compensation of our earthly journey, our works will be compensated by a perfectly just and magnificently merciful payment system in heaven. We will never be able to complain with regard to our heavenly wages. Our Father in Heaven is more gracious and generous in this regard than we could ever imagine.

Mormon obviously was inspired and directed in abridging the large plates of Nephi. He gave us some keen insights into what he was thinking and what he wanted us to learn from certain stories. He frequently wrote in summation of an experience, "and thus we see," as he did in this instance. He offered a brief summation and then had confidence that his readers would understand and receive their own insight. The phrase "and thus we see" is an absolute treasure and "doctrinal diamond" in the Book of Mormon. This phrase is used fifteen times by Mormon to introduce his insights. It is only used six other times in the Book of Mormon.

President Henry B. Eyring said, "What went before is what someone with spiritual sight will observe and then say, 'Oh, yes, now I see that.' And then follows, after the 'thus we see,' what that someone would see. When I understood that, I realized how gracious the word 'we' is in that phrase 'and thus we see.' The writer was saying, 'I include you with me among those who see.'"[12]

President Ezra Taft Benson once taught gospel teachers the following: "Your purpose is to increase testimony and faith. . . . Should you wonder how this is done, carefully study the Book of Mormon to see how Mormon did it with his 'and thus we see' passages."[13]

Going through these "and thus we see" passages throughout the Book of Mormon is a valuable, uplifting, and instructive practice. This particular "and thus we see" passage from Mormon about the inequality between the people of Ammon and the wicked Lamanites draws further attention to the inequality that resulted from their choices. Other gems are waiting to be unearthed as you study these passages.

BECOMING NEW CREATURES

Alma the Younger related his experience of repenting while he was struck dumb:

> And the Lord said unto me: Marvel not that all mankind, yea, men and women, all nations, kindreds, tongues, and people, must be born again; yea, born of God, changed from their carnal and fallen state, to a state of righteousness, being redeemed of God, becoming his sons and daughters;
>
> And thus they become new creatures; and unless they do this, they can in nowise inherit the kingdom of God. (Mosiah 27:25–26)

Going back to Alma 5:14, we are also asked if we have been spiritually born of God. A mighty change of heart is usually described in relation to being born again. As President Eyring said, God can "grant us a new heart and a new life."[14]

We all must be spiritually born again and rid ourselves of our carnal and fallen ways. We all must experience this mighty change of heart. President Ezra Taft Benson declared, "Can human hearts be changed? Why, of course! It happens every day in the great missionary work of the Church. It is one of the most widespread of Christ's modern miracles. If it hasn't happened to you—it should."[15]

President Spencer W. Kimball taught, "There are many people in this Church today who think they live, but they are dead to the spiritual things. And I believe even many who are making pretenses of being active are also spiritually dead. Their service is much of the letter and less of the spirit."[16]

If we are truly born again and experience a mighty change of heart, we will become disciples that live by the spirit of the law and not just the letter of the law. Those with whom we associate will see that we are spiritually alive and engaged. We will keep the commandments because we want to honor our God and express our love to Him. We will go to church because we desire to be spiritually fed and want to serve and uplift others. If we are merely checking off a list of things we have to do within the gospel, we are at risk of being spiritually dead, as President Kimball said. We have to show genuine excitement and enthusiasm for the gospel and the opportunity to be a member of Christ's Church here on earth.

With regard to our hearts, we should not get discouraged if we don't see necessary changes happening as quickly as we would like. If we stay on task, we will look back and it will become clear that the promises of the process have come to pass in our lives. We will find that our hearts are much more pure and clean than they were when we first tried to change. President Ezra Taft Benson said, "The Lord is pleased with every effort, even the tiny, daily ones in which we strive to be more like Him."[17] President Eyring promised, "Your habits of family prayer and scripture reading will create more lasting memories and greater changes of heart than you may realize now."[18] Sometimes, the change will be almost imperceptible, but it will be a positive change nonetheless.

While the story of the brother of Jared does not explicitly mention a mighty change of heart, we would like to bring up a couple of principles regarding repentance that relate to what we have been discussing. We have given examples in the Book of Mormon that illustrate how experiencing a mighty change of heart can be instantaneous. The people of Ammon, King Benjamin's people, Alma the Elder, and Alma the Younger and the sons of Mosiah fit this description. Many other individuals in the Book of Mormon further illustrate the same point, including Enos, Zeezrom, and King Lamoni's father, to name a few.

Elder Keith K. Hilbig said, "For most people in biblical and Book of Mormon times as well as today, this change of heart is not a singular event but rather a private and gradual process."[19] President Ezra Taft Benson said, "We must be cautious as we discuss these remarkable examples. Though they are real and powerful, they are the exception more than the rule. For every Paul, for every Enos, for every King Lamoni, there are hundreds and thousands of people who find the process of repentance much more subtle, much more imperceptible. Day by day they move closer to the Lord, little realizing they are building a godlike life."[20]

OLD HEARTS REMEMBERED NO MORE

At times, members of the Church are very hard on themselves. Sometimes, we want to be the judge of when our repentance is sufficient, but this is not our right. From the above examples, it is evident how quickly Heavenly Father wants to forgive us of our sins and how anxious the Savior wants to apply the grace and mercy afforded us through His Atonement. President Ezra Taft Benson said, "No one is more anxious to see us change our lives than the Father and the Savior."[21] He then referenced the Savior's invitation when He said, "Behold, I stand at the door, and knock: if any man hear my voice, and open the door, I will come in to him, and will sup with him, and him with me" (Revelation 3:20). The Savior is the one standing at the door and knocking, not us! He is that anxious to see us repent and return unto Him.

Complete forgiveness from repentance does not have a time limit set upon it unless dictated by priesthood authority. More importantly, it is the sincerity of our repentance and the follow through in making changes that determines our forgiveness. If we truly repent of our sins by confessing and forsaking them, we are forgiven and the Lord remembers our sins no more (see D&C 58:42–43).

Getting back to the brother of Jared, we read in Ether 2 that he and his people stayed upon the seashore for a space of four years. Apparently, the brother of Jared was not as diligent in keeping the commandments at this time as he should have been. The Lord stood before him in a cloud and chastened him for a space of three hours because he had not been calling on the name of the Lord (see Ether 2:14).

The brother of Jared had singular spiritual experiences with the Lord before this time. The Lord had been merciful unto him and his people when they pled to not have their language confounded. The Lord had stood in a cloud before the people and directed them where they should travel in the wilderness. The Lord had brought them all the way to the seashore in a very miraculous fashion.

Despite all of these miracles, the brother of Jared had stopped praying and had become slothful in his discipleship. After being chastened by the Lord, he repented and was forgiven. He was instructed to go to work and he did just that (see Ether 2:15–16). Not long after the brother of Jared had repented of his sins, the Lord appeared unto him in what is described as a way that never had man before been shown (see Ether 3:14–15). It is remarkably heartening that the brother of Jared could develop such mighty faith merely a couple of years after neglecting to call on the Lord for an extended period of time.

The brother of Jared could have had lingering doubts about his repentance. Instead, he had faith that the Atonement of Christ would allow him to be forgiven. He did not dwell on the years he lost that he might have been progressing—he forgave himself and committed to living the gospel more fully. He had faith that his sins were not remembered anymore and that every available gospel blessing could be his. And then he went to work! We take comfort in this story and the lesson it teaches us about the finality of repentance. We can repent and be forgiven of our sins and have faith that even the highest and most precious of gospel blessings can be ours.

This mighty change of heart, this spiritual rebirth, can only occur through the redeeming power of the Atonement and through the Holy Ghost's influence in this process. We can think of no greater blessing than to have the sanctifying power of the Holy Ghost and atoning blood of our Savior evident and working in our lives.

The Holy Ghost will be with us as we seek to rid our hearts of the natural man and become Saints. As we heed the Spirit's promptings, we will become something we never could otherwise become on our own. Our hearts will be cleansed and purified in ways only the Holy Ghost can bring about, by the power of the Atonement of Christ. Our lives will be richer in joy and happiness. We will walk how and where the Lord would have us walk. We will become more like Him, and our hearts will become more like His. Through the Atonement, our hearts can indeed become glorious, pure, and beautiful!

Chapter 6

PONDERING IN YOUR HEART

From the introduction to the Book of Mormon to its final chapters, pondering in our hearts to receive revelation is a frequently recurring, fundamental, and essential message. Pondering in the heart requires that the desires of the heart, the yearnings of the heart, the longings of the heart, and the cravings of the heart be focused toward the Lord in the search for answers. It is through this singleness of our heart's purpose and desire that pondering will invite the Spirit and bear the fruit of revelation.

TO PONDER IN OUR HEARTS OR MINDS?

Before we begin to study some of the examples described in the Book of Mormon, we want to first examine the significance of the phrase *pondering in our hearts*. Why is it that the Book of Mormon prophets chose to teach us about pondering in our hearts instead of pondering in our minds? Is there a difference between the two?

There are many subtle differences that can be drawn between matters of the heart and matters of the mind in scripture. Distinct enlightenment can come when we consider the differences, especially when trying to understand the act of pondering in our hearts. We are actually never instructed in the Book of Mormon to ponder things in our minds. Rather, we are taught to ponder things in our hearts. Modern revelation in the Doctrine and Covenants discusses this distinction between the heart and mind: "Yea, behold, I will tell you in your mind and in your heart, by the Holy Ghost, which shall come upon you and which shall dwell in your heart. Now behold, this is the spirit of revelation" (D&C 8:2–3).

This scripture is critical to our understanding of how the Holy Ghost operates in our lives. He can give us thoughts and ideas that enter our minds. Such thoughts and ideas "come upon us" as these verses indicate. He can also give us feelings and impressions that enter our hearts. These feelings and impressions don't just come upon us; they can actually "dwell in our hearts." Both thoughts and feelings are significant and critical aspects of personal revelation. However, in the Book of Mormon, we are provided evidence that the revelation we receive in our hearts may be more critical to the foundation and development of our personal testimonies of the gospel and our Savior, Jesus Christ than revelation we receive in our minds.

It is this relationship that allows people to become converted to Christ before they have a complete knowledge of basic gospel principles. President Harold B. Lee said, "When we understand more than we know with our minds, when we understand with our hearts, then we know that the Spirit of the Lord is working upon us."[1] This is not to say that understanding with our mind is not important; we are absolutely directed to seek knowledge with our minds too.

Can you think of the last time you tried to understand the gospel with your heart? Nephi taught that in addition to hearing the voice of the Spirit, we must *feel* the Holy Ghost's words (see 1 Nephi 17:45). In our experience, this type of revelation is much more frequent than hearing an actual voice. We feel the Spirit's words by identifying and listening to our feelings as we read the scriptures, pray, and go to church or the temple. We analyze how we feel when we keep a particular commandment or serve others. Spiritual things are often best understood by the heart. This is why the Book of Mormon teaches us so often to ponder things in our hearts. We should be pondering the feelings we experience as we strive to live the gospel. These feelings given by the Holy Ghost will never lead us astray.

The introduction to the Book of Mormon states, "We invite all men everywhere to read the Book of Mormon, to ponder in their hearts the message it contains, and then to ask God, the Eternal Father, in the name of Christ if the book is true." It is clear that prophets did not want us to get more than a page into the Book of Mormon before impressing upon us the importance of pondering in our hearts.

Moroni gave the following promise:

> Behold, I would exhort you that when ye shall read these things, if it be wisdom in God that ye should read them, that ye would remember how merciful the Lord hath been unto the children of men, from the creation of Adam even down until the time that ye shall receive these things, and ponder it in your hearts...And if ye shall ask with a sincere heart, with real intent, having faith in Christ, He will manifest the truth of it unto you, by the power of the Holy Ghost.
>
> And by the power of the Holy Ghost ye may know the truth of all things. (Moroni 10:3–5)

From this passage, we are taught that pondering in our hearts while remembering the Lord's mercies (feeling gratitude), and asking with sincerity of heart, real intent, and faith in Christ, will invite the manifestation of truth in our lives. Later in this chapter, we'll discuss other situations in the Book of Mormon where pondering in the heart is demonstrated and explained, but this seems like the perfect place for our discussion to begin.

Pondering in our hearts can be an intimidating subject for many of us. In the Guide to the Scriptures, to ponder means "to meditate and think deeply, often upon the scriptures or other things of God. When combined with prayer, pondering the things of God may bring revelation and understanding."[2] And how does this revelation come? "By the power of the Holy Ghost [we] may know the truth of all things (Moroni 10:5).

PONDERING IN OUR HEARTS BRINGS REVELATION

At those times in our lives when we are not feeling the Spirit with consistency or power, it can be very helpful to ask the question, "Why am I not feeling the Spirit more fully in my life?" Such vulnerable self-assessment is crucial to staying in touch with the Spirit. The Holy Ghost is remarkably willing at such times of humble self-reflection to show us those things that we need to work on to be more worthy of His companionship. As we wrestle to improve, the Spirit's influence will return to us and the experience will strengthen our testimony and resolve to sanctify ourselves.

The Church of Jesus Christ of Latter-day Saints is built upon personal revelation. Pondering in our hearts is one of the mightiest tools the Lord has given us to receive that revelation. God's children everywhere are called to the table of the Lord to feast upon that personal revelation. Nowhere is that better illustrated than the story of a lowly farm boy in upstate New York. Joseph Smith pondered upon James 1:5 and acted upon the prompting that came to him.

Joseph recounted, "Never did any passage of scripture come with more power to the heart of man than this did at this time to mine. It seemed to enter with great force into every feeling of my heart. I did reflect on it again and again" (Joseph Smith—History 1:12). We find it highly unlikely that Joseph's goal that day was to plow through and finish reading the five chapters of James.

Joseph reflected on this verse again and again. We love that from pondering a simple verse, the Restoration of the gospel commenced and a new dispensation was opened. Joseph did not just blow past this verse and keep going. He reflected on this particular verse again and again. As a result, he felt prompted to pray and ask

God for wisdom. If Joseph had not pondered upon this scripture and then acted as he did, where would we be today?

Pondering upon the things of God has led to many impactful and significant revelations received from the prophets of the Book of Mormon. When Lehi shared with his children his dream of the tree of life, it was his son Nephi that chose to ponder upon the things that his father had received. Nephi said, "For it came to pass after I had desired to know the things that my father had seen, and believing that the Lord was able to make them known unto me, *as I sat pondering in my heart* I was caught away in the Spirit of the Lord, yea, into an exceedingly high mountain, which I never had before seen, and upon which I never had before set my foot" (1 Nephi 11:1, emphasis added).

After Nephi pondered in his heart the things that his father had seen, the heavens opened, and he was shown the things his father had dreamed and was further shown *all* things (see 1 Nephi 14:24–26). This revelation would not have come to Nephi without a great deal of effort on his part, which included pondering in his heart upon the things his father taught him.

President Joseph F. Smith was pondering upon the scriptures in his room when he was given a magnificent revelation about the spirit world. He was shown Christ preaching the gospel to the spirits there. He was shown the organization of missionary work in the spirit world. In that vision, he saw Adam and Eve, Noah, Abraham, Isaac, Jacob, Moses, Isaiah, and many of the other noble and great ones that had lived upon this earth (see D&C 138). What a marvelous revelation that all began with the prophet pondering the scriptures in his heart!

At the end of the first day of the resurrected Savior teaching the Nephites, Jesus told the people to go home, ponder on what He had said, and pray to the Father for understanding. He knew they needed time to ponder and pray to gain this understanding, and He surely wanted them to go through this process to learn how to gain revelation in their lives (see 3 Nephi 17:2–3).

Alma told his son Corianton that he prayed for understanding of what happened to "the souls of men from the time of death to the time appointed for the resurrection" (Alma 40:7). Undoubtedly, Alma pondered upon this question in his heart. He said "he inquired diligently of God that he might know" (Alma 40:3). As a result of his diligence, pondering, and prayer, an angel came down and gave Alma this knowledge.

Joseph Smith and Sidney Rigdon were pondering upon a verse in the Gospel of John as Joseph was translating the New Testament. It reads, "And shall come forth; they that have done good, unto the resurrection of life; and they that have done evil, unto the resurrection of damnation" (John 5:29). As they pondered and meditated upon this scripture, one of the most glorious and significant visions since the Restoration of the Church came to them (see D&C 76).

Nephi's description of his love for the scriptures and the things of the Lord is worthy of our reflection. Nephi professed:

> And upon these things I write the things of my soul, and many of the scriptures which are engraven upon the plates of brass. For my soul delighteth in the scriptures, and my heart pondereth them, and writeth them for the learning and the profit of my children.
>
> Behold, my soul delighteth in the things of the Lord; and my heart pondereth continually upon the things which I have seen and heard. (2 Nephi 4:15–16)

The frequency and intensity with which we ponder determines the momentum we build toward receiving light and knowledge through the Spirit.

NEPHI AT THE GARDEN TOWER

Helaman 7–10 contains an extraordinary account of blessings poured out on the prophet Nephi as a result of his pondering in his heart. Though the events that led to his pondering were actually tumultuous and chaotic, a great spiritual outpouring was received in the quiet pondering that followed.

After finishing his prayer on his garden tower, Nephi preached to the gathered masses as one with great authority concerning the sins of the people and their need for repentance. Declaring our Father in Heaven's great condescension and His desire to mercifully bestow upon us every opportunity to change, a sign was given to the people through Nephi.

To demonstrate the power of his channel of communication with God, Nephi prophesied to the people that Seezoram had been murdered. Five messengers went to see for themselves if Nephi was speaking the truth. When they arrived and saw that Seezoram had indeed been murdered, they fell to the earth and were accused of the murder by those who later found them. Nephi was arrested shortly afterward and was brought before a number of judges.

We imagine a very emotionally charged scene in our minds, full of strong opinions and very vocal beliefs and judgments among the crowd and the judges. It was probably quite rancorous at different parts of the proceedings, filled with sharp contention and conflict. As the judges were intelligent people, they tried to trick Nephi into saying something that would incriminate himself. Nephi had to manage the questions they posed perfectly to avoid falling victim to their deceit and trickery.

Nephi eventually provided additional detail to the courts and announced that the chief judge Seezoram had been murdered by his brother, Seantum. Nephi was very specific in his prophesy of what Seantum would say when confronted. He also prophesied that Seantum would have blood on the skirts of his cloak, and even that Seantum's face would go pale to reveal his guilt. When the people went to question Seantum, Nephi's prophesy was proven in every particular. Seantum was taken into custody, and the five men were released, as was Nephi.

A very chaotic scene ensued as a great disagreement arose among the people. Some of the people believed Nephi to be a prophet at this point. Others went further and believed he was a god because of this miracle they had witnessed. And still others continued in their belief that he was not a prophet.

Here was Nephi, the focal point of an astonishing sequence of events, in the middle of a large group of people. Nephi may not have known at this point the Lord's will concerning him with his life hanging in the balance. It is likely that many in the multitude were seeking his death when he was bound and taken before the judges. It was just the day before that Nephi had called the people to repentance and prophesied that Seezoram had been murdered, laying the foundation for the adversity he would face over the next two days. The duration of these proceedings and the experience itself would have been emotionally draining.

It is a stunning scene to ponder. Mormon described it this way, "And it came to pass that there arose a division among the people, insomuch that they divided hither and thither and went their ways, leaving Nephi alone, as he was standing in the midst of them" (Helaman 10:1).

Eventually, after the crowd receded, Nephi was left standing there in wonderment, alone in the midst of a divided people. He then began the solitary journey to his own home. If you were Nephi at this point, wouldn't your mind be racing about what had just transpired? Would you be grateful for your safety and for the Lord's help in getting through this ordeal? Perhaps you would be thinking about the division of the people that still existed. Or might you be upset that there were still people too stubborn and hard-hearted to believe? Maybe Nephi was thinking about the tender mercies he had been given by God to have such things revealed unto him. Without question, Nephi was exhausted both physically and mentally from such an extended period of dramatic proceedings and ready for rest.

As he walked to his home, Nephi is said to have "pondered upon the things which the Lord had shown unto him" (Helaman 10:2). A voice came unto Nephi as "he was thus pondering in his heart" (verse 3). Again, a prophet of God is shown pondering upon the things of God in his heart, and a revelation is opened unto him. The Lord pronounced astonishing blessings upon Nephi, stating, "I will bless thee forever" (verse 5). Nephi was also given the sealing power that whatsoever he sealed on earth should be sealed in heaven, and whatsoever he loosed on earth should be loosed in heaven (verses 7–10).

As an aside, both of us relish the opportunity to take quiet walks to clear our minds and invite spiritual insight into our lives. Walking can be a very conducive activity for pondering and receiving revelation. The exercise is great for both the physical body as well as mental health, and wandering in God's majestic creations can train our thoughts on the things of the Lord. Many have gone into the mountains and other beautiful places in search of the divine.

It is important to scrutinize some of the things that Nephi did that led to this amazing moment and empowered his pondering. Nephi was able to push through fatigue and exhaustion, and continue wrestling for answers mentally. He was also cast down because of the people's works of darkness—his heart was grieving and open to comfort and consolation. Instead of being filled with hostility and focusing on the wrongs that had been committed, he instead pondered on the things that the Lord had shown unto him.

Finally, and absolutely vital to the receipt of revelation, Nephi demonstrated he was willing to act on the instructions he was given. Toward the end of his revelatory experience, he was told to go and declare these things to the people. In response, Nephi "did stop, and did not go unto his own house, but did return to the multitudes" (Helaman 10:12). He stopped dead in his tracks and immediately reversed course. He did not even go home to freshen up after such a draining experience. Surely, similar urgency in our response to the promptings we receive would clear the way for the receipt of additional revelation and instruction.

PONDERING THE SCRIPTURES

In a powerful sermon on revelation in 2 Nephi 32, Nephi expressed frustration with the people for not understanding how revelation works. After Nephi beautifully explained the doctrine of Christ in 2 Nephi 31, the people were not sure what they should do after they entered in by the way of baptism. Nephi was frustrated that the people were pondering what the next steps were.

Nephi responded that they needed to "feast upon the words of Christ; for behold, the words of Christ will tell you all things what ye should do" (2 Nephi 32:3). Nephi then promised that the Holy Ghost would show the people all the things they should do (see verse 5). In the verses that follow, Nephi once again expressed frustration that they were still pondering this in their hearts instead of searching the scriptures for knowledge. He then concluded by teaching the people that they should pray always and not perform anything unto the Lord without first praying that their performance be consecrated for the welfare of their souls. One of the takeaways from Nephi's frustrations may be that we should not get bogged down pondering over things for which we already have available answers. We need to search the scriptures for answers that are readily available before pondering in a search for more.

It is no coincidence that Nephi implores the people to feast upon the words of Christ and pray always. It is the perfect place to continue on the path toward Christ after entering through the gate of baptism. Prayer and feasting on the words of Christ will bring the Spirit into our lives, and the Holy Ghost will then teach us the things we should do. Elder Richard G. Scott said, "Pondering a passage of scripture can be a key to unlock revelation and the guidance and inspiration of the Holy Ghost. Scriptures can calm an agitated soul, giving peace, hope, and a restoration of confidence in one's ability to overcome the challenges of life."[3]

Among the greatest tools the Lord has provided to enrich our pondering are the holy scriptures. Great blessings will come to us if we are taking the time to ponder the scriptures in our hearts. Pondering, coupled with sincere prayer, as the Guide to the Scriptures states, can bring revelation and understanding to us.[4] President Thomas S. Monson stated, "As we read and ponder the scriptures, we will experience the sweet whisperings of the Spirit to our souls. We can find answers to our questions. We learn of the blessings which come through keeping God's commandments. We gain a sure testimony of our Heavenly Father and our Savior, Jesus Christ, and of Their love for us."[5]

Elder D. Todd Christofferson promised, "Study the scriptures carefully, deliberately. Ponder and pray over them. Scriptures are revelation, and they will bring added revelation."[6] How can we be more 'deliberate' in our study of the scriptures? Elder Quentin L. Cook said, "Pondering the scriptures regularly—rather than reading them occasionally—can substitute a superficial understanding for a sublime, life-changing enhancement of our faith."[7] Each of us needs life-changing enhancements of faith in this challenging and rebellious world.

The apostolic promises made to those who will diligently search the scriptures are legion: Added revelation; a life-changing enhancement of our faith; guidance and inspiration from the Holy Ghost; the calming of an agitated soul; and so much more are available to those that pay the price of diligent, personal scripture study. These are powerful promises that we have experienced in our own lives, and these blessing are attainable for all. But like so many other blessings of the gospel, the blessings of diligent scripture study only come after much effort on our part.

Some good questions to ask may be the following: Have I pondered the scriptures or other things of God regularly in the last week? Do I have a set amount of time each day when I make time to ponder, reflect, or meditate?

SPENDING A SET AMOUNT OF TIME

If your lives are at all similar to ours, it can be very difficult to make time to consistently ponder and do it properly. Yet both modern prophets as well as prophets of old have taught how vital this practice can be for our personal testimonies and spiritual understanding. President David O. McKay said, "I think we pay too little attention to the value of meditation; a principle of devotion. Meditation is one of the most secret, most sacred doors through which we pass into the presence of the Lord."[8]

One of the best things we have done with our scripture study is to set aside a certain amount of time each day. We push hard to study and ponder the Book of Mormon at least half an hour a day, in addition to time for the study of other scripture. While it is good to read a chapter a day or a certain number of pages (any time is better than no time!), we believe such a practice is "looking beyond the mark" in our scripture study (Jacob 4:14). When we determine a fixed amount that must be read, we tend to focus more on completion of the task than we do to listening to the Spirit as we seek revelation.

By setting aside a timeframe for study, we will not feel rushed to get through a chapter or set number of pages in the scriptures. Being taught what we need to learn about a doctrine or principle will not be limited to the number of verses we read. We can take as much time as is effective to learn more about a certain topic. We will be able to ponder and pray about what we have read.

If we set aside a specific amount of time, effort spent meditating and pondering will do as much to complete our goal as reading does! We might ponder how we are doing in our own lives with a particular commandment or situation we are studying. We may end up reading just a handful of verses and spending most of our time pondering those verses as well as quotes and other references in the scriptures on that topic. Such study can be fantastically effective!

President Henry B. Eyring described the difference between reading, studying, and pondering the scriptures. He said, "Reading, studying, and pondering are not the same. We read words and we may get ideas. We study and we may discover patterns and connections in scripture. But when we ponder, we invite revelation by the Spirit. Pondering, to me, is the thinking and the praying I do after reading and studying in the scriptures carefully."[9]

How would our scripture study measure on President Eyring's scale? Please do not misunderstand us. It is wonderful to read the scriptures. However, it is even better to study them. And it is far better yet to diligently ponder and pray about them as we read and study.

President Henry B. Eyring also said, "We may be nourished more by pondering a few words, allowing the Holy Ghost to make them treasures to us, than by passing quickly, and superficially, over whole chapters of scripture."[10] Personal revelation is much more apt to come to us if we are not in a rush. If we are taking the time to ponder and pray as a part of our scripture study, personal revelation will flow into us. What a tremendous blessing this can be in our lives!

Some helpful questions to ask may be: When was the last time I received personal revelation? What was I doing when I last received personal revelation? Where was I and what was the setting? How frequently do I receive such inspiration in my life? Do I write such occurrences down somewhere and ponder upon what I have learned?

WRITE IT DOWN

We are very grateful for edifying experiences we have had while pondering the scriptures in our hearts. As we have pondered the scriptures, revelation has come in many different ways. Often, excerpts from our patriarchal blessings have settled in our minds as we reflected on what we were reading. Such insights that come through pondering in our hearts can give much needed direction at defining moments in our lives, moments that will determine our eternal destiny.

We have learned that what we do with revelation we receive is just as critical as initially receiving revelation. Elder Richard G. Scott said, "Write down in a secure place the things you learn from the Spirit. You will find that as you write down precious impressions, often more will come. Also, the knowledge you gain will be available throughout your life."[11]

Elder Scott gave a wonderful example of how writing down revelation he had received had blessed his life. He related the following story of when he received some personal revelation:

Subsequently I prayed, reviewing with the Lord what I thought I had been taught by the Spirit. When a feeling of peace came, I thanked Him for the guidance given. I was then impressed to ask, "Was there yet more to be given?" I received further impressions, and the process of writing down the impressions, pondering, and praying for confirmation was repeated. Again I was prompted to ask, "Is there more I should know?" And there was. When that last, most sacred experience was concluded, I had received some of the most precious, specific, personal direction one could hope to obtain in this life. Had I not responded to the first impressions and recorded them, I would not have received the last, most precious guidance.

What I have described is not an isolated experience. It embodies several true principles regarding communication from the Lord to His children here on earth. I believe that you can leave the most precious, personal direction of the Spirit unheard because you do not respond to, record, and apply the first promptings that come to you.[12]

Those moments when revelation flows into our lives can be some of the most cherished experiences in our personal spiritual histories. In looking through the Notes app on his phone, Derek found a note that illustrates the reward of pondering in our hearts. A note on 2/17/17 states, "Reading at 12:00 at night. Learning much about Joseph Smith and 2 Nephi 3 as a chiasmus. Extra effort to complete my half hour is being rewarded by inspiration and learning!"

There have been other times where Derek has written down warnings he received from the Holy Ghost to avoid certain temptations that deprive us of His influence. On one occasion, he wrote the following: "We withdraw from the Spirit, not the other way around. He is anxious to be there for us." This one thought then led to further pondering on those things that we do to withdraw from the Spirit.

Once when Ryan was pondering faith in an effort to build faith and achieve a much-desired righteous goal, a somewhat contrary impression came to him: "Sometimes we are so busy developing the faith to get, we never know the faith to go without. We are so concerned with the faith to receive, we forget about the faith to accept. We are so consumed by the faith to do that we are oblivious of the faith required to be done unto. We are so desperate to cultivate faith unto deliverance that we miss the divinity of exercising faith in bondage." That highly personalized and applicable revelation provided a wealth of spiritual muscle at a time his strength was flagging.

We have also written down questions that have come into our minds as we study certain passages of scripture. We have then studied those questions and learned a great deal and strengthened our testimonies in the process. One of the greatest levers of being able to draw on the power of the Holy Ghost through pondering is beginning with the wonderfully right question. Frequently, we will simply feel the Spirit conveying our Savior's love as an answer to the right question. These sweet moments can be every bit as effective at helping shape our lives and drawing us toward the Savior as those moments where specific direction is given.

It is remarkable how often we can receive inspiration from the Spirit. We have felt through experience that our Father in Heaven is astonishingly willing to send His Spirit to help His children. He is no respecter of persons and desires to share as much as can be borne by all His children.

President Lorenzo Snow said, "It is the grand privilege of every Latter-day Saint to have the manifestations of the Spirit every day of our lives."[13] Mormon teaches us that the brothers Nephi and Lehi had "many revelations *daily*" (see Helaman 11:23, emphasis added). It is our privilege to have this same blessing in our lives. Learning the language of the Spirit and heeding His promptings in our lives is one of our greatest opportunities and duties as Latter-day Saints. As we write down the promptings we receive and follow them quickly, additional promptings will come, and they will begin to come more frequently and more distinctly.

How marvelous it is to consider the phrase *companionship of the Holy Ghost*. We are not blessed with the chance to feel the Spirit every now and then. We are not blessed with the Holy Ghost to be with us from time to time. We are blessed with the opportunity to have the constant companionship of the Holy Ghost. Companionship refers to friendship, fellowship, and attachment— a friendship that can be constant. The Holy Ghost can be the kind of friend to us that we hear from daily, even frequently throughout the day, if we do our part.

THE ROCK OF REVELATION

Personal revelation is so fundamental to the gospel that Moroni closed what he thought would be his final words in the Book of Mormon by speaking of revelation, miracles, and faith in Mormon 9. At this time, Moroni assumed this chapter would be the last thing he would share with us as he was planning to conclude with the abridgment of the Jaredites' account.

Moroni urged us:

And again I speak unto you who deny the revelations of God, and say that they are done away, that there are no revelations, nor prophecies, nor gifts, nor healing, nor speaking with tongues, and the interpretation of tongues;

Behold I say unto you, he that denieth these things knoweth not the gospel of Christ; yea, he has not read the scriptures; if so, he does not understand them. (Mormon 9:7–8)

Jesus shared a similar message while questioning His disciples. Jesus said:

He saith unto them, but whom say ye that I am?

And Simon Peter answered and said, Thou are the Christ, the son of the living God.

And Jesus answered and said unto him, Blessed art thou Simon Bar-jona: for flesh and blood hath not revealed it unto thee, but my Father which is in heaven.

And I say also unto thee, That thou art Peter, and upon this rock I will build my church; and the gates of hell shall not prevail against it. (Matthew 16:15–18)

What is this rock that the Church was to be built upon? Elder Bruce R. McConkie said that this is the rock of revelation. "And how could it be otherwise? There is no other foundation upon which the Lord could build His Church and kingdom. The things of God are known only by the power of His Spirit. God stands revealed or remains forever unknown. No man can know that Jesus is the Lord but by the Holy Ghost."[14]

The gospel of Jesus Christ is indeed built upon the rock of revelation, and such revelation was never intended to be limited to a select few. Pondering in our hearts is the key that unlocks this much-needed personal revelation. God is the same yesterday, today, and forever, and is He is no respecter of persons (see Mormon 9:9, Acts 10:34). Revelations have been given to people since the beginning, regardless of their socio-economic circumstances. Divine communication has flown unto God's children irrespective of their earthly prominence, status, or importance. It pours out on those who diligently seek it and follow the prescribed guidelines for its receipt. It is so today, and it will be so tomorrow.

Revelation is available to all of us. However, it is up to us to seek it—studying the scriptures, praying with all of our might, and persistently pondering these things in our hearts. It is then that a steadfast river of revelation will flow into our lives, bringing the heavenly peace that comes when we know we are communing with the Lord. May we consistently find a time to ponder upon the scriptures and things of God in our hearts. As we do so, revelation will come, and mighty blessings promised from prophets and apostles of the Lord will be ours.

Chapter 7

LOWLINESS IN HEART

While lowliness in our hearts or being poor in heart are phrases only mentioned thirteen times in the Book of Mormon, the doctrine is of vital importance for us on our path to a truly converted heart. Mormon taught his people, "For none is acceptable before God, save the meek and lowly in heart" (Moroni 7:44). Elder Neal A. Maxwell said in regard to this verse, "If we could but believe, really believe, in the reality of that bold, but accurate declaration, you and I would find ourselves focusing on the crucial rather than the marginal tasks in life."[1]

To be accepted before God, we must be lowly in heart! Jesus described himself in such terms when He said, "Learn of me; for I am meek and lowly in heart" (Matthew 11:29). So, what exactly does it mean to be lowly in heart? And how do we develop this virtue? There are a couple of great teaching moments in the Book of Mormon that exemplify lowliness in heart and how we can cultivate this characteristic. These teachings also detail great and mighty blessings promised to those who are lowly in heart.

The Zoramites in Antionum

We will begin our discussion with one of the greatest teaching moments in the Book of Mormon found in Alma chapters 32–34. Alma and a group of seven other missionaries are found trying to preach to the apostate Zoramites in Antionum at this time. Here again, there may be deeper meaning in the land being called Antionum. We previously wrote about Zeezrom in Antionah in the chapter on hardheartedness and mentioned that both *ezrom* and *antion* were units of silver and gold used by the Nephites. Here, the land of Antionum could also have deeper meaning by reference to the gold unit of an *antion* with "*–um*" being a commonly used geographical suffix. The Zoramites' "hearts were set upon gold, and upon silver, and upon all manner of fine goods" (Alma 31:24). The name of this city fits very well with the state of the Zoramites' hearts at the time.

Although they found no success preaching to those with worldly wealth, Alma and his companions began to preach and have success among the poorer class of people. As Alma was preaching upon the hill Onidah, a great multitude of people approached him from behind. They were poor in heart as a result of their poverty. Mormon describes this people as being "in a preparation to hear the word" because of their humility and lowliness in heart (Alma 32:6). The leader among this group further epitomized their lowliness in heart as he twice asked Alma, "What shall these my brethren do? . . . What shall we do?" (Alma 32:5). Surely great and mighty blessings await those who possess such lowliness in heart (see Alma 22:15; Acts 2:37)!

President Harold B. Lee said, "The poor in spirit means those who are spiritually needy, who feel so impoverished spiritually that they reach out with great yearning for help."[2] This is exactly what this group was doing! Alma quickly turned away from the group to whom he had been preaching and began to teach this group that was poor in heart.

Have you ever reached out with similar yearning for help or forgiveness in a moment of crisis? Picture someone hanging on by one hand on the edge of a cliff, reaching out with the other hand to a rescuer, with life itself hanging in the balance. We will all find ourselves in situations or moments in life when we need to reach out to Heavenly Father with such great yearning. While pride prevents us from asking for and accepting help, the lowly in heart are quick to ask and receptive and welcoming of counsel and answers. When we plead for forgiveness with intensity and purpose, when we understand our own nothingness before God and our dependence upon the Savior's Atonement and its accompanying mercy and grace, help and answers will come.

Alma recognized that these Zoramites were lowly in heart and even told them so. He said, "I behold that ye are lowly in heart; if so, blessed are ye" (Alma 32:8). Lowliness of heart is characterized by humility, gentleness, and the ability to be taught. The Zoramites were compelled to be humble because of their dire circumstances, but their lowliness of heart would be a great blessing to them going forward. They continued to ask questions of Alma as he taught them, and they accepted his answers as the pure truth that it was. They were converted to the gospel because they were initially lowly in heart and were prepared to receive the word of God.

Alma described "stubbornness of heart" as the opposite of lowliness of heart (Alma 32:16). People with stubbornness of heart would not have asked Alma for guidance about what they should do to worship God. People with stubbornness of heart would not have been receptive to the answers that Alma and Amulek offered. People with stubbornness of heart would not have chosen the gospel when faced with getting kicked out of the only home they had ever known.

THE SMALL FISH

We have both had many moments in our lives when we have needed to be lowly in heart, willing to reach out to others and particularly to Heavenly Father with great yearning. Derek had one such experience that has stuck with him through a lifetime. In his words:

141

At times, I've had medical issues arise that I couldn't endure or overcome on my own. I've reached out for priesthood blessings for comfort that could come in no other way. I've humbly pled for a business to be saved so I could provide for my family. I've reached out to be cleansed from sins I've shamefully committed.

One such moment of reaching out with great yearning for help in my life came when I was twelve years old. My dad had invited me to come along on a high adventure scouting trip with the older scouts in our ward. We camped up in the High Uintas for a week and had a great time. One day, my dad and I decided to go on a hike to a lake a few miles away. Looking back, I was particularly ill-prepared for this hike. We started off on what was a beautiful day and we were having a good time. We hiked for a couple of hours when I started to experience symptoms of stomach ulcers. I had stomach ulcers that caused severe pain from time to time and seemed to get worse without food. I continued forward for a while, but my condition and pain only worsened. I ended up telling my dad I couldn't continue hiking. As I said before, we were poorly prepared for potential problems on what was supposed to be just a day hike. We didn't even bring any food in our backpacks.

I felt completely helpless. I didn't have the strength to get back to camp on my own, and my dad didn't have the strength to carry me that far over the rough mountain terrain. Fortunately, we were next to one of the many lakes up in the High Uintas and had a fishing pole with us. My dad and I both prayed that he would be able to catch some fish that we could cook and eat to help me get feeling better. We yearned greatly for the Lord's help. We felt completely dependent on Him to help us out of this situation. I was physically debilitated and extremely needy at that time.

My dad was blessed to catch a fish on one of his first casts. It was a scrawny, little six-inch trout that you would never keep except under these circumstances. My dad started a fire and cooked that fish while he continued trying to catch a few more. He is a very good fisherman, and coupled with our many prayers, I figured he would catch a few more in short order, and I would start feeling better. Unfortunately, he never did catch another fish.

Once the small fish was cooked, we asked a blessing on it that it would fill me up so I could feel better and get back down the mountain to our camp. There must have been only two or three good little bites of meat on that fish. Miraculously, I was filled from that small fish. I remember that feeling well, even twenty-five years after it occurred. I felt better almost immediately and was able to hike back down the mountain to our camp without any issues. I will never read the stories of the Savior providing loaves and fishes miraculously to His followers in the same way. Heavenly Father taught us that we didn't need to catch a few large fish. Instead, He would provide for us in His own way.

As we reach out to our Heavenly Father in humble prayer for what we lack, He richly blesses us with what we need most. More important than being blessed physically, He can bless us with rich supply spiritually when we are poor in heart. The beauty of reaching out to others, or to Heavenly Father specifically, is in the blessings that we receive from this stretching of our souls. We learn how to pray with true sincerity of heart. We expand our faith in our Savior and His redeeming power. We learn to be more grateful for the power of the priesthood when we receive blessings. We learn to draw closer to the Lord by recognizing that we need Him to lift our burdens. We learn to be more sensitive to the influence of the Holy Ghost, and we learn to better recognize the things we do that keep the Spirit with us, as well as those that drive Him away.

PLANTING THE WORD IN OUR HEARTS

Alma's sermon on comparing the word unto a seed and how to increase our faith and gain knowledge takes on added significance and meaning when he teaches that we must give place that a seed may be planted in our hearts. If our hearts are not lowly, we simply cast the seed out due to our unbelief. If our hearts are stubborn, we will not give place for the seed. Hence, we will not progress in our testimonies and knowledge of the gospel. To emphasize this important doctrine, Alma and Amulek focused their teaching on planting the seed in our hearts four separate times (see Alma 32:28; 33:1, 23; 34:4).

Like stubbornness of heart, hardheartedness is also in opposition to lowliness in heart. Whereas hardheartedness repels the Spirit from entering into our hearts, lowliness of heart is akin to opening up our hearts and allowing the Spirit to enter. The lowly in heart are not concerned with people's perceptions regarding the imperfections and stains on their hearts. Rather, they open their hearts wide to say, "Hey, I need some help with all of this. I don't have all the answers, and I can't do it all on my own. Can you help me?"

Opening our hearts is mentioned twice in the Book of Mormon. In both of these instances, we are promised understanding if we open our hearts up to the Lord (see Mosiah 2:9; 3 Nephi 19:33). Those with open hearts have been promised great blessings by leaders of the Church. Elder Joseph B. Wirthlin promised, "If we would open our hearts to the refining influence of this unspeakable gift of the Holy Ghost, a glorious new spiritual dimension would come to light. We could know for ourselves things of the Spirit that are choice, precious, and capable of enlarging the soul, expanding the mind, and filling the heart with inexpressible joy."[3]

This new spiritual dimension of personal revelation and teachings from the Holy Ghost is attainable for all members of the Church. Instead of just going through the motions spiritually, we can receive indispensable personalized instruction and guidance at any moment we so need it. Too many members of the Church have never experienced this spiritual dimension and do not know how to tap into "the unspeakable gift of the Holy Ghost" (D&C 121:26).

How can we open up our hearts to the influence of the Holy Ghost? We need to listen to His promptings and follow them. If we desire to receive promptings from the Holy Ghost, we must ask Heavenly Father for the companionship of the Holy Ghost and then do our best to be worthy to receive such promptings. Then, when we receive a prompting, we need to write it down and act on it quickly! We need to show the Lord that we value and treasure these promptings and want to follow His will.

President Henry B. Eyring said, "When you demonstrate your willingness to obey, the Spirit will send you more impressions of what God would have you do for Him. As you obey, the impressions from the Spirit will come more frequently, becoming closer and closer to constant companionship."[4]

The thirteenth general president of the Relief Society, Sister Mary Ellen Smoot, said, "Service softens and opens hearts, for it is truly the gospel in action."[5] We feel this softening in our hearts every time we help out with a service project or do something kind for someone else. Not only does this service soften our hearts, but also it makes our hearts more receptive to the whisperings of the Spirit. We will be more prepared to hear the promptings of the Holy Ghost when we choose to serve others.

The seed or word that Alma and Amulek taught was Christ. The Zoramites recognized that the only way they could receive the word and nurture the seed was to open their hearts up to Him. By opening our hearts to Christ, we, too, can eagerly answer the "great question that Amulek posed—namely, is there really a redeeming Christ?" (see Alma 34:5).[6] The Book of Mormon resonates with a resounding yes to that great question. Yes, there really is a redeeming Christ! He has provided a way for us to return to live with Him and Heavenly Father. If we will keep our focus on our Savior and nourish the seed we have planted with faith, diligence, and patience, then it will become a tree springing up unto eternal life.

MEEKNESS, FAITH, HOPE, AND CHARITY

A second teaching moment about lowliness of heart is found in Mormon's exceptional sermon on faith, hope, and charity in Moroni 7. There is a vital characteristic in addition to faith, hope, and charity that often gets overlooked and goes unmentioned in speaking about this sermon. Mormon taught:

> And again, behold I say unto you that he cannot have faith and hope, *save he shall be meek, and lowly of heart.*
>
> If so, his faith and hope is vain, for none is acceptable before God, *save the meek and lowly in heart*; and if a man be *meek and lowly in heart*, and confesses by the power of the Holy Ghost that Jesus is the Christ, he must needs have charity; for if he have not charity he is nothing; wherefore he must needs have charity. (Moroni 7:43–44, emphasis added)

Elder Neal A. Maxwell said, "One cannot develop those other crucial virtues—faith, hope, and charity—without meekness. Meekness is often the initiator, facilitator, and consolidator."[7] Indeed, these verses indicate that meekness and lowliness of heart come before faith, hope, and charity. The only other necessary qualification to have charity is to confess by the power of the Holy Ghost that Jesus is the Christ.

In almost every reference to lowliness of heart in the Book of Mormon, this virtue is coupled with meekness. The word *meek* is defined as "patient, long-suffering, or submissive in disposition of nature; humble."[8] Elder Ulisses Soares defined meekness as "God-fearing, righteous, humble, teachable, and patient under suffering."[9]

Under these definitions, is there any wonder that Christ is the perfect example of meekness? He suffered incomprehensible agony and pain both in the Garden of Gethsemane and upon the cross at Golgotha. Yet the first three recorded sayings we have from Jesus while on the cross were for the benefit of others. While upon the cross, Jesus asked Heavenly Father to forgive those who did this to Him (see Luke 23:34). To the thief on his side, Jesus told him he would be in paradise with Him that day (see Luke 23:43). Jesus told His mother, Mary, that John would now be her son and would take care of her, and told John that Mary was now his mother, in essence telling John to care for his mother (see John 19:26–27). As the Atonement of Christ was happening, amidst intense suffering and pain, Jesus was still concerned about others more than Himself. Surely no one would be capable of demonstrating the same loving concern on the cross as did our Savior!

Jesus never murmured about His difficulties in life. He never complained about the brutal and unrelenting ironies He experienced on earth, a world that He Himself created. How easy it would have been—how tempting it could have been—to do just one thing for Himself. He could have shown his marvelous powers in a way to lift Himself above everyone. He could have easily thrown Himself from the pinnacle of the temple in dramatic fashion to prove to the people that He was indeed our Lord and Redeemer. Instead, Jesus always expressed His mission as following Heavenly Father's will in all things. He always did things for His Father, never for Himself. What an example of meekness and a lowly heart!

Elder Maxwell stated, "God has told us to be meek in order to enhance our enjoyment of life and our mortal education."[10] Have you ever thought of meekness and lowliness of heart being linked to an increased enjoyment of life? How does that work?

Elder Maxwell gave some examples of how these characteristics lead to increased enjoyment of life. He said:

> The meek are filled with awe and wonder with regard to God and His purposes in the universe. It is the observing meek who will contemplate the lilies of the field, will ponder the galaxies and see God moving in His majesty, will notice, and then lift up, those whose hands hang down.
>
> Because they make fewer demands of life, the meek are less easily disappointed. Meekness can also help us in coping with the injustices of life—of which there are quite a few. Among the meek there is usually more listening and less talking. Meekness permits us to be confident.[11]

These are all attributes that lead to a smoother, more enjoyable journey throughout life. Will the meek and lowly in heart be tested? Of course! But they will be more prepared to be tutored through life's experiences and become the people the Lord would have them be. They will stop to smell the roses and savor the beauty of His creations. They will humbly follow the prophet and other chosen servants of the Lord. They will confidently follow the Savior and will live fuller lives as a result.

MORONI AND PAHORAN

One of our favorite examples of this attribute of the heart is found toward the end of the book of Alma. At this point, Captain Moroni had been the Nephite commander for approximately twelve years. He was still out on the battlefront and must have been extremely fatigued by this point. He had seen countless people die under his command as well as the deaths of many fighting on the side of the Lamanites. No one had a better understanding than Moroni of what the wars had cost both the Nephites and the Lamanites.

In Alma 60, Moroni sent an epistle unto the chief judge, Pahoran. In a blow to the Nephite cause, the Lamanites had just taken the city of Nephihah. Moroni felt like that loss was preventable and was extremely direct and very emotional with Pahoran in an epistle. He used many cutting words and stinging phrases with the chief judge.

Some of the harsh rebukes of Moroni in this chapter include the following: "Great has been your neglect towards us" (Alma 60:5). "Can you think to sit upon your thrones in a state of thoughtless stupor?" (verse 7). "Ye have withheld your provisions from [our armies]" (verse 9). "The blood of thousands shall come upon your heads for vengeance" (verse 10). "The slothfulness of our government" (verse 14). "We know not but what ye yourselves are seeking for authority" (verse 18). "We know not but what ye are also traitors to your country" (verse 18). "Behold, I wait for assistance from you; and except ye do administer unto our relief, behold, I come unto you . . . and smite you with the sword" (verse 30). "Ye know that ye do transgress the laws of God, and ye do know that ye do trample them under your feet" (verse 33).

Can you imagine placing yourself in Pahoran's shoes? Imagine that you receive a letter from someone you consider a dear friend in which that person criticizes you, calls you a traitor, and says the blood of all those that died in the cause of the Nephites will be upon your head because of your lack of governing. This person even threatens to kill you if you don't do something about it. Obviously, Moroni did not fully know what was going on back home, just as we so often are not in possession of the whole story when we choose to criticize others.

Criticism is one of the most difficult things for people to handle without a meek and lowly heart. It is extremely challenging to be criticized and then react positively to that censure. Pahoran is a tremendous example for how he responded to Moroni's epistle. He was truly meek and lowly in heart in his response to Moroni.

In Pahoran's response to Moroni, we read, "And now, in your epistle you have censured me, but it mattereth not; I am not angry, but do rejoice in the greatness of your heart" (Alma 61:9). Pahoran goes so far as to say, "And now, Moroni, I do joy in receiving your epistle" (verse 19). And he closes his epistle with the words, "To my beloved brother, Moroni" (verse 21).

Pahoran's reaction is crammed with humility! How many of us would have reacted in the same way Pahoran did, instead of getting defensive and launching a counterattack? Much could be written and surmised from this exchange between Moroni and Pahoran. A case could be made that Pahoran was a passive leader who needed to hear this message in this fashion to feel a greater sense of urgency. However, even if Pahoran needed to hear this message, it wouldn't make it any easier for him to process it like he did. This story is definitely worth pondering in greater depth to gain more spiritual application from their exchange.

Captain Moroni was a huge hero of Mormon. Moroni was obviously greatly admired by Mormon, based on how much is said about him in the Book of Mormon. Mormon even named his son after this great captain. Mormon described Moroni in these words—"If all men had been, and were, and ever would be, like unto Moroni, behold, the very powers of hell would have been shaken forever; yea, the devil would never have power over the hearts of the children of men" (Alma 48:17). So, why is Mormon including these two epistles in his review and analysis of the war that had gone on for so long?

We believe one reason Mormon included these letters was to show the courage, strength, and leadership of Moroni. It does appear that Pahoran may have been quite passive as a leader, as we suggested above. Moroni uses quite a few statements in his epistle to Pahoran that would indicate such passivity. Some things he said to Pahoran include the following: "While [ye] sit upon your thrones and do not make use of the means which the Lord has provided for us . . . While ye sit in idleness . . . While ye sit still and behold these things . . . Begin to be up and doing" (see Alma 60:21–24).

When Pahoran first became chief judge, Moroni was allowed to execute king-men who were uprising against Pahoran and the government for treason. Why was Pahoran so apprehensive to go against these traitors in the same way at this time when Moroni had done so just five years earlier? He told Moroni he was worried about what he should do (see Alma 61:19). Why didn't Pahoran just treat these insurrectionists as traitors, as they had been dealt with before? Though it is interesting to ponder these circumstances, we cannot pass judgment; there could have been a variety of factors that led to this delay.

In Alma 59, Moroni sent a first epistle to Pahoran asking for more reinforcements, but Moroni apparently did not hear back from Pahoran. We do not know exactly why Moroni did not receive a response from Pahoran from the account that is given; there is not a great deal of detail. We do know Pahoran was forced out of Zarahemla and fled to Gideon, and his lack of a response may have occurred during this tumultuous time.

Whatever the reason for the lack of response, Moroni sent a second epistle, which was much more forceful. Perhaps Moroni chose to be this direct to get his point across with Pahoran. The

Nephite armies were in a very dire situation at this time and were about to perish with hunger. The cities the Nephites had miraculously regained were in peril and in danger of being lost again. The entire outcome of these wars hung in the balance. Moroni did not want to lose any of the momentum they had gained and have the war drag on any longer.

While we are not discounting the reaction Pahoran gave Moroni, we are also not ready to fault Moroni for his second epistle. Moroni received revelation which he shared with Pahoran. He said, "Behold, the Lord saith unto me: If those whom ye have appointed your governors do not repent of their sins and iniquities, ye shall go up to battle against them" (Alma 60:33). While we do not have all the details, this condemnation of the Lord seems to suggest that there were problems in ranks of the political leadership.

It can be spiritually productive to ponder these questions and others as we go about our study of the scriptures. We find that the more questions we ask as we read and study the scriptures, the more we are taught by the Spirit. As we have written down questions as they come to our minds when studying the scriptures, the search for answers has resulted in some of our most effective study sessions. The depth of learning available to us in the scriptures is inexhaustible or "unsearchable" as Jacob describes it (Jacob 4:8). Communion with the Spirit ensures we can always glean more from the scriptures, no matter how many times we have read them.

THE SERMON AT THE TEMPLE

The final teaching moment about lowliness of heart that we will discuss is from the Savior's sermon to the Nephites—the Sermon at the Temple, as it is widely called today. Jesus used the phrase "poor in spirit," which is synonymous with being poor in heart. In the Sermon on the Mount and in the Sermon at the Temple, Jesus taught the people the Beatitudes. To the Nephites, He taught, "Yea, blessed are the poor in spirit who come unto me, for theirs is the kingdom of heaven" (3 Nephi 12:3). This differs from the

Sermon on the Mount in which is recorded, "Blessed are the poor in spirit: for theirs is the kingdom of heaven" (Matthew 5:3).

Some people discount the Sermon at the Temple in the Book of Mormon by saying that it is basically the same thing as the Sermon on the Mount. There are actually many key differences between the two sermons. The somewhat subtle but very significant addition of the phrase "who come unto me" reminds us that suffering, hardship, or even just being poor in spirit are only beneficial if experiencing those things is accompanied with us coming unto the Savior.

The Savior's simple invitation "come unto me" is one of our favorite teachings in 3 Nephi 12. The King James Version of Matthew 5 does not include a single instance of the phrase "come unto me." 3 Nephi 12, however, includes this phrase six times! The Savior is very clearly pleading with us to come unto Him. This invitation was one of His central messages in this sermon that could otherwise have been lost. The Savior eagerly wants us to come unto Him, live like He would live, and do what He would do. He knows this is the way to find joy in this life and eternal life in the world to come.

It is very fitting that when the Savior is first heard speaking to the Nephites as well as in the last chapter of 3 Nephi, the Savior is pleading for us to come unto Him. Some of the Savior's first words to the people of Nephi were, "Yea, verily I say unto you, if ye will *come unto me* ye shall have eternal life. Behold, mine arm of mercy is extended towards you, and whosoever will come, him will I receive; and blessed are those who *come unto me*" (3 Nephi 9:14, emphasis added). The Savior's last recorded words in the book of 3 Nephi are, "Turn, all ye Gentiles, from your wicked ways; and repent of your evil doings . . . and from all your wickedness and abominations, *and come unto me*, and be baptized in my name, that ye may receive a remission of your sins, and be filled with the Holy Ghost, that ye may be numbered with my people who are of the house of Israel" (3 Nephi 30:2, emphasis added).

The primary invitation in the Book of Mormon is to come unto Christ. The Book of Mormon ends with a powerful final exhortation from Moroni to come unto Christ. He said, "Yea, come unto

Christ, and be perfected in Him, and deny yourselves of all ungodliness; and if ye shall deny yourselves of all ungodliness, and love God with all your might, mind, and strength, then is his grace sufficient for you, that by his grace ye may be perfect in Christ; and if by the grace of God ye are perfect in Christ, ye can in nowise deny the power of God" (Moroni 10:32). If we come unto Christ, we will be perfected in Him and our hearts will be perfected in Him through His grace.

The Lord promised Moroni, "And my grace is sufficient for the meek" (Ether 12:26). There could be no greater blessing promised to the meek and lowly in heart than this! Our Savior's grace will sufficiently make up all the difference and satisfy the deficit between who we are and who we need to become, even unto perfection. This promise demonstrates the confidence the Lord has in the meek and lowly in heart. He knows that such disciples will always return to Him. He knows that the meek and lowly in heart will always keep trying to improve and will be teachable and humble enough to recognize changes that need to occur in their lives. Christ will bestow sufficient grace upon them to someday be perfected in Him. What a glorious blessing!

Another powerful promise to those who are lowly in heart is found in Moroni: "And the remission of sins bringeth meekness, and lowliness of heart; and because of meekness and lowliness of heart cometh the visitation of the Holy Ghost, which Comforter filleth with hope and perfect love, which love endureth by diligence unto prayer, until the end shall come, when all the saints shall dwell with God" (Moroni 8:26). If we are lowly in heart, we will be visited by the Holy Ghost, the Comforter who fills us with hope and perfect love, even the pure love of Christ! Don't we all desire to be filled with charity? It can be ours if we are humble and teachable in all our doings.

Mormon's words in Moroni 8:26 contain a great key that teaches us how we can become lowly in heart. It says that a remission of sins brings us meekness and lowliness of heart. We must recognize our own sins and weaknesses and become dependent on the Savior to help us be forgiven. We must sincerely repent of our sins and do our best to move forward and have our hearts changed in such a way. We must give repentance a chance to change us through the Atonement. As we do so, we will find that our carnal, natural, and devilish tendencies can be swallowed up in Christ. Through the Holy Ghost, we can "become as a child, submissive, meek, humble, patient, full of love, willing to submit to all things which the Lord seeth fit to inflict upon us" (Mosiah 3:19).

FINDING REST UNTO OUR SOULS

When Alma was leaving his blessing upon his son, Helaman, he told his son to teach the people to be lowly in heart. He said:

> Preach unto them repentance, and faith on the Lord Jesus Christ; teach them to humble themselves and to be meek and lowly in heart; teach them to withstand every temptation of the devil, with their faith on the Lord Jesus Christ.
>
> Teach them to never be weary of good works, but to be meek and lowly in heart; for such shall find rest to their souls. (Alma 37:33–34)

It is enlightening to see humility and never being weary of good works coupled with being lowly in heart.

Those who are meek and lowly in heart will find rest unto their souls. The Savior gives us this simple invitation and marvelous promise:

> Come unto me, all ye that labour and are heavy laden, and I will give you rest.
>
> Take my yoke upon you, and learn of me; for I am meek and lowly in heart: and ye shall find rest unto your souls.
>
> For my yoke is easy and my burden is light. (Matthew 11:28–30)

When we carry the Savior's yoke upon us, we do not have to go it alone. Why carry our own burden throughout life when we have a loving Savior that would rather place on us a different yoke, an easier yoke that He promises to help us pull?

What does it mean in these scriptures to find rest unto our souls or to enter into the Lord's rest? This idea is mentioned frequently in the Book of Mormon and the Bible. This splendid blessing and its meaning is worth understanding in greater detail. President Joseph F. Smith taught us what it means to enter into the Lord's rest. He said, "It means entering into the knowledge and love of God, having faith in his purpose and in his plan, to such an extent that we know we are right, and that we are not hunting for something else; we are not disturbed by every wind of doctrine, or by the cunning and craftiness of men who lie in wait to deceive.' It is 'rest from the religious turmoil of the world; from the cry that is going forth, here and there—lo, here is Christ; lo, there is Christ.' The rest of the Lord, in eternity, is to inherit eternal life, to gain the fullness of the Lord's glory."[12]

Alma noted, "And thus being called by this holy calling, and ordained unto the high priesthood of the holy order of God, to teach his commandments unto the children of men, that they also might enter into his rest" (Alma 13:6). This verse states that a duty of high priests is to teach others about how to enter the Lord's rest as they themselves have done. Have we entered into the Lord's rest? Can we effectively explain and teach this doctrine to others? Are our testimonies so sure and firm that we constantly have peace? If not, we are not sufficiently meek and lowly in heart. Repentance that leads to a remission of our sins will bring us meekness sufficient to enjoy that rest.

Nephi approached the Lord in lowliness of heart to find out for himself if his family should leave Jerusalem. Because of his faith and lowliness of heart, he was visited with the Holy Spirit and received a confirmation that they were to leave Jerusalem and would be led to a land of promise. He was given confidence and sureness of his direction in life because he went to Heavenly Father in prayer for guidance. As towering obstacles presented themselves along the way, Nephi was sufficiently prepared to meet them because of the confirmation he received before he even left Jerusalem.

If we are to become lowly in heart, we need to humble ourselves and recognize that we are spiritually impoverished all the time. We depend upon the Lord for everything we have, both physically and spiritually. If we are to become lowly in heart, we need to be about the Lord's business always. Elder Neal A. Maxwell said that the meek and lowly in heart are "less concerned with their entitlements than they are with their assignments."[13]

We love that quote! Do we worry more about what we feel we deserve in life or about helping others around us? Are we more worried about the title of our calling than the people we are called to serve? Do we become weary of performing good works? It's interesting to note that when we do good works, we have the opportunity to find rest unto our souls instead of being weary. The Spirit can sanctify us unto the renewing of our bodies (see D&C 84:33). Every time we serve, our hearts have the opportunity to be humbled just a little bit more.

Can we become like the Savior and take someone else's yoke upon us? Can we lighten the burdens of those around us by bearing them ourselves? He who was meek and lowly in heart provides the example for us. We are under covenant to follow His example once we are baptized members of His Church. The gospel is infinitely more about what we can give than what we can take. We must help lighten the burdens of others to truly become lowly in heart.

As we go through life and experience pain and suffering meekly, we will be comforted as we trust in the Lord and His purposes for us. How we handle our pains and sufferings will determine in large part the measure of peace that we are given on our journey. Do we become bitter and murmur because of the lot we are given? Our Savior never complained about His lot in life, nor did He protest the injustices He suffered. He never once expressed regret about the pains and sins He took upon Himself. As we learn to be like the Savior in our relatively modest pains and sufferings, we will find rest for our weary souls.

SECTION 3

Hearts Prepared for the Temple

Jesus taught Nicodemus, "Except a man be born again, he cannot see the kingdom of God. Except a man be born of water and of the Spirit, he cannot enter into the kingdom of God" (John 3:3, 5).

The Prophet Joseph Smith taught, "It is one thing to see the kingdom of God, and another thing to enter into it. We must have a change of heart to see the kingdom of God, and subscribe the articles of adoption to enter therein."[1] These articles of adoption are the saving ordinances of the gospel accompanied by covenants we enter into with the Lord. Section Two focused on the mighty change of heart that allows us to *see* the kingdom of God. In this section, we will focus on characteristics of the heart that will allow us to *enter into* the kingdom of God.

The Psalmist wrote, "Who shall ascend into the hill of the Lord? Or who shall stand in his holy place? He that hath clean hands and a pure heart" (Psalm 24:3–4).

If we are to ascend into the hill of the Lord and realize the blessings of temple worship, our hearts must be pure! This was known and taught in Old Testament times and is our focus today as well.

The Book of Mormon gives special prominence to the temple and the conditions of the heart we must develop to be worthy to attend the temple, participate in sacred ordinances, and enter into sacred covenants. Our hearts must become celestial if we are to one day receive exaltation and live with our Heavenly Father and His Son, Jesus Christ. As we study the following conditions of the heart, it will be readily apparent that the temple is expressly linked to all of these conditions.

While the temple is not our final destination, it allows us to experience "the fullest blessings of the Atonement" in our lives and will lead to our exaltation.[2] That is not to say that these conditions of the heart do not have other applications in our lives, but our main focus in this section will be on developing celestial hearts to get on or stay on the covenant path as President Nelson describes and receive a new heart from the Savior.[3]

Elder James E. Faust said, "In the temples of the Lord, we learn obedience. We learn sacrifice. We make the vows of chastity and have our lives consecrated to holy purposes. It is possible for us to be purged and purified and to have our sins washed away so that we may come before the Lord as clean, white, and spotless as the newly fallen snow."[4] We can think of no better summary than that given by Elder Faust of what we must learn in the temples of the Lord.

We will examine the following conditions of the heart in this section: having a broken heart and contrite spirit, being pure in heart, doing things with full purpose of heart, and turning our hearts to our children and fathers. It is our hope that you will reflect on President Faust's message and relate these conditions of the heart to what you need to learn and what you covenant to do in the temple. In so doing, we know you will be blessed to recognize an even greater importance of the temple in your life and a greater determination to become or stay temple worthy. President Thomas S. Monson said, "No sacrifice is too great, no price too heavy, no struggle too difficult in order to receive [temple] blessings."[5] As such, the work we perform on our hearts in this section is worth every ounce of effort we have to give.

Chapter 8

A BROKEN HEART AND a CONTRITE SPIRIT

Developing a broken heart and a contrite spirit is the first characteristic necessary for us to enter into the kingdom of God. A broken heart is mentioned ten times in the Book of Mormon, with eight of those mentions paired with a contrite spirit. The prophet Jacob gives the other two mentions in reference to people's hearts breaking because of others' wrongdoings.

Many people think of a broken heart and a contrite spirit as being a commandment from our Savior that He first gave to people after His Resurrection. However, the principle of having a broken heart and a contrite spirit was well established prior to the Savior's mortal ministry. Nephi mentions having a broken heart and a contrite spirit hundreds of years before the birth of Christ. He said, "May the gates of hell be shut continually before me, because that my heart is broken and my spirit is contrite!" (2 Nephi 4:32).

Old Testament prophets also taught about having a broken heart and a contrite spirit. The Psalmist wrote, "The sacrifices of God are a broken spirit: a broken and a contrite heart, O God, thou wilt not despise" (Psalm 51:17). The Psalmist also taught, "The Lord is night unto them that are of a broken heart; and saveth such as be of a contrite spirit" (Psalm 34:18). People in Old Testament times knew that they needed to put up their sacrifices and offerings unto the Lord while also giving unto Him their hearts.

When the Savior appeared to the Nephites, He declared that the Law of Moses was fulfilled in Him. He then declared what the law of sacrifice would be going forward. He said, "And ye shall offer for a sacrifice unto me a broken heart and a contrite spirit. And whoso cometh unto me with a broken heart and a contrite spirit, him will I baptize with fire and with the Holy Ghost" (3 Nephi 9:20). With the Savior's words, the sacrifices and burnt offerings of the past were supplanted with offering unto Jesus a broken heart and a contrite spirit.

SMASHED AND SHATTERED

So, what exactly does it mean to have a broken heart and a contrite spirit? We often think of a broken heart as a humble heart and a contrite spirit as a repentant or remorseful spirit. Sometimes learning from the ancient languages sheds additional light when studying the scriptures. In Hebrew, *broken* means not just to break, but also to smash or shatter; *contrite* means to crush.[1,2] Our hearts must be smashed or shattered before the Lord can give us a new heart. We cannot harbor in our old hearts any remaining pretenses that we can do anything on our own. Our spirits must be crushed in the sense that we know we have fallen short and depend completely on the Savior to lift us up and save us. With a crushed spirit, we will recognize our own nothingness before God and understand that we are unprofitable servants without Him.

The Savior provided the perfect example to us of having a broken heart and a contrite spirit. He did this in two magnificent and miraculous ways as we learn from His suffering in Gethsemane and Golgotha. First, the Savior's spirit was crushed in the Garden of Gethsemane, the place of the olive press. What a humbling and incredible thought this is! So agonizing was His suffering for us, so excruciating was His pain, and so intense was His love that His spirit was literally crushed from the stress and pressure of it all.

Second, Jesus Christ, our Savior and Redeemer, literally died of a broken heart on the cross in Golgotha. The Psalmist prophesied, "Reproach hath broken my heart; and I am full of heaviness: and I looked for some to take pity, but there was none; and for comforters, but I found none. They gave me also gall for my meat; and in my thirst they gave me vinegar to drink" (Psalm 69:20–21). This prophecy provides details of Jesus's heart actually breaking during His atoning sacrifice as well as the vinegar the soldiers offered Jesus to drink on the cross.

Elder Bruce D. Porter said, "In Gethsemane, the Savior 'descended below all things' as He bore the burden of sin for every human being (D&C 88:6). At Golgotha, He 'poured out his soul unto death,' and His great heart literally broke with an all-encompassing love for the children of God (Isaiah 53:12). When we remember the Savior and His suffering, our hearts too will break in gratitude for the Anointed One."[3] Have you ever felt or expressed gratitude to your Heavenly Father for the Savior and His Atonement to the point your heart aches?

Elder James E. Talmage, in his book *Jesus the Christ*, believed that a broken heart was the cause of Jesus's physical death. He wrote:

> The strong, loud utterance, immediately following which He bowed His head and "gave up the ghost," when considered in connection with other recorded details, points to a physical rupture of the heart as the direct cause of death. If the soldier's spear was thrust into the left side of the Lord's body and actually penetrated the heart, the outrush of "blood and water" observed by John is further evidence of a cardiac rupture; for it is known that in the rare instances of death resulting from a breaking of any part of the wall of the heart, blood accumulates within the pericardium, and there undergoes a change by which the corpuscles separate as a partially clotted mass from the almost colorless, watery serum. Similar accumulations of clotted corpuscles and serum occur within the pleura.[4]

The temple being rent in twain was symbolic of Jesus passing through the veil of death to return to His Father. It can also be said that when the temple was rent in twain, the temple's heart was broken as well. The imagery of the temple being torn asunder is remarkably moving and poignant! The Lord of the whole earth, our Creator, broke His heart for us and asks for our spiritually broken hearts in return.

The second way Jesus showed us how to have a broken heart and a contrite spirit was in how He lived His life. Elder Porter said, "Though Jesus of Nazareth was utterly without sin, He walked through life with a broken heart and a contrite spirit, as manifested by His submission to the will of the Father."[5]

The scriptures are filled with instances of Jesus submitting to the will of His Father. Jesus declared, "I seek not mine own will, but the will of the Father that sent me" (John 5:30). We have the Savior as the supreme example of giving Himself wholly to Heavenly Father's purposes. His submission to the Father was perfect and the scriptures do a beautiful job of emphasizing and articulating the surrender of His will to the Father.

Jesus told the Nephites, "I have suffered the will of the Father in all things from the beginning" (3 Nephi 11:11). This one statement defines the entire focus of our Savior's life. The most important events in His life were capped with this declaration. From the premortal existence to His death, Christ always made it clear that His mission was to do the will of the Father that sent Him. The first recorded words in our scriptural account of Jehovah in the premortal existence are during the grand council in heaven. When He accepted His role in the plan of salvation as our Savior and Redeemer, He said, "Father, thy will be done, and the glory be thine forever" (Moses 4:2).

Some of Jesus's first words we have recorded of His mortal life include the time He was found preaching in the temple at twelve years of age. He proclaimed, "I must be about my Father's business" (Luke 2:49).

Throughout His mortal ministry, Christ repeatedly reminded His disciples that He was sent not to do His own will, but the will of the Father. On the shores of Galilee, while teaching the disciples how to pray, in the temple, and during the Sermon on the Mount, we find Jesus constantly teaching His disciples to do Heavenly Father's will. He teaches us in the Sermon on the Mount, "Not everyone that saith unto me, Lord, Lord, shall enter into the kingdom of heaven; but he that doeth the will of my Father which is in heaven" (Matthew 7:21).

During His time of great agony and pain in Gethsemane, our Savior prayed, "Father, if thou be willing, remove this cup from me; nevertheless, not my will, but thine be done" (Luke 22:42). Then, on the cross, after completing His mission here on earth, before giving up the ghost, Christ's last words were, "Father, it is finished, thy will is done" (Matthew 27:50, footnote a; from JST Matthew 27:54). How fitting it is that with His last mortal breaths, the Savior uttered the same words He used in the premortal existence!

This principle truly envelops the gospel of Jesus Christ. Christ perfectly summarized His life when He visited the Nephites. He said, "Behold I have given unto you my gospel, and this is the gospel which I have given unto you—that I came into the world to do the will of my Father, because my Father sent me" (3 Nephi 27:13).

THE ONLY THING TRULY OURS TO GIVE

We too may witness our appreciation to our Heavenly Father by giving ourselves wholly to His purposes by doing His will. Elder D. Todd Christofferson said, "You can offer the Lord the gift of your broken, or repentant, heart and your contrite, or obedient, spirit. In reality, it is the gift of yourself—what you are and what you are becoming."[6]

Elder Neal A. Maxwell said, "The submission of one's will is really the only uniquely personal thing we have to place on God's altar. The many other things we 'give,' brothers and sisters, are actually the things He has already given or loaned to us. However, when you and I finally submit ourselves, by letting our individual wills be swallowed up in God's will, then we are really giving something to Him! It is the only possession which is truly ours to give!"[7]

King Benjamin spoke about how we needed to put off the natural man and become submissive like a little child. He said we must be "willing to submit to all things which the Lord seeth fit to inflict upon [us], even as a child doth submit to his father" (Mosiah 3:19). Are we ready to be this submissive, this brokenhearted? Are we ready for difficult, stretching, and maybe even painful tutorials from the Lord? If we go through life with broken hearts and contrite spirits, these experiences will indeed be tutorials and not just painful, bitter experiences. We will become more like our Heavenly Father and will eventually be given a new heart like our Savior's.

We love the imagery of our hearts being made of clay. An old Protestant hymn, "Have Thine Own Way, Lord," has the following lyrics:

> Have Thine own way, Lord!
> Have Thine own way!
> Thou art the Potter;
> I am the clay.
> Mould me and make me
> After Thy will,
> While I am waiting,
> Yielded and still.
>
> (Lyrics by Adelaide A. Pollard)[8]

We begin to show cracks and flaws in our hearts of clay as we sin. Our hearts become hardened, prideful, and set upon the things of the world. The only way for us to fix those flaws in our hearts is to break up the hardened clay with a hammer, pound it into dust, and start over. Indeed, we cannot say we are even as much as the dust of the earth (see Mosiah 2:25). It takes our Savior's intervention to receive a newly transformed heart. A broken heart allows the Atonement of Christ to change and transform our hearts at the hands of the Potter.

Sister Neill F. Marriott, second counselor in the Young Women general presidency, said, "Paradoxically, in order to have a healed and faithful heart, we must first allow it to break before the Lord. . . . *The result of sacrificing our heart, or our will, to the Lord is that we receive the spiritual guidance we need.*"[9] From the examples that follow, you will see that in every instance, spiritual guidance is granted to those who come to the Lord with a broken heart.

THE WEIGHT OF HELPLESSNESS

While there are many experiences and examples that could be shared of what it is to feel a broken heart, Derek has felt the unmistakable involvement from a loving Father in Heaven through his particularly difficult challenge with depression and anxiety. In Derek's words:

As I mentioned earlier, I have struggled with anxiety and depression for about six years now. I have tried therapy. I have tried numerous medications. I have tried meditation. I have visited with numerous doctors and therapists. I have had priesthood blessings. None of these efforts have produced significant fruits of improvement. I frequently feel helpless and hopeless. It's been especially humbling to have simple and mundane tasks that used to be very easy for me to complete become extremely overwhelming. I have wondered at times if I'm even really sick or if I'm just making it all up in my head. I have felt the weight of guilt for the burden that these sicknesses have placed on the rest of my family.

This experience over the past six years has changed me in many ways, but more than anything it has helped me start to cultivate a broken heart. It's extremely difficult for me to ask for help from a doctor or therapist and talk about such intimate problems with strangers. It's been very hard for me to talk to my immediate and extended family and close friends about my struggles. It's hard to help them understand what I'm feeling and experiencing when I know it doesn't make sense to a normal, rational person. It's especially hard to describe to them why I struggle with commonplace assignments and activities as simple as making an ordinary phone call.

Not a day goes by, and if I'm being honest, not a waking hour goes by, without me battling my anxiety. I offer countless prayers each day for help to stand up to the challenges of the day. As challenges arise, I pray even more frequently and fervently for courage, strength, and comfort. I try my best to exercise faith in the ability to be healed. I also try my best to exercise faith to continue to press forward and battle these diseases if I am not healed.

One wonderful blessing that has resulted from my anxiety and depression has been the constant remembrance of my Savior. As Ammon said, "I know that I am nothing, as to my strength I am weak" (Alma 26:12). I depend upon my Savior to get through each and every day. It's impossible for me to forget my Savior from day to day and even from hour to hour because I don't know how else to handle things. This is perhaps the greatest blessing that has come from my illness.

I do better on some days than others, but in the end I know that I have been given these challenges for a reason and I hope "that these things [will] give me experience, and [will] be for [my] good" (D&C 122:8). My anxiety and depression have definitely chipped away at my heart—and that's not to say that it doesn't need further breaking. I am grateful that I have been humbled from being unable to do simple things on my own and for being completely dependent on the Lord and those around me.

Bruce Hafen, in his book *The Broken Heart*, said, "Part of the sacrifice of a broken heart and a contrite spirit is a willingness to sacrifice the love affair so many of us have with our own egos."[10] It is difficult to have a big ego when you have anxiety and depression. Instead, you have to keep reminding yourself that you are worth something, that there are those out there in the world that value you. "Remember the worth of souls is great in the sight of God"

(D&C 18:10). It is instructive that this verse starts off with the word *remember*. There are definitely times when we all need to lean on the remembrance that our worth is great in the sight of God.

HIGHLY PERSONALIZED TRIALS

Mortality seems to ensure that all will be given certain experiences in life that are designed to help us be humble and dependent on the Lord. We will be given individualized, specific trials to help us develop broken hearts and contrite spirits. It would be a daunting task to develop our hearts to be sufficiently broken and our spirits sufficiently contrite without such trials and difficulties. We need to find out, if we do not know already, that we don't have all the answers, that we are truly nothing without the Savior. At some point, we all have to go to Him in humble prayer and ask for the help, wisdom, and direction we need.

After his father's death, Nephi, in what's often referred to as Nephi's Psalm, beautifully described various attributes of having a broken heart. He lamented:

> Nevertheless, notwithstanding the great goodness of the Lord, in showing me his great and marvelous works, my heart exclaimeth: O wretched man that I am! Yea, my heart sorroweth because of my flesh; my soul grieveth because of mine iniquities.
>
> I am encompassed about, because of the temptations and the sins which do so easily beset me.
>
> And when I desire to rejoice, my heart groaneth because of my sins; nevertheless, I know in whom I have trusted. (2 Nephi 4:17–19)

After the death of his father, Nephi was in a highly emotional and tender state. Not only had his dad died, but his brothers had escalated their feud with Nephi again and they wanted to kill him. Nephi had to separate himself from his wicked brothers for his own safety. Worse yet, Nephi knew from his visions that even after an amazing journey to the promised land, his people would eventually be destroyed from the face of the land.

The death of a loved one, personal tragedy, and disappointment are all things we may have to deal with on this earth, just as Nephi did. These tragedies bring us heartbreak as it is known in a temporal context, as well as the opportunity to experience spiritual heartbreak. Spiritual heartbreak is one of the great purposes of the troubles, suffering, and anguish we experience while in mortality.

Those with spiritual eyes to see are continually taught that they are not meant to be in charge in this life. We may pray to have certain burdens taken from us, but often the Lord's will is that we carry them for a time and learn from them. We are promised that He will visit us in our afflictions, not withhold from us all afflictions or keep us from experiencing any afflictions (see Mosiah 24:14). Without tribulation of some sort, it would be almost impossible for us to learn to have spiritually broken hearts. We would not feel the need to plead to our Heavenly Father and learn to depend upon Him.

It is not surprising that Nephi mentions his heart so often in 2 Nephi 4. We have already discussed verse 32, where Nephi describes his heart as broken and his spirit contrite. However, it was already evident that this was the case just from reading verses 17–19. His heart sorrowed, his soul grieved, and his heart exclaimed what a wretched man he thought he was. Remember, this "wretched man" had been visited by the Savior and had performed many mighty miracles in His name.

Often, it seems, as Elder Gerrit W. Gong describes, "The harder we try, the further we may feel from the perfection we seek."[11] This was definitely the case with Nephi at this time in his life. Nephi was doing so many things right in his life. The more he sought to keep the commandments and do Heavenly Father's will, the more sins and imperfections he saw within himself. Nephi's heart was truly sufficiently humble and broken to learn even more from the Lord and draw ever nearer to Him.

Alma the Younger is another great example of having a broken heart. Although it is not described in these exact words, his heart was broken from the experience he had with the angel calling him to repentance. Alma later described this experience to his son Helaman:

> When I heard the words—If thou wilt be destroyed of thyself, seek no more to destroy the church of God—I was struck with such fear and amazement lest perhaps I should be destroyed, that I fell to the earth and I did hear no more.
>
> But I was racked with eternal torment, for my soul was harrowed up to the greatest degree and racked with all my sins.
>
> Yea, I did remember all my sins and iniquities, for which I was tormented with the pains of hell. . . . The very thought of coming into the presence of my God did rack my soul with inexpressible horror.
>
> Oh, thought I, that I could be banished and become extinct both soul and body, that I might not be brought to stand in the presence of my God, to be judged of my deeds.
>
> And now, for three days and for three nights was I racked, even with the pains of a damned soul. (Alma 36:11–16)

While guilt and pain were primary feelings that Alma felt on this occasion from all the sins he had committed, he also recognized his own nothingness before the Lord. He saw his sins for what they were, and he did not want to go before his God with such iniquities still unresolved. His heart was shattered and broken by his past actions. His ground had been harrowed, and he was sufficiently humbled. Only then was he ready for the Lord to work through him.

Alma continued, "I cried within my heart: O Jesus, thou Son of God, have mercy on me, who am in the gall of bitterness, and am encircled about by the everlasting chains of death" (verse 18). At this most humble and desperate time, Alma reached out to the Savior in faith to receive a forgiveness of his sins.

King Benjamin's people also had broken hearts and contrite spirits after they were taught at the temple. They "viewed themselves in their own carnal state, even less than the dust of the earth. And they all cried aloud with one voice, saying: O have mercy, and apply the atoning blood of Christ that we may receive forgiveness of our sins, and our hearts may be purified; for we believe in Jesus Christ, the Son of God, who created heaven and earth" (Mosiah 4:2). The Spirit had touched their hearts and awakened them to a sense of their own nothingness and their worthless and fallen state (see Mosiah 4:5).

Again, an important characteristic of a broken heart from these examples is that we must seek out our Savior, knowing that we are nothing on our own. We can receive forgiveness and the comfort and peace we seek only after coming unto the Savior.

There are many other examples in the Book of Mormon of people that suffer through disappointment, pain, and earthly injustice. It is interesting to study the effects that trials and tribulations had on people. Sometimes, the trials people faced helped their hearts become broken and their spirits contrite, while in other instances very similar challenges further hardened their hearts. The brokenhearted were able to exercise faith and trust that the Lord had a plan for each one of them and that these things were for their good. They were able to keep an eternal perspective that allowed them to learn from any earthly injustices they experienced.

THE SACRIFICE OF ALL THINGS

The Book of Mormon depicts a remarkable legacy of sacrifice in addition to providing more detail about the Atonement of Christ than any other book of scripture. Abinadi suffered death by fire for the Savior and His gospel. The sons of Mosiah were called to endure incredible hardships and sacrifice while preaching the word. On multiple occasions, some of the people of Ammon were murdered for their beliefs after burying their weapons of war. Mormon and Moroni endured great tribulation as they led the Nephite armies hopelessly against the Lamanites and witnessed the entire destruction of their people. They spent many lonely years watching out for their lives, knowing that they would be killed for declaring themselves followers of Christ.

Amulek left his life of comfort and a rich family heritage to preach to the wicked people of Ammonihah as Alma the Younger's companion. He sacrificed tremendously for the gospel. He and Alma witnessed one of the most heartbreaking scenes in the Book of Mormon when saints, including children, along with their holy scriptures, were burned in a great fire. It is very possible that Amulek had members of his family in that fire and was told to refrain from using the priesthood to save them. After this, Amulek and Alma were bound in strong cords, cast into prison, stripped of their clothes, smitten, and spit upon, all because they believed in Christ and preached His gospel.

So many other examples could be listed here from the Book of Mormon that illustrate disciples of Christ sacrificing their all in His name. It comes as no surprise then that we too are asked to sacrifice in behalf of the Savior and His Church.

The *Lectures on Faith* state, "Let us here observe, that a religion that does not require the sacrifice of all things never has power sufficient to produce the faith necessary unto life and salvation; . . . it is through the medium of the sacrifice of all earthly things that men do actually know that they are doing the things that are well pleasing in the sight of God. When a man has offered in sacrifice all that he has for the truth's sake, not even withholding his life, and believing before God that he has been called to make this sacrifice because he seeks to do his will, he does know, most assuredly, that God does and will accept his sacrifice and offering, and that he has not, nor will not seek his face in vain."[12]

Joseph Smith gave the ultimate sacrifice a mortal can give and died in behalf of the gospel and the Lord. Since the Restoration of the gospel, Church members have offered stirring sacrifices in behalf of the Savior. Some have given their lives for their faith, including many pioneers that came west. Others have been disowned by their parents or other family members for the gospel. Some have made huge financial sacrifices to join the Church. Others have used all of their energy and efforts to further build the kingdom of God here on the earth, at the expense of temporal achievement.

The Savior repeatedly taught during His earthly ministry about the magnitude of the sacrifice we must make for the gospel. He taught this clearly in both the Parable of the Hidden Treasure and the Parable of the Pearl of Great Price. In these two accounts, the man and merchant sell all that they have for the treasure and pearl, respectively. If we have the opportunity to inherit the kingdom of God, we need to be willing to sacrifice everything as well.

John Rowe Moyle

The early pioneers made life-altering sacrifices to become members of the Church and move to the Salt Lake Valley. They have left us such a tremendous heritage of sacrifice for the kingdom of God! Our great-great-great-great-grandfather is John Rowe Moyle. He was an early pioneer who settled in Alpine, Utah. John migrated with his family from England and came to Alpine via the first handcart company. After settling in Alpine, John was called to be a stonecutter on the Salt Lake Temple that was being built.

He walked weekly from Alpine to Salt Lake, beginning his journey around 2:00 a.m. on Monday, staying the week with his son, leaving around 5:00 p.m. on Friday, and arriving home around midnight. He did this for almost twenty years until tragedy struck. One day, John was out milking the family cow and got kicked in the leg. His leg suffered a compound fracture, and the decision was made to amputate his leg just below the knee.

John ended up carving his own wooden leg, and when his leg had healed sufficiently, he decided it was time to go back to work on the temple. He walked the twenty-two miles with his wooden leg and continued to work on the temple. He had the honor of engraving the inscription, "Holiness to the Lord, the House of the Lord," on the outside of the temple. We think often of this inscription on the temple and of our ancestor's incredible sacrifice that he made for the Savior's Church. We often think about his wife, Phillippa, and her weighty sacrifice to take care of the children, the house, and all of the chores and work on the farm while her husband was gone during the week.[13]

A TEST OF FAITH IN RUSSIA

Young eighteen- and nineteen-year-old boys and girls offer a great sacrifice of time and effort to go on missions for one and a half to two years. Older couples also offer similar sacrifices to go on missions and be away from their families and loved ones. Members of the Church all across the world sacrifice valuable time and resources while fulfilling their church callings. We are also called upon to sacrifice by paying tithing. We both served missions among faithful members that experienced scarcity and saw the weight of this sacrifice. It is one thing to pay tithing when you have enough to live on, or even a surplus, but the faith necessary to sacrifice and pay tithing when you don't think you even have enough to live on is awe-inspiring.

While tracting one day in Novocherkassk, Russia, Derek met an older man and his wife. In his words:

They weren't particularly religious, but they were anxious to hear what we had to teach them. We asked them to read the Book of Mormon, and they accepted that challenge. They also accepted our challenge to come to Church, which at the time was being held in the hotel at which we were staying. We were in a city of approximately 180,000 people and had exactly zero members of the Church there. When it came time to talk about the Word of Wisdom, they were ready to put aside bad habits that had been with them for decades. They did it happily. We felt like this was a "golden couple" that was ready to come into the Church.

When we went back to teach them the law of tithing, the discussion started to have a troubling feel to it. I could see the stress that the principle of tithing was causing them. This couple explained to me that they only got about $12 per month and couldn't afford another expense.

If they had to pay tithing, they quite literally wouldn't have enough to live on. We tried our best to address their concern, but we knew this would be a huge test of faith for them. At the end of the discussion, we challenged them to pray about tithing.

I look back at this experience now and am even more amazed at what we were asking them to do. We were asking them to believe what these two very callow American missionaries taught them about this Church that had a handful of people attending at the time in a hotel we were renting out, but had zero actual members. We then wanted them to give 10% of their income to the Lord, which I'm sure they were maybe thinking would end up back in America somewhere or perhaps even in our own pockets. The faith that was required of them was astonishing.

When we went back to talk to them, the husband opened the door slightly and handed us back the Book of Mormon we had given them. He said they just couldn't obey the law of tithing because they wouldn't have enough on which to live. I could see the hurt in this man's face as he was saying this. His eyes were very red. I could tell that they had thought a lot about this and that their decision wasn't being taken lightly. I was devastated by their decision.

I know that this couple will be blessed for their actions up to this point. I'm still amazed at their faith and willingness to learn how to pray, to read the scriptures, and to go to church. The gospel is a plan of mercy and grace. The Savior will ensure that they are given every opportunity permitted to them to accept the gospel and come unto Him. My prayer is that they will be able to have the faith sufficient to accept our Savior's sacrifice and be prepared to give Him an acceptable offering in return.

We will all be asked to make sacrifices for the gospel. Such sacrifices can come in many different forms and many will be demanding. It is easier said than done, but we need to keep an eternal perspective in regard to sacrifice. We will more readily sacrifice what is necessary when we know the eternal rewards that are to come.

THE BLESSINGS OF A BROKEN HEART

The Savior taught:

> He that loveth father or mother more than me is not worthy of me: and he that loveth son or daughter more than me is not worthy of me.
>
> And he that taketh not his cross, and followeth after me, is not worthy of me. (Matthew 10:37–38)

He who sacrificed all has given us the invitation to sacrifice greatly as we are called upon to do so. For most of us, we will not be called upon to sacrifice our lives in the service of the Church. We will, however, be called upon to sacrifice our time, talents, and efforts in various ways for the building up of the kingdom of God on the earth.

Amazing blessings are promised to those who live the law of sacrifice and do their best to live with broken hearts and contrite spirits. The Lord promised, "But blessed are the poor who are pure in heart, whose hearts are broken, and whose spirits are contrite, for they shall see the kingdom of God coming in power and great glory unto their deliverance; for the fatness of the earth shall be theirs" (D&C 56:18). What beautiful promises! We all seek the deliverance of our Lord to be able to live with Him again. And who does not welcome the promise that the fatness of the earth will be theirs?

Lehi taught:

> Wherefore, redemption cometh in and through the Holy Messiah; for he is full of grace and truth.
>
> Behold, he offereth himself a sacrifice for sin, to answer the ends of the law, unto all those who have a broken heart and a contrite spirit; and unto none else can the ends of the law be answered. (2 Nephi 2:6–7)

Only those with broken hearts and contrite spirits can receive the greatest blessings of the Atonement of our Savior. Christ has been sent "to bind up the brokenhearted" (Isaiah 61:1). As we offer Him our broken hearts, He has promised to bind them up and make them whole again. We must come to the Lord in the spirit of sacrifice and prove to Him that we want nothing more than to have eternal life and will do whatever He requires of us to receive of His mercy and grace.

As we come to the Lord in this spirit of sacrifice, the Holy Ghost will reveal additional ways for us to give an acceptable offering to the Lord. We may be prompted to spend more time in His service, visiting with our ministering families or widows in our wards. We may be inspired to serve in the temple more often. We may be prompted to give a more generous fast offering. We may be encouraged to better keep the Sabbath Day holy. We may be prompted to murmur less in the trials we are currently facing. The variety of ways that we can sacrifice for the Lord is limitless. We know that promptings will come if we seek them.

As we humbly come before the Lord to receive a remission of our sins and do our best to live the law of sacrifice, we will develop sufficiently broken hearts and contrite spirits. Every time we humbly kneel and ask forgiveness of the sins we have committed, our hearts will become more fit for the kingdom. Every decision we make in an effort to sacrifice for the Lord will bring us closer to having the broken hearts we need to be accepted before Him. As we become more brokenhearted, an increase in compassion and empathy will inevitably develop within us along this journey. With that increased compassion and empathy, we will become a great blessing to our fellow man.

CHAPTER 9

PURE IN HEART

Becoming pure in heart is the second characteristic necessary for us to enter into the kingdom of God. The Book of Mormon mentions the pure in heart specifically on seven different occasions. There are an additional seventeen mentions of "thoughts," "intents," "desires," "wishes," and "affections of our heart." Our thoughts, desires, and wishes must also be pure and aligned with the will of God.

Usually, we think of purity in terms of being clean, without fault or blemish, and free of any contamination or filth. The scriptures and modern-day prophets and apostles provide additional insight into what it means to be pure in heart. Twice, Jacob speaks of the pure in heart as having firm minds (see Jacob 3:1–2). President Dallin H. Oaks said, "If we act for the right motives and if we refrain from forbidden desires and attitudes, we have pure hearts."[1] D&C 41:10 mentions that the pure in heart have "no guile." While serving as second counselor in the Presiding Bishopric, Elder Vaughn J. Featherstone said, "Pure connotes the absence of foreign substance. The individuals whose minds and hearts are pure have removed from their lives foreign thoughts and passions."[2] The Savior told Joseph Smith the pure in heart "seek counsel, and authority, and blessings constantly" from the prophet or from the Lord (D&C 122:2).

Clearly, there is greater depth to the meaning of *pure in heart* than first meets the eye. Several components and facets of being pure in heart will be identified and studied throughout this chapter. While being pure in heart can relate to the law of chastity specifically, it also relates generally to keeping high moral standards in all behavior and thought. Such is our call to be pure in heart.

JACOB'S SERMON ON THE PURE IN HEART

From the Book of Mormon, the prophet Jacob spoke about many different conditions of the heart, but he was particularly concerned about the pure in heart. After Nephi died, Jacob gave a powerful sermon to the Nephites and admonished them to keep the commandments. He lamented the fact that women and children who were pure in heart had to listen to Jacob chastise their husbands and fathers who had not lived up to their covenants. These men had many wives and concubines and had broken their wives' hearts and lost the confidence of their children because of their bad examples before them (see Jacob 2:35). This is one of the most damning descriptions that could possibly be given in regard to familial relationships. Still, there was a way back for these men. There is always a way back. That's why Jacob was trying to reach them and call them to repentance.

The Lord said, "For I, the Lord God, delight in the chastity of women. And whoredoms are an abomination before me" (Jacob 2:28). These husbands were anything but pure in heart. These men's spiritual situation was dire and the Lord's fair daughters were crying out to Him for help. The Lord had heard the sobbing of their hearts, and in response, He promised curses and destruction upon these men if they did not change their ways.

Jacob turns his attention in Jacob 3 by now directly speaking to those who were pure in heart, to those women and children who had suffered so greatly. Jacob provided comfort as well as some beautiful promises to them. He said:

But behold, I, Jacob, would speak unto you that are pure in heart. Look unto God with firmness of mind, and pray unto him with exceeding faith, and he will console you in your afflictions, and he will plead your cause, and send down justice upon those who seek your destruction.

O all ye that are pure in heart, lift up your heads and receive the pleasing word of God, and feast upon his love; for ye may, if your minds are firm, forever. (Jacob 3:1–2)

Here, Jacob promises the pure in heart certain blessings that are undoubtedly some of the greatest our Savior can give us. It is worth an in-depth study of these blessings one by one. First, the pure in heart will be consoled in their afflictions. Great blessings of comfort and consolation were needed for these women and children that had suffered because of the sins of their husbands and fathers. Such suffering led the women and children to have broken and sobbing hearts. Jacob even says that "many hearts died, pierced with deep wounds" (Jacob 2:35). Surely, only Christ could revive such dead hearts.

Elder Neal A. Maxwell said, "Today we move among so many of the walking wounded and the casualty list grows."[3] Sexual immorality pierces both the heart of the offended and the offender with deep wounds. We should cultivate an awareness of the wounded among us and do our best to lift them up. We also need to ensure that our choices do not become the swords that pierce others' hearts.

Jacob's second promise to the pure in heart was that the Savior would plead their cause before Heavenly Father. Jesus Christ is our Advocate with the Father. What a tremendous blessing! Christ has put Himself in the position where He can advocate for us. He took upon Himself our sins and broke the bands of death. Because of His Atonement, "He shall make intercession for all men" (2 Nephi 2:9).

In the Doctrine and Covenants, the Savior gives us a powerful synopsis of how He will advocate in our behalf with Heavenly Father. He said:

Listen to him who is the advocate with the Father, who is pleading your cause before him—

Saying: Father, behold the sufferings and death of him who did no sin, in whom thou wast well pleased; behold, the blood of thy Son which was shed, the blood of him whom thou gavest that thyself might be glorified;

Wherefore, Father, spare these my brethren that believe on my name, that they may come unto me and have everlasting life. (D&C 45:3–5)

The Savior is not advocating for us with the Father by focusing on and describing our works. He is advocating for us by focusing on and describing *His* glorious Atonement and *His* works. If we believe on *His* name, He will plead our cause before the Father. He will ask the Father that His suffering for our sins be used "to appease the demands of justice" (Alma 42:15).

It seems members of the Church at times mistakenly associate the Savior primarily with mercy, while associating Heavenly Father primarily with justice. The Savior is indeed merciful and Heavenly Father is indeed just, but Heavenly Father is equally merciful and the Savior is equally just. They have exactly the same attributes and virtues. They are one!

Our Heavenly Father wants us to be redeemed every bit as much as the Savior does. We should be grateful to our Heavenly Father for His mercy as well as our Savior's mercy. However, it is the sacred responsibility and privilege of our Savior to be our Advocate with the Father. And He will plead our cause before our Father if we are pure in heart, just as Jacob promised (see Jacob 3:1).

Jacob's third promise is that the pure in heart will also be able to feast upon the Savior's love forever (see Jacob 3:2)! His love is abundant; His love is infinite. His arm of mercy is always extended towards us (see Jacob 6:5). To feast upon His love, we must take notice of all the blessings He gives us on a daily basis through His atoning sacrifice. If we feast upon His love, our hearts can be filled to the brim with love. And the promise is that we may do so forever.

The magnitude of the pain and suffering that sexual immorality causes others is often incomprehensible to anyone outside of the people affected and our Savior, Jesus Christ. Our Savior is the only one who can revive and renew such dead hearts. He can become our Father in a few ways. We become Christ's children when we are spiritually born again. The same can be said when He revives and restores our hearts. He is not only the Master Healer, but also the Father through whom we can receive new hearts.

After Jacob detailed a few of the blessings promised to the pure in heart, he then provided a strict warning to those who are not pure in heart. He said, "But, wo, wo, unto you that are not pure in heart, that are filthy this day before God; for except ye repent the land is cursed for your sakes; and the Lamanites, which are not filthy like unto you, nevertheless they are cursed with a sore cursing, shall scourge you even unto destruction" (Jacob 3:3).

It is interesting to note that Jacob stated that the Lamanites were more righteous than the Nephites at this point in time because they were loyal to their wives and did not commit the whoredoms of which the Nephite husbands were guilty. The Lamanites were blessed with the promise that their seed would not be destroyed because of this devotion to their wives. They were blessed with God's mercy and would one day become a blessed people.

Jacob summarized this beautifully and simply by saying, "Behold, their husbands love their wives, and their wives love their husbands; and their husbands and their wives love their children" (Jacob 3:7). We should all be striving for familial relationships that can be summarized in such a way as was attributed to these Lamanites. What a stark contrast to the description given to Nephite husbands who had broken their wives' hearts and lost the confidence of their children! If we are not shaken by these two descriptions, we should be! Elder Parley P. Pratt said that the pure in heart "know how to prize" familial relationships in life.[4] Now is a good time to take stock of our relationships with our spouses and children and ensure that we prize our relationships with them.

"They Shall See God"

The blessings promised by Jacob to the pure in heart are some of the greatest in all of scripture. The Savior promised an even greater blessing when He visited the Nephites. He said, "And blessed are all the pure in heart, for they shall see God" (3 Nephi 12:8). President Gordon B. Hinckley said that this "is a covenant, made by Him who has the power to fulfill."[5] This is no idle promise. If we are pure in heart, we can and will see God.

The Savior added an extra qualifier to seeing Him when He said, "Yea, and my presence shall be there [in the temple], for I will come into it, and all the pure in heart *that shall come into it* shall see God" (D&C 97:16, emphasis added). What a call for all of us to attend the temple! What a thrilling promise to those who serve frequently in the temple! Our Savior will come into the temple and allow the pure in heart to see Him.

There are additional meanings to this promised blessing of seeing God. Elder David B. Haight said "see" can be defined as "coming to know Him, discerning Him, recognizing Him and His work, perceiving His importance, or coming to understand Him."[6] As we try to purify our thoughts and actions, we will become more like Him and will get to know Him better.

Elder L. Whitney Clayton said, "The condition of our heart determines how much evidence of divinity we see in the world."[7] The pure in heart shall see God in more and more places as their spiritual eyes become more opened and attuned. One of our favorite poems is by Elizabeth Barrett Browning. She wrote the following:

> Earth's crammed with heaven,
> And every common bush afire with God,
> But only he who sees takes off his shoes.[8]

The purer we become, the more divinity we will recognize in the Lord's creations. Not only will we see divinity in the Lord's creations on earth, but we will also see the divinity in all people with whom we come in contact. Even the darkest souls have a spark of divinity within them because of their divine heritage. It is our duty to look for this spark in others.

The more we have the Holy Ghost with us, the purer we can become; the purer we become, the more we will have the Holy Ghost with us. Purity and virtue start with our thoughts. Virtuous, clean thoughts are vitally important to becoming pure in heart.

PURITY IN OUR THOUGHTS

President Ezra Taft Benson said, "Thoughts lead to acts, acts lead to habits, and habits lead to character—and our character will determine our eternal destiny."[9] A famous proverb states, "As he thinketh in his heart, so is he" (Proverbs 23:7). We may be able to entertain a random thought or two in our minds that will not lead to an action, but eventually our thoughts will always win us over and will lead to actions based on those thoughts. We cannot naively believe that our thoughts are of no consequence to what we become.

The prophet Alma said, "And our thoughts will also condemn us" (Alma 12:14). Temptations are all around us and often launch their attack with our thoughts. Bad thoughts will inevitably come into our minds. It is what we choose to do with these thoughts that will define us. As Jacob taught, we must have "firm minds." We have been given counsel to rid ourselves of bad thoughts that come to us and to ensure we keep our minds firm.

President Boyd K. Packer counseled us to sing a hymn to get rid of bad thoughts that have entered into our minds. He said, "Because the music is uplifting and clean, the baser thoughts will slip shamefully away. For while virtue, by choice, will not associate with filth, evil cannot tolerate the presence of light. In due time you will find yourself humming the music inwardly, almost automatically, to drive out unworthy thoughts."[10] Have you tried this simple practice? This is not an idle promise from President Packer. If we sing a hymn, degrading thoughts will indeed slip shamefully away.

Elder Bruce R. McConkie used a different tactic. He was known to preach sermons to himself in his mind to try to keep his thoughts centered on the Savior.[11] The Lord said He hates "an heart that deviseth wicked imaginations" (Proverbs 6:18). We simply cannot think that our thoughts have less bearing on our spiritual salvation than our actions. We need to "let virtue garnish [our] thoughts unceasingly" (D&C 121:45).

We appreciate learning about the work and effort that apostles of the Lord have given to uphold virtuous thoughts in their lives. Their tremendous examples can be very instructive if we look to them. If these great men worked at it this hard, we should assume that we will have to work every bit as hard. Are there other ways you can think of to keep your thoughts clean and pure and focused on the Savior?

Another approach that will help in keeping our thoughts clean and pure is avoiding places and situations where temptations frequently arise. Often times, the battle can be won early on by avoiding certain websites, TV shows, movies, music, and groups of people. If you know you struggle keeping your thoughts clean when you go to a certain website, block that website! If you know you withdraw from the Spirit when you watch a certain TV show, don't ever watch it again! We cannot just pray for strength in temptation. We also have to remove ourselves from temptation as best we can.

Once we succumb to watching a bad movie, it will become more difficult for us to resist temptation and have virtuous thoughts. A certain picture or scene from a bad movie can linger with us for a very long time. As we spend more and more time in evil environments, any impure thoughts that are entertained will more quickly lead to impure actions.

THE "DOCTRINAL DIAMOND" IN HELAMAN 4:12

Helaman 4 describes the Lamanites' success in taking the land of Zarahemla and many other lands from the Nephites. Mormon attributes this to the wickedness of the Nephites at this time. At the end of verse 12, there is a subtle lesson to be learned about the Nephites that has significant application today. This is another "doctrinal diamond" from the Book of Mormon. Some of the Nephites are described as "deserting away into the land of Nephi, among the Lamanites" (Helaman 4:12).

One of the reasons the Nephites were so wicked was because they put themselves in wicked environments. They wanted to be right in the middle of it all. It was not enough for some of them to do wickedly among their own people. It was not enough for some to merely "mingle with the Lamanites" (Alma 50:22). Many Nephite dissenters were even more comfortable in the very heart of wickedness, fleeing their homes to live among the Lamanites by their own free will. Once we place ourselves in such an environment, it may be too difficult for us to resist certain temptations. We suffer the consequences of choosing to go into that evil environment in the first place.

We may find that as we enter the great and spacious building, we cannot easily find the door that leads back out (see 1 Nephi 8:26–27). We may find that if we start down a strange road and proceed to make a few turns, it is very difficult to trace our steps back (see 1 Nephi 8:32). We may find that if we go down forbidden paths, we will become lost and expend a lot of time and energy to find the right path again (see 1 Nephi 8:28). If we go down certain paths, there will be consequences. There will be pain and disappointment and suffering. "Wickedness never was happiness" (Alma 41:10). We cannot afford to take even one step toward the great and spacious building, along a strange road, or down a forbidden path.

By no means are we saying that once we go down a forbidden path in life, we cannot find our way back. Through the Atonement, we can always find our way back. There is always hope. However, it would be so much better for us if we just stayed on the right path in the first place. The scary reality is that some people do not return once they go down strange roads or forbidden paths. We cannot allow this possibility, and we cannot afford to leave our exaltation to the least bit of chance.

"Look unto Me in Every Thought"

Instead of focusing our discussion solely on how to rid ourselves of bad thoughts, of even greater importance is embracing *good* thoughts. King Benjamin taught, "For how knoweth a man the master whom he has not served, and who is a stranger unto him, and is far from the thoughts and intents of his heart?" (Mosiah 5:13). The Savior commanded us, "Look unto me in every thought" (D&C 6:36).

How can we look to the Savior in every thought? We can do this by focusing on that which is "true, honest, just, pure, lovely, and of good report" as Paul taught the Philippians (Philippians 4:8). These are all characteristics of our Savior, and by so doing we are looking unto Him in our thoughts. Consistent scripture study and prayer will also help us look to the Savior. If we notice that we are not doing things daily to help us remember the Savior or feel of His Spirit, we will drift further and further away from Him.

This practice of looking to the Savior in every thought is of paramount importance to us in our discipleship. As we partake of the sacrament each week and renew our covenants, we commit to remember the Savior always. If we are successful, we are promised to always have His Spirit to be with us. The Savior gave us another blessing when He quoted Malachi, "And a book of remembrance was written before him for them that feared the Lord, *and that thought upon his name*. And they shall be mine, saith the Lord of Hosts, in that day when I make up my jewels" (3 Nephi 24:16–17, emphasis added). If we ensure that our thoughts are focused on the Savior, we will receive eternal life and become one of His jewels.

Our quest to be pure in heart is so much more than just avoiding temptations and evil environments. Being pure in heart requires us to seek after wholesome, uplifting environments and activities. There is no more effective way to keep our thoughts pure than to spend our time in positive, inspiring, and uplifting places. By so doing, our hearts will be filled with the Spirit and His fruits—love, joy, peace, longsuffering, gentleness, goodness, faith, meekness, temperance—so there will be no room in our hearts for that which is impure and unholy (see Galatians 5:22–23).

THE HIGHER LAW OF CHASTITY— TAKING UP OUR CROSS

After promising the pure in heart that they shall see God, our Savior gave us a higher law in regard to chastity. He said:

> Behold, it is written by them of old time, that thou shalt not commit adultery;
>
> But I say unto you, that whosoever looketh on a woman, to lust after her, hath committed adultery already in his heart.
>
> Behold, I give unto you a commandment, that ye suffer none of these things to enter into your heart;
>
> For it is better that ye should deny yourself of these things, wherein ye will take up your cross, than that ye should be cast into hell. (3 Nephi 12:27–30)

We have often pondered upon the loyalty that is necessary in a celestial marriage. This commandment from our Savior shows to what extent we must be loyal to our spouses. We must be loyal to our spouses in every thought, word, feeling, and action. Elder L. Whitney Clayton said, "Loyalty is a form of respect. Prophets teach that successful marriage partners are 'fiercely loyal' to each other. They never do or say anything that approaches the appearance of impropriety, either virtually or physically. Watch and learn: terrific marriages are completely respectful, transparent, and loyal."[12] If we feel our thoughts drifting toward places we should not go, remember this principle of loyalty and the Savior's command He has given us to help strengthen our marriages.

Jesus taught us what it means to take up our cross. He said, "And now for a man to take up his cross, is to deny himself all ungodliness, and every worldly lust, and keep my commandments." (Matthew 16:24, footnote d; from JST Matthew 16:26).

We love the imagery of Saints taking up the cross. While members of the Church generally do not wear crosses, we have the opportunity to take up His cross and carry it daily. When we have a lustful thought come into our minds, we can think of the Savior and what He did for us on the cross. To honor Him, we can determine to carry our crosses by denying ourselves of such lusts. To honor Him, we can deny ourselves of all ungodliness that may be tempting to us. Such acts are much more important than actually wearing a cross around our neck.

Sister Neill F. Marriott of the Young Women General Presidency, provides some hope for us on this challenging journey. She said, "Can you become clean and stay clean in an unclean world? Yes, you can! You know the truth and have the support of the Holy Ghost, parents, leaders, and the living prophet. As you look to Jesus Christ, you can and will remain clean before Him. Asking Heavenly Father to create a clean heart in you is an act of faith. He has all power; turn to Him often and humbly ask for His divine help to keep your feelings pure—even sexually pure."[13] We must ask Heavenly Father to create a pure heart in us and ask in faith. Every prayer of faith requires action on our part. Each time we are faced with a choice to entertain an impure thought, a prayer to our Heavenly Father can provide us with greater resolve to remain pure and clean.

ALMA'S TEACHINGS—BEING MADE PURE

Another powerful example given in the Book of Mormon concerning the pure in heart is found in Alma 13. Here, Alma taught the people of Ammonihah about the priesthood and about high priests, specifically. Alma taught that high priests are prepared from the foundation of the world on account of their exceeding faith and good works.

Alma taught:

> Now, as I said concerning the holy order, or this high priesthood, there were many who were ordained and became high priests of God; and it was on account of their exceeding faith and repentance, and their righteousness before God, they choosing to repent and work righteousness rather than to perish;
>
> Therefore, they were called after this holy order, and were sanctified, and their garments were washed white through the blood of the Lamb.
>
> Now they, after being sanctified by the Holy Ghost, having their garments made white, being pure and spotless before God, could not look upon sin save it were with abhorrence; and there were many, exceedingly great many, who were made pure and entered into the rest of the Lord. (Alma 13:10–12)

All of us can be sanctified and be made clean through the blood of the Lamb and through the Holy Ghost. Our hearts can be made pure. Significantly, as made clear in scripture, we cannot make our own hearts pure. These verses say their garments were "made white." Much like Sister Marriott said, the Psalmist prayed, "Create in me a clean heart, O God" (Psalm 51:10). We cannot make our hearts pure on our own. The Spirit must sanctify and purify our hearts through the power of the Atonement of the Savior.

It is a comforting thought to us that there were many, exceedingly great many, who were made pure. As we repent, our hearts will change. Our garments can be washed white through the blood of the Lamb. There is hope for all of us. We can be made clean. We can be made pure.

"If This Be the Desire of Your Hearts"

The desires of our hearts must also be pure and much like our thoughts, desires lead to actions as well. President Dallin H. Oaks said, "Desires dictate our priorities, priorities shape our choices, and choices determine our actions."[14] We are told that we will be judged according to the desires of our hearts (see D&C 137:9).

One of the best examples in scripture about the desires of people's hearts is the story of the people of Alma the Elder at the waters of Mormon. Alma had been teaching the people faith, repentance, and redemption through the Lord.

Alma then said:

> Behold, here are the waters of Mormon and now, *as ye are desirous to come into the fold of God*, and to be called his people, and are willing to bear one another's burdens, that they may be light;
>
> Yea, and are willing to mourn with those that mourn; yea, and comfort those that stand in need of comfort, and to stand as witnesses of God at all times and in all things, and in all places that ye may be in, even until death, that ye may be redeemed of God, and be numbered with those of the first resurrection, that ye may have eternal life—
>
> Now I say unto you, *if this be the desire of your hearts*, what have you against being baptized in the name of the Lord, as a witness before him that ye have entered into a covenant with him, that ye will serve him and keep his commandments, that he may pour out his Spirit more abundantly upon you?
>
> And now when the people had heard these words, they clapped their hands for joy, and exclaimed: *This is the desire of our hearts.* (Mosiah 18:8–11, emphasis added)

Before Alma baptized these 204 believers, he wanted to make sure they understood the covenant associated with baptism and had aligned the desires of their hearts with these covenant obligations. The people were extremely enthusiastic in their response to

Alma's question about their desires and elated at the opportunity for baptism. They gave such a pure and faithful reply! They clapped their hands for joy and excitedly said that this was the desire of their hearts.

The people were thrilled to get baptized, but they were even more excited to be called God's people and to serve others around them. They had received a testimony of the blessings that awaited them if they were true to their baptismal covenants and desired nothing more than to have the Spirit with them more abundantly in their lives.

Improving our thoughts and desires is not doomed to be a fruitless endeavor. We *can* change our thought patterns. Our thoughts *can* become more refined. We *can* align our desires with the will of the Lord! While these commandments may seem overwhelming, we *can* commit to them and keep them. We *can* do it!

We take great solace in the words of Alma. Alma testified, "For I know that [God] granteth unto men according to their desire, whether it be unto death or unto life . . . but he that knoweth good and evil, to him it is given according to his desires, whether he desireth good or evil, life or death, joy or remorse of conscience" (Alma 29:4–5). We will receive from the Lord according to our righteous desires.

President Dallin H. Oaks gave us this promise in regard to these verses: "This means that when we have done all that we can, our *desires* will carry us the rest of the way. It also means that if our desires are right, we can be forgiven for the mistakes we will inevitably make as we try to carry those desires into effect. What a comfort for our feelings of inadequacy!"[15]

HARSH DOCTRINES

Some might say that there are some harsh doctrines associated with the thoughts, intents, and affections of our hearts. Mormon taught:

> For behold, God hath said a man being evil cannot do that
> which is good; for if he offereth a gift, or prayeth unto

God, except he shall do it with real intent it profiteth him nothing.

For behold, it is not counted unto him for righteousness.

For behold, if a man being evil giveth a gift, he doeth it grudgingly; wherefore it is counted unto him the same as if he had retained the gift; wherefore he is counted evil before God.

And likewise also it is counted evil unto a man, if he shall pray and not with real intent of heart; yea, and it profiteth him nothing, for God receiveth none such. (Moroni 7:6–9)

This sounds like a harsh doctrine. Can we really pray in such a way that our prayers do not benefit us? Yes! Further, such prayers offered without real intent are actually counted as evil unto us!

We have to pray with real intent of heart, as Mormon taught us, to receive any benefit from prayer. The same can be said about going to church, or serving others, or doing anything in the gospel! How often do we give a gift to the Savior grudgingly in such a way? Do we grudgingly go to the temple in a hurry because we have other "more important" things to do? Do we unenthusiastically fulfill our callings and assignments just to say that we did them? We imagine that most, if not all of us, have struggled with something similar to this from time to time. We might get discouraged and think that it is hard enough to go to church, study the scriptures, pray, and keep the commandments; so if we do not even profit from doing some of these things or even have them counted as evil in the eyes of the Lord, then why even try?

The secret, however, lies in this very doctrine of doing things with real intent, with proper desire in our hearts. As we give gifts righteously, it actually becomes *easier* for us to study the scriptures, pray, go to church, magnify callings, and keep the commandments. Through our righteous intent, we come to enjoy and love doing these things.

Alma counseled his son Helaman, "Yea, and cry unto God for all thy support; yea, let all thy doings be unto the Lord, and whithersoever thou goest let it be in the Lord; yea, let all thy thoughts be directed unto the Lord; yea, let the affections of thy heart be placed upon the Lord forever" (Alma 37:36). What a beautiful phrase: "the affections of [our] heart." The question of where we place our affections is worth asking at regular intervals of self-reflection. Are our affections upon riches? Are our affections upon the honors of women and men? Or are our affections upon the Lord?

The prophet Joseph Smith once said, "Our affections should be placed upon God and His work, more intensely than upon our fellow beings."[16] The prophet was speaking at a funeral at the time he said this. This too may sound like harsh doctrine given at a particularly difficult time for some of those to whom it was given. But this viewpoint gives us great eternal perspective. If we will place our affections upon the Lord and His work, everything else will take care of itself. We will be able to live again with our loved ones in the Lord's marvelous presence and enjoy magnificent blessings eternally.

Elder Parley P. Pratt said, "The gift of the Holy Ghost quickens all . . . affections; and adapts them, by the gift of wisdom, to their lawful use. It inspires, develops, cultivates, and matures all . . . affections of our nature."[17] As He can with all conditions of the heart, the Holy Ghost can do more to develop, inspire, quicken, and cultivate our hearts than can be done in any other way. Those who are falling short and sense their affections, thoughts, and desires are moving further away from the Lord must pray for the Spirit to return to them and do things that will help them feel of His influence.

Being pure in heart is a continuous effort waged on multiple fronts. We are bombarded today by temptations to be impure in our thoughts, words, and actions. We are inundated with crude entertainment options and salacious websites. There has never been a time in which such things were as easily accessible. If we go near such evil environments, we must move away quickly. Never go near such places. Do not allow yourself to linger there if you do find yourself in such a place. Rather, we are commanded to stand in holy places (see D&C 45:32). As Elder Bruce R. McConkie promised, "We gain purity of heart by obedience."[18] Every positive choice we make with regard to our thoughts, words, and actions will result in additional purity in our hearts.

One last area that deserves consideration on our part in the effort to develop a pure heart is service to our fellow men. While a member of the Seventy, Elder Dale E. Miller said, "Those willing to serve are invited to labor in the vineyard of the Lord, steadily transforming themselves to become the pure in heart."[19] A multitude of blessings are promised to those who serve others. This particular blessing from service deserves emphasis and reflection. We will become the pure in heart as we serve others.

Elder Royden G. Derrick said, "When one extends mercy to others, he develops purity in heart."[20] Those that extend a helping hand to others and are constantly on the lookout to serve will be blessed with purity of heart. Those that are merciful and forgiving of others, remembering the spark of divinity that is within all of us, will be blessed with purity of heart. Focusing on these things will effectively and rapidly purify hearts. Alma posed a deeply introspective question to the people of Zarahemla. He asked, "Can we look up to God at that day with a pure heart and clean hands?" (Alma 5:19).

President Dieter F. Uchtdorf summed things up perfectly when he said, "[The Savior's] Atonement allows us to leave the past behind and move forward with a pure heart."[21] When the Atonement of Christ is applied in our lives, our hearts will be purified. To apply the Atonement of Christ, we can work to clean up our thoughts and ensure they are directed toward the Savior. We can take up our cross daily, denying ourselves of all ungodliness. We do this by removing anything in our lives that is foreign to our Savior and His gospel. Taking advantage of the miraculous gift of the Atonement of Christ, our hearts can be made pure as we perform our critical labors while on the earth.

Chapter 10

FULL PURPOSE OF HEART

Joseph Smith said, "I told the brethren that the Book of Mormon was the most correct of any book on earth, and the keystone of our religion, and a man would get nearer to God by abiding by its precepts, than by any other book" (introduction to the Book of Mormon). Within its pages, the Savior pleads with us to come unto Him or return to Him almost forty times in many different settings! He also instructs us on *how* we can come unto Him.

The Savior repeatedly used the phrase "with full purpose of heart" in his supplications for the Nephites to come unto Him. Interestingly, this phrase "full purpose of heart" is not found anywhere in the Bible. The Book of Mormon contains so much magnificent imagery and such a beautiful narrative of the heart that can be found in no other place.

"COME UNTO ME"

The Lord spoke to those who were spared from the widespread destruction that swept across the Nephites' lands after His Crucifixion. He said, "O ye house of Israel whom I have spared, how oft will I gather you as a hen gathereth her chickens under her wings, if ye will repent and return unto me with full purpose of heart" (3 Nephi 10:6). The Savior taught the Nephites at the temple in Bountiful, "Come unto me with full purpose of heart, and I will receive you" (3 Nephi 12:24). Jesus reminded His disciples to not cast out those who were unworthy to partake of the sacrament, "For ye know not but what they will return and repent, and come unto me with full purpose of heart, and I shall heal them" (3 Nephi 18:32). The Savior sees the divine potential in everyone, that they might cast off their sins and come unto Him with full purpose of heart.

There are ten specific references in the Book of Mormon that use the phrase "full purpose of heart" or speak of doing something "with all our hearts." Joseph Smith taught that we must subscribe to certain articles of adoption to enter into the kingdom of God.[1] On our personal covenant-path journey, in developing a Christlike heart, coming to the Lord with full purpose of heart is one of those articles of adoption necessary to enter into the kingdom of God.

What exactly does it mean to do something with full purpose? Something is "full" when it has no empty space or when it is not lacking or omitting anything.[2] "Purpose" is defined as the reason for which something is done or created or for which something exists.[3] These definitions bring added meaning to what the Savior and prophets meant when they employed this phrase. The reason for our existence on Earth is to learn to follow and emulate the Savior, and this is to be done with complete and singular devotion on our part.

Coming to Christ with "full purpose of heart" is akin to living the law of consecration. The Lord is asking for us to fully give our hearts to Him, not merely a portion. Hearts must be fully consecrated to His purposes for us to be able to most effectively serve Him and do His will. There are plentiful examples of people who have properly developed this condition of the heart in the Book of Mormon, as well as examples of others whose behavior lacked a full purpose of heart.

Elder Patrick Kearon of the Seventy described what it means to have full purpose of heart in this way: "We must cease fighting against God and instead give our whole hearts to Him, holding nothing back. Then He can heal us. Then he can cleanse us from the venomous sting of sin."[4]

Are we holding anything back in regard to the gospel and the commandments we have been taught to keep? Are we "pressing forward with a steadfastness in Christ, having a perfect brightness of hope, and a love of God and of all men, and feasting upon the word of Christ?" (2 Nephi 31:20). Amaleki teaches us to "come unto [Christ], and offer [our] whole souls as an offering unto Him" (Omni 1:26). We cannot afford to leave any of the affections of our heart with Satan and that for which he stands.

HALF-HEARTEDNESS

Half-heartedness is in stark contrast to doing something with full purpose of heart. Have you ever done anything half-heartedly? Have you ever worked on a school project half-heartedly and noticed a large drop in the quality of the finished product as a result? Have you ever done the bare minimum in a job and just tried to skate by? Have you half-heartedly sat in a church meeting just waiting for it to end so you could say you were there? It is possible that an honest assessment of our daily activities will reveal that a great deal of half-heartedness has infected our efforts.

Elder Neal A. Maxwell said, "It is so easy to be half-hearted, but this only produces half the growth, half the blessings, and just half a life, really, with more bud than blossom."[5] We cannot imagine half a heart would be ideal for peak physical performance. Maybe half a heart would lead to us being half-alive, and that condition sounds remarkably unappealing.

Elder Mark E. Petersen said, "There is no reward for half-hearted obedience. We must become vigorous and enthusiastic about living our religion, for God commands that we serve him with *all* our heart, with *all* our might, with *all* our strength, and with the very best of our intelligence. With Him there can be no halfway measures. We must be fully *for* him or we may be classed with those who are *against* him."[6]

President Gordon B. Hinckley said, "There is a tendency on the part of some to become indifferent. There are those who drift off seeking the enticements of the world, forsaking the cause of the Lord. I see others who think it is all right to lower their standards, perhaps in small ways. In this very process they lose the cutting edge of enthusiasm for this work."[7]

Both of the above quotes from Elder Petersen and President Hinckley discuss enthusiasm. Enthusiasm is a natural byproduct of living the gospel with full purpose of heart. While the word *enthusiasm* is not mentioned in the scriptures, there are several similar synonyms that are mentioned, such as zeal, diligence, and dedication.

THE ENTHUSIASM OF THE PEOPLE OF AMMON

The people of Ammon are one of the best examples of enthusiasm in the Book of Mormon. Mormon referred to the zeal of the people of Ammon on three separate occasions in his abridgment. Obviously, their zeal had a profound impact on Mormon and was an attribute that Mormon highly esteemed. Mormon first described them thus: "And Ammon did preach unto the people of king Lamoni; and it came to pass that he did teach them all things concerning things pertaining to righteousness. And he did exhort them daily, with all diligence; and they gave heed unto his word, and they were zealous for keeping the commandments of God" (Alma 21:23).

Mormon was impressed by the zeal the people of Ammon had for keeping the commandments of God. He provided further insight into this zeal when he observed, "And they were among the people of Nephi, and also numbered among the people who were of the church of God. And they were also distinguished for their zeal towards God, and also towards men; for they were perfectly honest and upright in all things; and they were firm in the faith of Christ, even unto the end" (Alma 27:27).

The zeal that the people of Ammon exhibited toward God in keeping His commandments was constantly reflected in their interactions with others. They were strict in keeping the commandments, and their discipleship was set apart by its exactness. Any interactions they had with others were governed by these principles, and others took notice.

On the third occasion, Mormon noted, "They were a zealous and beloved people, a highly favored people of the Lord" (Alma 27:30). Is there any surprise that the Lord would favor or bless those who possessed this distinctive characteristic? The Lord has said on multiple occasions that He is a jealous God (see Exodus 20:5, Mosiah 11:22, Mosiah 13:13). The Lord wants a zealous people, a people excited and exuberant for His law, His plan, and His atoning sacrifice with its resultant grace and mercy.

We can think of no better description of enthusiasm and zeal than Mormon's words here. The people of Ammon lived the gospel with full purpose of heart. They were firm in the faith of Christ, even unto death. Sadly, there were many that did suffer death by the Lamanites, yet they remained steadfast in Christ and to the covenants they had made with the Lord.

BE ENTHUSIASTIC!

One of our dad's favorite missionary stories that he liked to share with us growing up is about enthusiasm. He served in the New England States Mission. He remembers being invited by an Episcopalian church to share some information about the Church. He accepted the invitation and attended with his district leader at the time. His district leader was a short elder that made up for any lack of height with an abundance of enthusiasm. My dad recognized that when this missionary spoke, people lit up and were attracted to what he had to say because of his enthusiasm. Enthusiasm both for the gospel and in his manner of communication qualified him to act as a very effective ambassador for the Church.

Every district meeting run by this district leader concluded in the same manner. The missionaries would repeat a quote attributed to Dale Carnegie. They would excitedly say, "If you want to be enthusiastic, you have to act enthusiastic!" They repeated it three or four times, getting louder with each repetition. This gave them "the cutting edge of enthusiasm," as President Gordon B. Hinckley called it, that they needed to perform their labors that day and week.[8]

Derek had a memorable experience learning the importance of enthusiasm during his mission in Russia. In his words:

One of the fondest memories from my mission was at a time when I was doing my best to work with full purpose of heart. I had a newer missionary as my companion at the time. We were working in an area that hadn't seen much success or teaching in it for a long time. As such, we had to knock on a lot of doors to try to find people to teach. I remember one week in particular in which we knocked on over six hundred doors and just did not have any success. It was rare to not have at least someone interested in listening to the first discussion or wanting to at least talk to some foreigners.

I remember it raining pretty hard as that week came to a close. It was dark, and we easily could have gone back to our apartment a couple of hours early to rest. However, we chose to press on and kept knocking on doors. I would love to end this story by saying that we found a "golden investigator" eager to learn more about the Savior and His Church when we knocked on our final door that night, but that is not what happened.

Disappointingly, we did not have any more success in finding people to teach with those last doors to end the week than we did with the first doors of that week. However, we had done our missionary work with full purpose of heart and with zeal. We strongly felt the Spirit sustain us in our efforts. That tangible, sustaining feeling we felt from the

Holy Ghost that night has not dimmed with me over the last almost twenty years.

Enthusiasm is contagious. Our enthusiasm can have an enormous impact on others when we attend church meetings, participate in a service project, or even read scriptures as a family. On the other hand, we can be a destructive drain of energy to others in these same situations. What type of people do we want to be?

"THE PERIL OF THE CENTURY"

Have you ever done anything in your life with full purpose of heart? We are convinced that many of life's most satisfying moments occur when we do something with great conviction and determination. President David O. McKay said, "The peril of this century is spiritual apathy."[9] This prophet of the Lord could see that there were many within the Church that did not have their hearts fully invested in the Savior's gospel. This prophet of the Lord saw the danger of us not coming unto Christ with full purpose of heart.

The apathy President McKay spoke about can be seen in many walks of life. There seems to be an epidemic of apathy toward that most precious commodity—time—in our world today. It is regularly and excessively wasted on degrading and demoralizing activities. The minutes we are given are finite and limited. Are we zealously using those minutes to be of service to those around us? Are we apathetic in our relationships with others, or do we give them our full focus and attention? Do we take loved ones for granted? Do we strive for greatness in all that we do, or do we gladly put up with mediocrity in many areas of life? Life is much more exhilarating and fulfilling when we are striving to maximize our time in worthy pursuits.

Lehi described himself as a "trembling parent" when he gave some final instruction to his rebellious sons, Laman and Lemuel, before he died (2 Nephi 1:14). He said, "O that ye would awake; awake from a deep sleep, yea, even from the sleep of hell, and shake off the awful chains by which ye are bound, which are the chains which bind the children of men, that they are carried away captive down to the eternal gulf of misery and woe" (2 Nephi 1:13). Lehi told his sons seven times in this chapter to either awake or arise!

That deep sleep, those awful chains, will come upon all of us if we invite that influence into our lives. This theme is of such importance that it is frequently alluded to throughout the Book of Mormon. One of the most prominent phrases cited along these lines is "dwindling in unbelief."

DWINDLING IN UNBELIEF

Ryan received the following inspiration in regard to this principle. In his words:

> This past summer I've had several chances to take in several peaceful campfires in the mountains of Utah and Idaho. There is something captivating and gripping about looking into a campfire. For me, campfires are marvelous tools for self-reflection and introspection. I like to think eternal truths can gently wash over me while looking into the soft flames on a quiet evening—if I will search for them and if I am willing to receive them.
>
> It struck me this year that there are few things in the world that make for a better example of what it means "to dwindle" than a good campfire. A campfire is either growing in intensity and strength due to the addition of fuel, or it is ebbing, waning, fading, and dying. There is no middle ground in the life of a campfire, and yet the changes that take place when one is weakening are subtle and almost imperceptible.
>
> Second to second, there are indistinguishable differences in the amount of light and warmth a campfire produces. In the moment, it is difficult to tell that there is any progress or change taking place at all. If we are unaware of the process, we will miss seeing any difference at all until a substantial change has already taken place. This slight

and almost indiscernible weakening and diminishment of warmth and heat can also be described as dwindling.

There is value in looking at some of the definitions of the term *dwindle*. A few definitions include the following: "to become gradually less until little remains;" "to grow or cause to grow less in size, intensity, or number; diminish or shrink gradually;" and "to become smaller and smaller; shrink; diminish, to fall away, as in quality; degenerate."[10,11,12] Other common synonyms include the words decline, sink, weaken, shrink, decay, whither, shrivel, peter out, reduce, and taper.

The word *dwindle* is used twenty-seven times in the Book of Mormon, within nine different books, and is nearly always paired with the words "in unbelief." We've attempted to highlight throughout this book the prophets in the Book or Mormon who frequently remind us of the divine providence they received in directing and targeting their teachings for us in our day (see Mormon 8:35 and 3 Nephi 26:12). I have decided that the Book of Mormon prophets' repeated warnings with regard to dwindling ought to cause myself caution—and maybe even alarm.

We are told that when the written scriptures and commandments of God aren't before our eyes, we will dwindle (see Mosiah 1:5). Mormon showed that faithfully keeping the commandments leads us to deliverance, while not doing so will lead to dwindling (see Alma 50:22). Mormon stated that because of iniquity the Church dwindled and testimonies of Christ faltered (see Helaman 4:23). In the book of 4 Nephi, Mormon spoke of a people that dwindled "from year to year" (4 Nephi 1:34).

Can I look back at my life and see days, months, and even years that I didn't grow as much as I should have because I was actively dwindling? Yes, sadly I can. Dwindling in unbelief is paralleled with departing from the right way and not knowing the God in whom we should trust (see Mormon 9:20). And we are warned that

God's miracles in our lives cease when we dwindle. I need His miracles in my life!

I have been thinking about what "dwindling in unbelief" would look like in today's world and in my life. It may be found in slightly shorter and less heartfelt prayers each day, or even skipping prayers here and there altogether. It may be in almost imperceptibly weaker fasts month to month. It may be a little less focus on the Savior in my life and a little less effort to have His Spirit with me. It may be more and more time on social media or surfing the Internet, seeking the world's validation. It may be a little less diligence studying the scriptures each day, or more and more time passing by without studying at all. It may be an increasing focus on the world and material things, and less focus on things of the Spirit. It may be frittering away precious time sitting in front of the television, overindulging in hobbies, or just plain spending time on things that won't help me grow closer to Christ.

Words like *casual*, *periodic*, *sporadic*, and *irregular* seem to describe dwindling in today's world. Dwindling in unbelief can be remarkably subtle, gradual, and difficult to recognize. Before we know it, we can find ourselves on the outside looking in, or worse yet, on the outside throwing rocks in frustration.

The campfire of our testimony is in constant need of rekindling. Testimonies are either growing or they are diminishing! A fiery redetermination and continual recommitment to serve the Lord is the antithesis of dwindling. An effort to actively grow our testimony will fight the fade. Diligently, patiently, faithfully nourishing the word will defeat the decay. Praying with all the energy of our heart and doing things with full purpose of heart will reverse the decline in our spirituality. It may be that the remedy to dwindling is found in words like intensity, passion, might, and strength. The long-term solution to overcoming the danger of dwindling is found in Christlike habits, routines, and patterns.

Though dwindling is hard to see in the moment, looking back on my life, it is easy to see chunks of time that are bigger than I want to admit that were dwindled away. I have dwindled more than enough in my life to know its terrible cost, and I am trying to better recognize dwindling and more quickly beat it out of my life. Dwindling happens when I am least prepared to recognize it. I have also felt periods of intense spiritual feasting, and I am trying to better recognize what it takes to prolong and intensify those periods as much as possible.

REPENTING WITH FULL PURPOSE OF HEART

The antithesis of dwindling in unbelief or being in a state of deep sleep with regard to the gospel is living the gospel with full purpose of heart. In almost every instance, the phrase "full purpose of heart" in the Book of Mormon is coupled with repentance. Nephi declared, "If ye shall follow the Son, with full purpose of heart, acting no hypocrisy and no deception before God, but with real intent, repenting of your sins, witnessing unto the Father that ye are willing to take upon you the name of Christ, by baptism . . . behold, then shall ye receive the Holy Ghost" (2 Nephi 31:13).

President Howard W. Hunter said:

There must be genuine effort, *wholehearted effort*, if change is to come. Consider this aspect of resolve, of genuine resolution. There is a phrase common in the Book of Mormon that describes what our efforts should entail. The phrase "full purpose of heart" is used by Nephi in his final counsel to our generation. He promises that if we will follow the Son of God with "full purpose of heart," *then* the promised blessings will flow to us. Nephi clarifies the phrase by adding "acting no hypocrisy and no deception before God, but with real intent, repenting of your sins, witnessing unto the Father that ye are willing to take upon you the name of Christ" (2 Nephi 31:13). The "full purpose of heart" Nephi describes is much more fixed and determined than are the usual New Year's resolutions with many people.[13]

We need to repent to experience a mighty change of heart. However, there is additional meaning given to repentance when considered in terms of repenting with "full purpose of heart." Going back to the Savior's counsel, He said we must "return and repent, and come unto [Him] with full purpose of heart" (3 Nephi 18:32). We are commanded to repent with full purpose of heart. How does repentance happen in such a way? Sins surely must be forsaken and confessed, but this must also be accompanied with a complete return unto the Savior (see D&C 58:43). Backs must be completely turned to sin and the return unto Christ must be made with an eye steady on Him. It is not sufficient to take a few steps forward and then turn around for a quick gaze on Babylon before continuing forward again. A process like that does not constitute repentance with full purpose of heart.

Hugh Nibley said, "Repentance isn't complete until we have really meant what we are doing."[14] The Bible Dictionary says repentance "comes to mean a turning of the heart and will to God, and a renunciation of sin to which we are naturally inclined."[15] Have you ever tried to repent of something without full purpose of heart? Though we may feel we want forgiveness at that particular moment, on such occasions our heart is not quite ready to turn away from that wrongful act completely, and we often fall back into the same sin.

CLEAVE UNTO GOD

Jacob implored his people, "Wherefore, my beloved brethren, I beseech of you in words of soberness that ye would repent, and come with full purpose of heart, and cleave unto God as he cleaveth unto you. And while his arm of mercy is extended towards you in the light of the day, harden not your hearts" (Jacob 6:5). Again, Jacob counseled us to repent and come unto the Savior with full purpose of heart. Jacob was encouraging the Nephites to put forth effort to become clean and draw nearer to God. There is great power in Jacob's exhortation to cleave unto God as He cleaves unto us. Hyrum Smith, brother to the prophet Joseph Smith, was similarly exhorted to cleave unto God with all his heart (see D&C 11:19).

"To cleave" means to adhere firmly and closely to something.[16] A Church Handbook indicates that to "cleave means to be completely devoted and faithful to someone."[17] As the definitions indicate, it is possible to cleave to something and or someone. Are we completely devoted to our God? Do we try to stick closely and firmly to Him? We will unavoidably perish if we do not cleave unto Him! (see Helaman 4:25).

The scriptures and latter-day Church leaders give us several directives in regard to our cleaving. We are commanded to cleave unto our spouse and none else (see Genesis 2:24). We are instructed to lift up our hearts and rejoice and cleave unto our covenants (see D&C 25:13). We will cleave unto every good thing if we have faith in Christ (see Moroni 7:28). We are instructed to cleave unto charity (see Moroni 7:46). The Jaredites provided an example of cleaving unto material possessions and the dangers inherent with this practice (see Ether 14:2). Elder Robert D. Hales said, "The eternal plan includes holding fast to the iron rod—cleaving to God's word and the word of his prophets. We need to tighten our grip on the rod that leads us back to Him."[18]

We rejoice in the fact that our Savior cleaves unto us! His arm of mercy is ever extended toward us. He is fully devoted to helping us come unto Him and return to live with Him and our Heavenly Father. He performs His work with full purpose of heart. We know that He fully and completely gave His heart to us in His atoning sacrifice. Now, He asks us to respond in kind by coming unto Him with full purpose of heart. Sister Anne C. Pingree, second counselor in the Relief Society general presidency testified, "When we do come to the Savior with full purpose of heart, we will feel His loving touch in the most personal ways."[19] His outstretched arm and the grace and mercy offered to us through His atoning sacrifice will indeed bless us.

The Great Commandment

The Pharisees asked Jesus, "Master, which is the great commandment in the law? Jesus said unto him, Thou shalt love the Lord thy God with all thy heart, and with all thy soul, and with all thy mind" (Matthew 22:36–37). Moroni called upon those who did not believe in Christ, "Come unto the Lord with all your heart" (Mormon 9:27).

Both of these scriptures express the degree to which we must come unto Christ and love Him. It has to be with all our hearts! Anything less will not suffice, nor will it be acceptable to Him. We cannot allow ourselves to believe that we can hold onto one or two things that go contrary to his commandments. We cannot hold anything back from the Savior to receive His full blessings. However, in return for our complete love and devotion, Heavenly Father and Jesus will give us everything they have. Their grace and mercy far, far outweigh anything we think we deserve from our own works.

We challenge you to examine your hearts and see if you are holding anything back from the Lord. Are you hesitant to put your time and talents into your calling to do your best job possible? Do you minister with full purpose of heart? Are there certain things you are currently doing in your life that you know are wrong or are maybe just not as good as something else you could be doing? Do you really, truly extend yourselves to sacrifice of your means to the poor and needy? You will find ways that you can serve the Lord with greater purpose of heart as you honestly answer these questions.

PROMISED BLESSINGS

We will receive healing and relief under the watchful care of "the Great Physician, our Savior, Jesus Christ" as we repent with full purpose of heart.[20] The Savior promised us that He will gather us, He will receive us, and He will heal us if we come unto Him with full purpose of heart (see 3 Nephi 10:6, 12:24, 18:32). Elder Richard G. Scott testified that "Satan's temptations lose power in our lives" as we serve our Savior and fellow man with full purpose of heart.[21]

We will be filled with charity in our hearts as we pray with full purpose of heart, with all the energy of our hearts. This type of prayer is characterized by exercising our faith in Heavenly Father's ability to answer our prayers. Such prayer is distinguished by going to work to bring about such fulfillment as best we can on our own and by focusing on the needs of others.

Elder Gene R. Cook said, "When we pray with fervency we pray with real intent. We pray from the heart. We really mean what we say, and we say what we feel. This brings an added humility, an increased power to our prayers that we never have when we pray in a surface manner only, perhaps only speaking words."[22] Elder Cook was speaking about praying with all the energy of our hearts (see Moroni 7:48). We cannot afford to just speak words when we pray. We need to pray with energy and with real intent. Then, we will see the full blessings come to us from our prayers.

All available blessings of the Atonement of Christ can be ours as we cleave unto Him. We will not only be forgiven of our sins and be cleansed, but we will also receive added strength and power to be more effective servants of His on this earth. What a marvelous journey we will have as we move onward with full purpose of heart in the gospel of the Lord! There is no grander, nobler pursuit than this.

Chapter 11

TURN HEARTS OF THE CHILDREN TO THEIR FATHERS

The three previous conditions of the heart we have reviewed in this section have clear ties to the temple and are necessary qualifications to enter into the kingdom of God. It is fitting to conclude this section with a study of turning our hearts to our fathers as well as turning our hearts to our children. While the mention of this particular condition of the heart is from a single verse in the Book of Mormon, its impact and meaning are significant enough to merit further discussion and study in this book. The Book of Mormon includes strong examples of families that turned their hearts to their children and to their fathers. President Howard W. Hunter called on Church members to "establish the temple of the Lord as the great symbol of our Church membership."[1] In order for this to happen, we must turn our hearts to our fathers and to our children. Joseph Smith taught, "We without [our ancestors] cannot be made perfect; neither can they without us be made perfect" (D&C 128:18).

MALACHI'S PROPHECY

Malachi's prophecy was so critical to the Nephites' understanding of the plan of salvation that the Savior quoted it to them and had them include it in their record. He then expounded the prophecy unto them. He said:

> Behold, I will send you Elijah the prophet before the coming of the great and dreadful day of the Lord;
>
> And he shall turn the heart of the fathers to the children, and the heart of the children to their fathers, lest I come and smite the earth with a curse. (3 Nephi 25:5–6)

What can we understand and learn from this prophecy? Joseph F. Smith said:

> The fathers are our dead ancestors who died without the privilege of receiving the gospel, but who received the promise that the time would come when that privilege would be granted them. The children are those now living who are preparing genealogical data and who are performing the vicarious ordinances in the temples.
>
> The turning of the hearts of the children to the fathers is placing or planting in the hearts of the children that feeling and desire which will inspire them to search out the records of the dead. Moreover the planting of the desire and inspiration in their hearts is necessary. This they must have in order that they might go into the house of the Lord and perform the necessary labor for their fathers.[2]

The prophet Joseph Smith said, "The word *turn* here should be translated *bind*, or seal."[3] Our ancestors who did not have the opportunity to have the gospel preached unto them in mortality will have this opportunity. They will also have the chance to accept ordinances performed by proxy in their behalf. Their hearts are bound to ours. They are dependent on us to do this work. They cannot do the work and receive these ordinances on their own.

This particular prophecy from Malachi is quoted in each of the standard works, adding to its supernal significance. Moroni quoted Malachi's prophecy when he visited Joseph Smith in 1823, but he used slightly different wording. Moroni used the word *plant* instead of *turn*. He said, "And he shall plant in the hearts of the children the promises made to the fathers, and the hearts of the children shall turn to their fathers" (D&C 2:2). Moroni added the phrase, "the promises made to the fathers," which signifies the Abrahamic covenant.

Moroni's visit to Joseph Smith and subsequent instruction quoting Malachi's prophecy is also recorded in Joseph Smith—History 1:37–39 in the Pearl of Great Price. This account is consistent with the wording recorded in D&C 2. Why is this particular prophecy of such weight that it is included so frequently in the scriptures?

We are blessed to remember the promises made to our ancestors regarding the gospel. They, like us, were given certain promises through the Abrahamic covenant. Our ancestors, if faithful, were promised a numerous posterity and that their seed would receive the gospel and bear the priesthood. Our ancestors were also promised that all the families of the earth would be blessed, even with the greatest blessings of the gospel, which are the blessings of salvation and eternal life because of their ministry.

We are blessed to have these promises brought to our remembrance. They will be planted in our hearts. The Abrahamic covenant, studied frequently, will remind us of the wonderful blessings the Lord has in store for all of us. We will come to know that the only way our ancestors are assured of these great blessings is by doing their temple work. The urgency of this great work will then be impressed upon our hearts and lead us to action.

After Nephi obtained the brass plates, Lehi began to study them and found a genealogy of his fathers on them. This was one of the greatest blessings that Lehi received from reading the brass plates. He discovered that he was a descendant of Joseph, who was the son of Jacob. Nephi observed, "And now when my father saw all these things, he was filled with the Spirit, and began to prophesy concerning his seed" (1 Nephi 5:17). Lehi was inspired and filled with the Spirit through learning about his ancestors.

WHO WAS ELIJAH?

The scriptures teach that Elijah would come again to earth and begin this work. Who was Elijah? Why was he foreordained and selected to be the one to come to turn our hearts to our fathers? Elijah is first introduced to us in a conversation he had with King Ahab. Elijah told the king that there would not be any more rain for years to come, only according to his word (see 1 Kings 17:1). Elijah had been given the sealing power on earth.

Elijah also performed miracles with a widow and her son. Elijah asked the widow to bring him a little cake and some water. The widow only had enough flour and oil at home for herself and her son to eat one more meal, and then she assumed they would die. She demonstrated extraordinary faith in giving Elijah all of her food instead of choosing to meet not only her own needs, but also the needs of her son in such a dire situation. The widow was given the blessing that her flour and oil would never run out until rain came again on the earth, as a result of her transcendent faith. The widow's son fell sick and died after being blessed with this miracle. Elijah raised him from the dead (see 1 Kings 17:10–24).

Elijah called down fire from heaven when he confronted the priests of Baal in 1 Kings 18. He had all the priests of Baal killed and then asked for the Lord to send rain again upon the earth after a three-and-a-half-year drought. Elijah fasted for forty days and forty nights as he went to Horeb (see 1 Kings 19).

Finally, we are told Elijah was taken up by a whirlwind into heaven in a chariot of fire and was translated (see 2 Kings 2:11). Elijah held the sealing power of the Melchizedek Priesthood. The Bible Dictionary teaches us, "He appeared on the Mount of Transfiguration in company with Moses and conferred the keys of the priesthood upon Peter, James, and John. He appeared again on April 3, 1836, in the Kirtland Temple and conferred the sealing keys upon Joseph Smith and Oliver Cowdery."[4]

This is the Spirit of Elijah that is commonly referenced. President Russell M. Nelson further explained that the Spirit of Elijah is "a manifestation of the Holy Ghost bearing witness of the divine nature of the family."[5] We strongly believe and know that families can be together forever. There would be no motivation for millions of Saints to perform temple ordinances for the dead if we did not have faith in this precious truth.

The spirit of seeking out our dead and performing ordinances for them vicariously has grown tremendously since the time Elijah appeared in the Kirtland Temple. This spirit is also manifest throughout the world with people who are not members of the Church. President Henry B. Eyring said we will feel "a tug on [our] heart" as we get involved in this work.[6] This is the Spirit of Elijah working in our hearts through the Holy Ghost.

SAVIORS ON MOUNT ZION

Obadiah in the Old Testament prophesied there would be "saviors on Mount Zion" (Obadiah 1:21). Joseph Smith instructed us on how we can be saviors on Mount Zion. He said, "How are they to become saviors on Mount Zion? By building their temples, erecting their baptismal fonts, and going forth and receiving all the ordinances . . . in behalf of all their progenitors who are dead."[7]

This is a monumental task that will not be completed in our lifetimes. Temple work will carry on throughout the Millennium. Despite the magnitude of this task, we can recognize the urgency of the work and do our part through the Spirit of Elijah. It is no coincidence that the technological advances of late and the many tools now at the Church's disposal have increased the ability and the desire to do more work for our kindred dead.

Elder David A. Bednar invited the youth in a general conference address in 2011 to learn and experience the Spirit of Elijah.[8] It has been extraordinary to see the increase of involvement by youth in temple and family history work since that time. The youth of the Church have been given gifts of ability and knowledge needed to use this technology to accomplish this great work. Just in the past seven years since Elder Bednar gave this address, tens of thousands of youth have joined in this great work and have shown a remarkable aptitude and love for it.

There have been recent changes within the temples to allow young women the opportunity to work in the baptistry and assist with tasks that were only performed by adult sisters in the past. Young men that hold the office of priest in the Aaronic Priesthood are now allowed to perform baptisms for the dead. The youth of the Church are more actively engaged in temple work than ever before. Their hearts are turned to their fathers more so than any other generation since the Restoration of the Church in these latter days.

HENRY WOOD, OUR PIONEER ANCESTOR

We love to learn more about our ancestors. We love to read about them and hear their stories. As we have written earlier, we are enormously grateful for our pioneer heritage—for people like John Rowe Moyle that have taught us how to live by faith and work hard. We are also encouraged by finding records of ancestors who need their temple work done and going to the temple to do their work.

We had a wonderful experience not very long ago. We had the opportunity to go and look at some first editions of the Book of Mormon. We saw one that had a signature from Henry Wood on the inside cover. Being curious, we went home and looked this person up to see if we were related somehow. We went on to FamilySearch and were shocked to find that he is our sixth-great-grandfather through our mother's line. Not only that, our dad's great-great-great-grandfather was Henry Wood's brother-in-law! It was exciting to identify so many connections to our family.

It was thrilling to look up details of Henry's life and learn more about him. He and his wife, Elizabeth DeMille, had fifteen children. One of them, Daniel Wood, was converted to the gospel in

1833 and was baptized by Elder Brigham Young. Daniel became a steadfast pioneer and missionary. He and his wife sold everything they had to leave Canada and go to Kirtland to be with the Saints. They were driven out of Kirtland and left behind a forty-acre farm to go to Davis County, Missouri. They subsequently moved to Far West and then to Nauvoo as mobs and persecution plagued the Saints. Daniel's family ended up being one of the first six families to settle the Bountiful/Woods Cross area of Utah. Woods Cross is named after the Daniel Wood family.

Many of you have such fun and interesting family history stories to tell. Others having no story to tell are blessed with the exciting opportunity to be the pioneer of their family! If you are the pioneer, you will be blessed with strength and faith on your journey above your own. You will feel the Spirit of Elijah in your life. You will be blessed to realize the magnitude of the decisions you make and know that they will affect generations and generations to come.

AMULEK, THE PIONEER

The Book of Mormon is full of stories about pioneers who had the courage to accept the word of God and come into the fold of God. Amulek was such a pioneer in his family. Mormon records the following, "And it came to pass that Alma and Amulek, Amulek having forsaken all his gold, and his silver, and his precious things, which were in the land of Ammonihah, for the word of God, he being rejected by those who were once his friends and also by his father and his kindred" (Alma 15:16). The examples of Saints who have been disowned by their parents for accepting the gospel and being baptized into the Church are abundant. We cannot imagine the enormity of the sacrifice that Amulek was asked to make. His father and other kindred rejected him for accepting the gospel. We are not told what kindred rejected him in addition to his father, but we can be confident that these were people very close and dear to Amulek.

Amulek mentioned earlier that Alma had blessed his entire household when he dwelt with them (see Alma 10:11). The subsequent rejection of Amulek apparently came after the horrific incident described in Alma 14 in which women and children were burned to death because they believed in the word of God. It is hard to overstate the trauma that such an experience would have on family relationships.

Amulek and Alma had to watch the Saints burn to death, and their scriptures with them. Amulek likely had women and children near to him that were consumed in that fire, and he was forced to watch them burn to death. We cannot begin to comprehend how awful and traumatic that experience would have been to witness. Amulek and Alma were bound with strong cords and put in prison to be tortured for their beliefs and teachings. They were spit upon and mocked and smitten on their cheeks. Their clothes were taken from them. They went days without food and drink.

Why did Amulek go through this? He had come from wealth and a comfortable and prosperous station in life. He'd had good relationships with his family up to this time and had many friends. Amulek chose to go through this because the Holy Ghost witnessed to him that Alma was preaching the actual word of God. He had received a witness and knew he had to follow God's commandments and the counsel from this prophet of the Lord.

So, how does this relate to Amulek turning his heart to his children? It may seem backward in this example since his own children likely died in the fire, but it is not. It could appear to readers that Amulek lost his family by accepting the gospel. He may have lost some of his family temporally as they burned in the fire, but this faithful act ensured these believers received the gift of eternal life (see Alma 14:11). Amulek knew if he lived faithfully, he would see them again. He knew that family relationships exist forever through the gospel, but those ties would be severed if the gospel were not lived by those family members.

Amulek was unquestionably a pioneer. He was the one person in Ammonihah that initially listened to Alma in the land of Ammonihah. He understood the impact the gospel could have on each member of his family. What a rich heritage Amulek, the pioneer, left behind to his descendants!

The Great Symbol of Our Church Membership

Something special happens when we choose to ponder on the lives of our ancestors. The Spirit of Elijah enters into our hearts. We begin to feel closer ties to our ancestors. Our love for them deepens the more we learn about them. As members of the Church, our hearts quickly turn to thoughts of ensuring our dear ancestors receive necessary temple ordinances so that they may be blessed if they choose to accept the gospel in the spirit world. We inevitably begin to ponder our own lives and actions and strive to bring honor to our ancestors in all that we do.

So much of the Spirit of Elijah is centered on the temple. We cannot measure our individual progress in having our hearts turned to our fathers without examining our testimony of, and our participation in, the temples of the Lord. We must make the temple "the great symbol of our membership" in the Church, as President Howard W. Hunter declared.[9]

Our ultimate goal in this work is to go to the temple for ourselves and our kindred dead. A necessary element in the achievement of this goal is to do everything we can to bring our lives into harmony with the gospel and be worthy to go to the temple. Pictures of temples in our homes help remind us daily of the blessings of the temple and the covenants we make there.

Attending the temple on a regular basis will keep the Spirit of Elijah close to our hearts. Efforts should be made to take our own family names to the temple to do their work, if possible. Consideration might be taken to become a temple worker if it is the right season of our lives to do so. This could be a potential goal to work toward for the future if the time is not right. The blessings of the temple are powerful and real.

President Thomas S. Monson promised:

As we attend the temple, there can come to us a dimension of spirituality and a feeling of peace which will transcend any other feeling which would come into the human heart. We will grasp the true meaning of the words of the Savior when He said: 'Peace I leave with you, my peace I give unto you. . . . Let not your heart be troubled, neither let it be afraid. Such peace can permeate any heart—hearts that are troubled, hearts that are burdened down with grief, hearts that feel confusion, hearts that plead for help.[10]

We love how these blessings of temple attendance from a prophet of God involve our hearts. The temple is truly a place where the Holy Ghost can accomplish some of the best work in our hearts through sanctification. Our hearts can be relieved of heavy burdens, grief, and confusion. Our hearts' pleadings for help will be heard, and guidance and instruction will be given to us. Our eternal perspective expands the more we visit the temple. As this perspective is enlarged, it helps us through our challenges and trials and reminds us of things we must learn as we work through them.

It is important for family history work to become a higher priority in our lives. Classes are readily available to learn how to do family history if we do not know how to do it. There are many more resources at our disposal in the Church in this regard than there used to be. We should schedule time on a consistent basis to work on our family lines. These activities will richly carry the Spirit of Elijah into our lives. The responsibility is ours to pray for the Spirit of Elijah to be with us and to have our hearts turned to our fathers. Our hearts will be purified and sanctified each and every time we participate in this great work.

TURNING FATHERS' HEARTS TO THEIR CHILDREN—ALMA THE YOUNGER

Up to this point, we have primarily discussed ways that children can turn their hearts to their fathers, but this promise from Malachi also states that the hearts of the fathers shall turn to their children.

One instance we have brought up in which fathers and mothers turn their hearts to their children is the opportunity to be the family's pioneer into the gospel. This sacred responsibility, once studied and fully understood, immediately turns the heart of the pioneer to his or her children. There are many other ways that mothers and fathers can turn their hearts to their children.

Alma, the son of Alma, is an inspiring example of someone who turned his heart to his children. His father, and undoubtedly his mother, were loving examples in this regard and never gave up on their once wayward son. Alma the Younger gave some final counsel to his three sons in Alma 36–42. These chapters are some of the most doctrinally rich, beautifully written chapters in the Book of Mormon. It is very interesting to see how Alma spoke so differently with each son. Alma's children were all at different levels of spiritual maturity and needed very personalized counsel. His teachings to his children illustrate a remarkable lesson for parents. A single approach to parenting without allowing for the individual differences of each unique child will not work. Every child must be thought of individually and prayerfully to know how to best help and teach him or her. That seems to be precisely the pattern that our own Father in Heaven uses in parenting us.

We can begin to understand how long Alma must have pondered on what he would teach his sons by studying Alma 36. This may be the most famous chiasmus in the Book of Mormon. Much study can be done of Alma's literary masterpiece in this chapter. We are impressed by how much time and effort Alma spent choosing and composing these heartfelt words for his son Helaman. By putting the counsel to Helaman into this literary form, it would have become far more memorable and impactful for Helaman. Alma took his role as a father very seriously. Alma was guided by the Spirit to give each of his sons personalized messages that would benefit them throughout their lives. We are confident that Helaman would have considered this chiasmus a personal treasure for the remainder of his life.

Alma's lengthiest counsel was reserved for his son, Corianton, who had lost his way in the gospel while serving a mission. Alma patiently taught his son doctrines of the gospel about which Corianton was worried. He implored Corianton to accept counsel from his brothers and learn from their examples. He pleaded with Corianton to repent and to once again become an effective missionary. It is impossible not to feel Alma's love and concern for his son rise from these pages. Alma wanted desperately for Corianton to live the gospel and enjoy its richest blessings that are reserved for the righteous.

Like Alma, we can leave a legacy of faith with all of our children. It does not all have to happen right before we die. We can make sure that our children receive father's blessings every school year and at other significant moments in life. Mothers play a vital role in bringing the blessings of the priesthood into the home. Mothers should join fathers and be actively involved in ensuring that the home is a refuge where priesthood power is felt. It is ideal when fathers invite and welcome a mother's input in regard to father's blessings. We enjoy asking our wives what inspired thoughts they have had regarding our children. Such thoughts and discussion between spouses puts us in the proper frame of mind to give the blessing the Lord would have our children receive.

We can make sure our children hear our testimonies of the gospel and of the Savior not only at church, but also during family home evenings and regular, everyday teaching moments that often arise. We can also write letters to our children expressing thoughts that we might find hard to express in other ways.

JOURNAL WRITING—OUR SMALL PLATES AND LARGE PLATES

One of the most important ways mothers and fathers can turn their hearts to their children is to keep a personal journal and to work on keeping a family history. Elder Hartman Rector Jr. of the Seventy said:

> I personally believe that the writing of personal and family histories will do more to turn the hearts of the children

to the fathers and the fathers to the children than almost anything we can do. I am sure you will never turn your own children's hearts more to you than you will by keeping a journal and writing a personal history. They will ultimately love to find out about your successes and your failures and your peculiarities. It will tell them a lot about themselves, too.

Also, I seriously doubt that you will ever turn your own heart more to your own fathers than by writing your family history. You must know a lot about them before you can write it. This will lead to much in-depth research. I promise you will love them when you become acquainted with them.[11]

Keeping a personal journal blesses the writer's life in many ways. The gift of truly turning your heart to your children and being impressed to write for their benefit and learning is one of these great blessings. You will think about your children and their individual challenges and strengths as you write. You will write down your experiences, trials, and feelings. Once you have passed on, your children will read your journals and they will see how you dealt with life's struggles and find additional strength to meet the challenges of the day. We would encourage you to share some of your journals before you pass away too. You will know when the right time is to share certain experiences with your family.

President Spencer W. Kimball was a stalwart journal writer. He had dozens and dozens of large volumes that he filled throughout his lifetime. He said:

> I promise you that if you will keep journals and records, they will indeed be a source of inspiration to your families, to your children, your grandchildren, and others, on through the generations. As our posterity read of our life's experiences, they, too, will come to know and love us.
>
> What could you do better for your children and your children's children than to record the story of your life, your triumphs over adversity, your recovery after a fall,

your progress when all seemed black, your rejoicing when you had finally achieved?[12]

President Kimball counseled us as a prophet of God: "A word about personal journals and records: We urge every person in the church to keep a diary or a journal from youth up, all through his (or her) life."[13] He stated on another occasion, "Every person should keep a journal and every person can keep a journal. It should be an enlightening one and should bring great blessings and happiness to the families. If there is anyone here who isn't doing so, will you repent today and change—change your life?"[14]

What a simple way to turn our hearts to our children and allow our children's hearts to be turned to us! If we are striving to have our hearts turned in such a manner, we have the key to be able to do so. We have the prophet's command to keep a personal journal. As with all other conditions of the heart, it will take effort to turn our hearts to our ancestors and to our children. It is so with all aspects of the gospel. But we can do it!

Derek relates the following:

> I haven't been the best example of journal writing over the years, but I cherish the passages I have written. I smile just thinking of some of the journals I kept when I was ten or twelve years old. I love to refer to the journal I kept on my mission to be reminded of difficulties and blessings that came to me from that experience. I've shared journal entries with my children and have seen them light up and laugh with some of the stories. It's easy to see the impact it has on them. The power of journal writing is real. It's true what President Kimball said. Our sacred duty is to be a record-keeping people. We can change our lives through journal writing. The blessings associated with this practice are that meaningful.

We love the idea of keeping a blessings journal like President Henry B. Eyring does. Before writing, he always asks himself this question, "Have I seen the hand of God reaching out to touch us or our children or our family today?"[15] He's maintained this practice for years. A great time to write and ponder is before we start our prayers at night.

President Kimball said, "Those who keep a book of remembrance are more likely to keep the Lord in remembrance in their daily lives. Journals are a way of counting our blessings and of leaving an inventory of these blessings for our posterity."[16] We are commanded to remember the Savior always, as stated in the sacrament prayers. Journal writing can help us keep this covenant.

There are many different ways to keep a journal today. We like to think of there being a "large-plates journal" and a "small-plates journal." Day-to-day activities are often recorded on Facebook or other social networks. That is more of a "large-plates" type of journal (and please know that we are not discounting the actual large plates at all). Our children and families love to see what we are busy doing on a day-to-day basis, what we consider important enough to comment about, etc.

Keeping a spiritual journal based on the testimonies and the blessings we receive in our lives will be much more valuable to our children and families than details of our day-to-day activities. This is more of a "small-plates journal." This type of journal detailing our spiritual journey through life is absolutely priceless. By recording such spiritual moments, we demonstrate to the Lord that we value the blessings and revelation we receive in our lives enough to write them down and ponder them.

A journal entry may take just a handful of minutes if you use a computer. It would not require nearly the time it would if you were to do it by hand. It has been fun, however, to go back and read our ancestors' own handwriting, but we know this is becoming a lost art. Either method will be a great blessing to your posterity, but if a computer is used, regular and careful backing up and storage is vital.

INVITING THE SPIRIT OF ELIJAH

Heartfelt prayer to have the Spirit of Elijah enter into our hearts is critical. Our hearts will be sanctified as we are involved in any of the activities we have mentioned in this chapter to turn our hearts. The Spirit of Elijah involves much more than just genealogy work. It includes journal writing, writing family histories, and attending the temple more frequently. It involves more active parenting and spending time to get to know our children better. It requires living in such a way that we become worthy pioneers for our progeny. It necessitates spending more time learning about our ancestors and remembering their contributions. As we engage in these uplifting activities, we will truly become saviors on Mount Zion for those we love, and our hearts will be saved in the process.

CONCLUSION

Chapter 12

CHEER UP YOUR HEARTS

There is no more fitting way to conclude this book than to review something of which we need more of in our hearts—joy, rejoicing, and cheer! In this book, we have studied the diseases of the heart and the influence Satan tries to wield on our hearts. We have likewise examined conditions of the heart that are associated with conversion to the Savior and His gospel and the gateway to such conversion—baptism. Lastly, we have looked at conditions of the heart that go hand in hand with temple covenants that help us enter the kingdom of God and receive exaltation with our Heavenly Father. To conclude our examination of the heart in the Book of Mormon, we are excited to address the importance of cheering up our hearts, rejoicing and having joy in our hearts, and having thankful hearts after all the hard work we have previously done to develop our hearts.

We love the hymn "You Can Make the Pathway Bright" for its powerful message of a joyous heart, particularly the first and fourth verses.

1. You can make the pathway bright,
   Fill the soul with heaven's light,
   If there's sunshine in your heart;
   Turning darkness into day,
   As the shadows fly away,
   If there's sunshine in your heart today.

Chorus:
   If there's sunshine in your heart,
   You can send a shining ray
   That will turn the night to day;
   And your cares will all depart,
   If there's sunshine in your heart today.

4. You can live a happy life
   In this world of toil and strife,
   If there's sunshine in your heart;
   And your soul will glow with love
   From the perfect Light above,
   If there's sunshine in your heart today.[1]

Cheer, joy, and gratitude help extinguish the diseases of the heart. There is not enough room for the diseases of the heart to prosper and grow when the heart is filled with such feelings. Who on this earth has more reason to rejoice and be cheerful and thankful than members of The Church of Jesus Christ of Latter-day Saints? We know of our Heavenly Father's plan for us. We know that He sent His Son to earth to die for us that we might live again. We know that we have prophets upon this earth and the gift of the Holy Ghost to help guide us today. A knowledge of such glorious gifts and blessings should cause us to continually rejoice.

AMMON SPREADS THE CHEER

There are more than twenty verses in the Book of Mormon that describe a cheerful, thankful, rejoicing, joyful, or glad heart. Our favorite example in the Book of Mormon of a cheerful, joyful heart is the story of Ammon as a missionary among the Lamanites. Ammon is initially bound and taken before King Lamoni when he enters their land. He eventually convinces King Lamoni to allow him to become his servant, and he is asked to watch the king's flocks. Ammon had only been in the king's service for three days before complete mayhem ensued. He was out with other servants tending the flocks when a group of Lamanites came to cause trouble. They scattered the king's flocks with the intent to steal them. The other servants with Ammon wept and were terrified at the consequences that awaited them for having lost the king's flocks. These servants knew if they lost the sheep the king would likely kill them.

How did Ammon react to this unfolding, disastrous scene? His *"heart was swollen within him with joy*; for, said he, I will show forth my power unto these my fellow-servants . . . in restoring these flocks unto the king, *that I may win the hearts of these my fellow-servants"* (Alma 17:29, emphasis added). Ammon was a fantastic, unceasing, and inspirational optimist! He was convinced the glass was half-full. Actually, he considered the glass completely full and overflowing. Ammon would have lacked experience with how the servants went about their work after only two or three days on the job and very limited training. He did not know the lay of the land as well as he would have liked either.

What were Ammon's first words he spoke to his fellow servants? "My brethren, be of good cheer" (Alma 17:31). Can you imagine being in Ammon's shoes, seeing all your flocks scattered by a substantial number of Lamanites, understanding that death was a distinct possibility if the flocks were not recovered? We humbly acknowledge that we may find it far easier to relate to the feelings and reactions of Ammon's servants than the courage and cheer of Ammon if we were placed in this situation. The Lamanites who scattered the flocks would represent a very intimidating danger. It would be easy to think of how difficult or impossible it would be to gather sheep that had been scattered. The prospect of being killed by the king for not doing the job well would be terrifying. Those are very natural initial reactions. The first words of Ammon, however, told his fellow servants to be of good cheer in this precarious position.

Ammon obviously had a cheerful heart. He truly accentuated the positive and saw opportunities in his most difficult challenges. Many of us are familiar with how this story ends. Ammon took the lead in gathering the flocks back to the waters of Sebus. Then, Ammon miraculously defended himself against this entire group of Lamanites when they came again. King Lamoni agreed to listen to Ammon's teachings of the gospel and was converted along with his people because of Ammon's example. None of this would have transpired, however, except that Ammon first displayed a cheerful, joyful heart to lead his fellow servants.

Ammon quickly decided to act and tried to change his circumstances instead of complaining about his plight. An entire people's history could have looked much different if Ammon did not look joyfully upon the situation in which he was placed. Ammon's cheerful disposition turned out to be infectious, as cheerful dispositions are often wont to be. King Lamoni's people, later known as the people of Ammon, became famous for their zeal in living the gospel. The people were exposed to Ammon's excitement for living the gospel, and they wanted to be like him. Ammon's passion and joy rubbed off on them.

There is also a great deal to learn from the symbolism of Ammon tending to the flocks of the Lamanites in this story! He was truly a missionary tending to the Lamanite people that had all been scattered about. He was able to cheerfully gather them together just like the sheep. Then, when the Lamanites tried again to scatter the flocks, Ammon told the servants to encircle the sheep about so they would not flee (see Alma 17:33). The people were gathered safely in because of Ammon's efforts, much like the sheep that were under his care. Ammon was saved spiritually in the process of the great missionary work he had undertaken, much like he and the other servants were saved from death by the king for performing their labors!

You may read this chapter and start thinking to yourself, "Boy, these brothers sure like using exclamation marks! In fact, they need to calm down a little bit and get back into the rhythm of using a bunch of periods. They are overdoing it here." These exclamation marks are merely used to show how excited and joyful we get when talking about the gospel. It could be said that Ammon's enthusiasm was known to result in his communication being laced with inferred exclamation marks, even when they were not spelled out.

It is no surprise to see Ammon rejoicing as he reflects on his mission in Alma 26. This chapter could aptly be named the "reveling in rejoicing" chapter! Ammon begins his revelry in rejoicing by saying to his brethren, "How great reason have we to rejoice" (Alma 26:1). You will notice a couple exclamation marks as he starts his address in this chapter. It is probably a good thing we were not the ones to add punctuation to the Book of Mormon after it was translated. We would have thrown in a dozen or two more exclamation marks in this chapter alone!

Ammon reveled, "Now have we not reason to rejoice? Yea, I say unto you, there never were men that had so great reason to rejoice as we, since the world began; yea, and my joy is carried away, even unto boasting in my God; for he has all power, all wisdom, and all understanding; he comprehendeth all things, and he is a merciful Being, even unto salvation, to those who will repent and believe on his name. Now, if this is boasting, even so will I boast; for this is my life and my light, my joy and my salvation" (Alma 26:35–36).

Ammon was such a joyful missionary. Alma shared similar feelings while reflecting on his missionary efforts in Alma 29. He shared another marvelous missionary message, a jubilantly joyous journaling, for bringing some souls to repentance. Alma used the word *joy* seven times in these seventeen verses alone. Maybe you can get on us for some dubious alliteration, but the exclamation marks have to stay! These two chapters can do much to lift and bless us when we find ourselves in need of some joy in our own lives.

THE PLAN OF HAPPINESS, THE GOSPEL OF JOY

The gospel is a gospel of joy. It is frequently spoken that gospel literally means "good news." Lehi taught, "Men are, that they might have joy" (2 Nephi 2:25). Alma calls Heavenly Father's plan "the great plan of happiness" (Alma 42:8, 16). We have been blessed with a Savior that has redeemed us from physical death and from the first spiritual death that we may stand again before Him to be judged. Moreover, the Savior has given us the blessing to be redeemed from the second spiritual death through His Atonement and His accompanying mercy and grace if we will repent. Through His sacrifice, we can return to live with our Heavenly Father and Savior once more. We need to "give thanks unto his holy name by night" and "let [our] hearts rejoice" for what the Savior has done for us (2 Nephi 9:52).

President Russell M. Nelson said, "When the focus of our lives is on God's plan of salvation and Jesus Christ and His gospel, we can feel joy regardless of what is happening—or not happening—in our lives."[2] Our joy is not dependent upon our circumstances. The better we live the gospel, the greater our joy will be. This is our privilege here on earth.

President Dieter F. Uchtdorf proclaimed, "Walking in the path of discipleship does not need to be a bitter experience. It is 'sweet above all that is sweet.' It is not a burden that weighs us down. Discipleship lifts our spirits and *lightens our hearts*. It inspires us with faith, hope, and charity. It fills our spirits with light in times of darkness, and serenity during times of sorrow. It gives us divine power and lasting joy."[3]

Do we look at living the gospel as a burden? It is easy to make a checklist of all the things we need to do to live the gospel. It is easy to get overwhelmed thinking about all the commandments we are to keep and all the things we must do to fulfill our Church callings. It is a daunting and impossible task if we think of achieving perfection in our hearts today. However, our Heavenly Father has created a perfect plan, and our Savior, Jesus Christ, has made it perfectly possible for us to be successful within this plan.

We gladly agreed to come down to earth for this mortal experience when we first learned details of Heavenly Father's plan. We even all "shouted for joy!" (Job 38:7). While we focus a lot of our time and efforts on the trials of life and are indeed here on earth to be tested, we are also commanded to have joy while on this earth. We will all have difficult experiences during our mortal sojourn, but we are to balance the heartache with joy through the Savior. Do you remember the last time you experienced joy in your life? Periods without experiencing joy are common to man on this mortal journey, but hopefully it has not been too long since you last felt joy through the peace and promises of our Savior.

Jacob pled with the Nephites, "Therefore, *cheer up your hearts,* and remember that ye are free to act for yourselves—to choose the way of everlasting death or the way of eternal life" (2 Nephi 10:23, emphasis added). What a blessing it is to be able to choose for ourselves here on earth and to have such magnificent promises awaiting us if we are faithful, even eternal life! It is important to note that Jacob did not ask the people to find somebody else to cheer up their hearts, or find a new situation or circumstance that would cheer up their hearts. He told the people to cheer up their own hearts. We can choose to be cheerful and joyful.

There are so many scriptures about rejoicing in our hearts for various blessings of the gospel. Many will be mentioned in this chapter, but there are many more that we could cite that further teach the importance of rejoicing in our hearts. It is a good exercise to read through the scriptures and mark all the joyful, cheerful, positive verses. You will find that your scriptures will become heavily marked with such passages.

One of our favorite verses in all of scripture is found in the book of 3 Nephi. Quoting Isaiah, the Savior promises, "For the mountains shall depart and the hills be removed, but my kindness shall not depart from thee, neither shall the covenant of my peace be removed, saith the Lord that hath mercy on thee" (3 Nephi 22:10). With strikingly beautiful language, the Savior defines His covenant of peace. We know how unlikely it is for mountains to depart from before us and for hills to be removed. And still, though mountains may depart and hills may be removed, our Savior's kindness will never depart. What a comforting, reassuring blessing! We rejoice in this peace-giving blessing of kindness that is given to us. It makes us want to be that much kinder to those around us, knowing that our Savior is infinitely kind despite our flaws and imperfections.

REJOICE IN CHRIST

This brings us to what we should rejoice in more than anything else, the Savior. Nephi succinctly states, "We rejoice in Christ" (2 Nephi 25:26). How do you individually rejoice in Christ? To rejoice in Christ, we first need to come to know Him and understand His life and mission here on earth. Do we spend sufficient time in the New Testament learning about the Savior's walk here on earth? Do we spend sufficient time in the Book of Mormon learning about the Savior's time amongst the Nephites? Do we spend sufficient time in the other standard works learning about the prophecies and testimonies that are given of our Savior? Can we say that we truly rejoice in Christ because we have come to know who He is?

We love the cheerful hymn, "Rejoice, the Lord is King." The first verse is as follows:

> Rejoice, the Lord is King!
> Your Lord and King adore!
> Mortals, give thanks and sing
> And triumph evermore.
> Lift up your heart! Lift up your voice!
> Rejoice, again I say, rejoice!
> Lift up your heart! Lift up your voice!
> Rejoice, again I say, rejoice![4]

We will have you know that we merely copied these lyrics as they are written. Notice the exclamation marks! Rejoicing is a series of exclamation marks! If we go about living the gospel ending our days with a bunch of periods and semicolons, we are living it incorrectly. There should be many moments of reflection and joy that bring exclamation marks into our lives.

We will naturally want to rejoice in what the Savior has done for us as we understand and learn more about Him, His infinite Atonement, and His infinite love for each of us. Elder Dieter F. Uchtdorf asked, "My dear brothers and sisters, aren't the restored gospel of Jesus Christ and our membership in His church great reasons to rejoice?"[5] We are members of The Church of Jesus Christ of Latter-day Saints, the Lord's Church restored again here upon the earth! We have been given and understand truths and doctrines about the plan of salvation that are precious above any earthly treasures! We know why we are here! We know where we came from! We know where we can go after this life and that all does not end here!

As the prophet Jacob puts it, "Come unto the Holy One of Israel, and feast upon that which perisheth not, neither can be corrupted, and let your soul delight in fatness. Behold, my beloved brethren, remember the words of your God; pray unto him continually by day, and give thanks unto his holy name by night. *Let your hearts rejoice.* And behold how great the covenants of the Lord, and how great his condescensions unto the children of men" (2 Nephi 9:51-53, emphasis added). We should rejoice in our hearts for the covenants we have entered into or will yet be able to enter into. We should rejoice in our hearts that the Savior came down to this earth to die for us and atone for our sins. Our souls should truly delight in fatness and overflow with rejoicing possessing this great knowledge!

REJOICE IN THE WORDS OF CHRIST

Nephi included many of Isaiah's writings on the small plates, "that whoso of my people shall see these words may *lift up their hearts and rejoice for all men*" (2 Nephi 11:8, emphasis added). Do we view Isaiah's words and other prophets' words as able to lift up our hearts and help us rejoice? Jeremiah gloried, "Thy words were found, and I did eat them; and thy word was unto me *the joy and rejoicing of mine heart*" (Jeremiah 15:16, emphasis added). To rejoice in God's word, we must eat His word, as Jeremiah says. We must feast upon His word. Reading, studying, and pondering God's word will invite the companionship of the Holy Ghost into our lives, which in turn will allow the Atonement to enter into our hearts! We cannot afford to leave this blessing of scripture on the table, not even a leftover crumb. We must eat it all! And then, oh what joy we will feel in our lives!

OTHER THINGS WE REJOICE OVER

The scriptures and latter-day prophets have counseled us to rejoice over many different things in our hearts.

We are to rejoice in our hearts over the temples with which we have been blessed. When the Lord appeared to Joseph Smith and Oliver Cowdery in the Kirtland Temple, He said, "*Let the hearts of thy brethren rejoice*, and *let the hearts of all my people rejoice*, who have, with their might, built this house to my name" (D&C 110:6). How do we manifest our rejoicing for the temple?

We are to rejoice in our hearts over our children and spouses. The author of Ecclesiastes wrote, "Live joyfully with the wife whom thou lovest all the days of the life of thy vanity" (Ecclesiastes 9:9). The First Presidency, in a letter dated April 14, 1969, declared, "We have been commanded to multiply and replenish the earth that we may have joy and rejoicing in our posterity."[6]

We are told to rejoice over today, this very day that we are living! The Psalmist wrote, "This is the day which the Lord hath

235

made; we will rejoice and be glad in it" (Psalm 118:24). Do you wake up and rejoice in the day that lies before you?

President Gordon B. Hinckley said, "Walk with faith, rejoicing in the beauties of nature, in the goodness of those you love, in the testimony which you carry in your heart."[7] Do we ever think about our own testimonies and rejoice in the things we know to be true? Unfortunately, it is sometimes an easier practice to dwell on all the things we do not know about the gospel. We need to be grateful for all that we do know, and take comfort that additional knowledge will be given line upon line, precept upon precept, here a little and there a little" (2 Nephi 28:30). Do we rejoice in the beauty of this earth and all of the Lord's creations? Do we rejoice in the goodness of those around us and express gratitude for all the kindnesses that are rendered in our behalf?

WHO WILL WE ALLOW TO REJOICE OVER US?

The Lord proclaimed, "Nevertheless, ye are blessed, for the testimony which ye have borne is recorded in heaven for the angels to look upon; and they rejoice over you, and your sins are forgiven you" (D&C 62:3). It is heartening to think of angels actually rejoicing over us! It is very easy to fall into the trap of inordinately dwelling on our shortcomings and imperfections. While we need to work on making our weak things strong, we need not magnify our weaknesses. There is harm in doing so. It is easy to think that angels should never have reason to rejoice over us, but bearing our testimonies is a reason we can all give them to rejoice. Such angels will assuredly include our own ancestors that watch over us.

There are other scriptures that speak of the devil rejoicing. He wants us to "be miserable like unto himself" (2 Nephi 2:27). Enoch saw the devil laughing and his angels rejoicing (see 3 Nephi 9:2; Moses 7:26). Why were they rejoicing? They were rejoicing because of our sins! President Spencer W. Kimball taught Elder

Robert D. Hales the following: "Robert, the adversary can never have joy unless you and I sin."[8]

The choice is then ours. We can choose to rejoice in Heavenly Father's plan of happiness and in the Savior's infinite love He has given us through His atoning sacrifice. We can choose to bear our testimonies, giving angels in heaven cause to rejoice. We can choose to live the gospel and obtain joy in our hearts. We can also choose to sin and allow the devil and his angels to rejoice over us. Who will we allow to rejoice over us?

An optimistic heart is closely related to a rejoicing heart. One of our favorite examples of optimism was President Gordon B. Hinckley. You couldn't help but smile every time he walked up to the pulpit. He fittingly taught, "The gospel is a thing of joy. It provides us with a reason for gladness. Of course there are times of sorrow. Of course there are hours of concern and anxiety. We all worry. But the Lord has told us to *lift our hearts and rejoice.* I see so many people . . . who seem never to see the sunshine, but who constantly walk with storms under cloudy skies" (emphasis added).[9]

On a separate occasion, he continued with this theme. "I am asking that we stop seeking out the storms and enjoy more fully the sunlight. I am suggesting that as we go through life we 'accentuate the positive.' I am asking that we look a little deeper for the good, that we still voices of insult and sarcasm, that we more generously compliment virtue and effort."[10]

Do we stop to smell the roses? Do we consider the marvelous creations of our Lord and remember they are here for us to admire and enjoy? Like other conditions of the heart, it takes effort on our part to cultivate a rejoicing heart, but we can do it!

There are some in this life that find great joy and inspiration in nature, and we like to consider ourselves part of that group. Some are able to see and process things during the day that many others don't. They can be found in complete awe when viewing a sunset. They recognize and rejoice in the sound of the birds singing. They love seeing the fruit trees blossom and leaves miraculously reappear after a long winter. They love watching the magic of wildlife around them. Some even notice small insects and think of what intricate, profound creations they are. They delight in looking at the mountains, rivers, and streams the world sets before them. They bask in the majesty of wind and storms. The more time we spend in nature and contemplate our Creator, the more joyful will be our hearts.

Thankful Hearts

We have also been instructed to have thankful hearts in addition to cheerful, joyful, rejoicing hearts. Being thankful is much more about what we do to show thanks than by how often we say thanks. Jacob hoped that we would have thankful hearts for the scriptures the prophets left for us (see Jacob 4:3). Do we show Jacob and our Heavenly Father our thanks for the scriptures by spending time reading, studying, and pondering them on a regular basis? We express our gratitude for the scriptures by treasuring up their words.

We all know the words of our Savior, "If ye love me, keep my commandments" (John 14:15). The Savior could just as easily have said, "If ye are grateful for me, keep my commandments." The best way we can express gratitude to our Savior is to keep His commandments, apply His Atonement in our lives, and follow Him.

Captain Moroni was described as "a man whose heart did swell with thanksgiving to his God, for the many privileges and blessings which he bestowed upon his people" (Alma 48:12). He experienced great trials and suffering. He witnessed thousands upon thousands of people killed on the field of battle, and yet he had a thankful heart. He recognized this experience on earth as being for his good. He was grateful. Most importantly, Moroni expressed his gratitude by his works.

Moroni's reward for his thankful heart is summarized as follows, "And he who receiveth all things with thankfulness shall be made glorious; and the things of this earth shall be added unto him, even an hundred fold, yea, more" (D&C 78:19).

Most of us have been around people who have abundantly thankful hearts. We each worked as nursing home administrators for a few years. Patients' thankful hearts always humbled us. Many of these patients were in otherwise dire circumstances of failing health. Some did not have families or friends around to provide comfort and support. Yet, they were thankful for the smallest thing that was done for them or for whatever health they still had. Frequently, expressions of thanks were given to us for wheeling them over to the dining room or getting supplies for them from the activities room. Every simple gift (such as a pen or a can of soda) they were given seemed to be treasured for months on end. It was humbling to learn from such excellent examples of thankfulness regardless of circumstances. Our experience is that there are humbling and beautiful examples of gratitude in whatever nursing home in which you serve and come to know the residents.

Alma taught, "Counsel with the Lord in all thy doings, and he will direct thee for good; yea, when thou liest down at night lie down unto the Lord, that he may watch over you in your sleep; and when thou risest in the morning *let thy heart be full of thanks unto God*; and if ye do these things, ye shall be lifted up at the last day" (Alma 37:37, emphasis added).

Do we specifically follow this counsel that Alma gave to his son Helaman? Specifically, we are taught to express our gratitude to the Lord each morning we wake up. This is a great practice to get into if you aren't doing this already. This attitude of gratitude can stay with us throughout the day. We need to study commandments we are given in a detailed and specific manner. We cannot simply say that we are thankful when we pray. This is not the commandment Alma is relaying to us. Alma specifically counseled us to pray in the morning with a heart full of thanks. This then is what we should do.

President Ezra Taft Benson said, "There is a great tendency for us in our prayers and in our pleadings with the Lord to ask for additional blessings. But sometimes I feel we need to devote more of our prayers to expressions of gratitude and thanksgiving for blessings already received."[11]

Some of our most impactful prayers have been when we have tried to only express gratitude for what we have been given. The Holy Ghost can actually help us in this regard. The Savior taught, "The Holy Ghost . . . shall teach you all things, and bring all things to your remembrance" (John 14:26). We are commanded to have thankful hearts (see Jacob 4:3; Alma 37:37). The Holy Ghost can bring blessings to our remembrance and remind us to express our gratitude for them.

OUR SAVIOR AND REDEEMER'S GLORIOUS ATONEMENT

Above all else, we should express our gratitude for our Savior and His loving sacrifice for us. President Gordon B. Hinckley said, "No other act in all of human history compares with it. Nothing that has ever happened can match it."[12]

Expressing our gratitude for the Atonement, and being thankful in our hearts for the Atonement, involves much more than simply saying thanks in our prayers, although we should definitely do that. President Joseph Fielding Smith said:

> One of the greatest sins, both in magnitude and extent . . . is the sin of ingratitude. When we violate a commandment, no matter how small and insignificant we may think it to be, we show our ingratitude to our Redeemer. It is impossible for us to comprehend the extent of his suffering when he carried the burden of the sins of the whole world, a punishment so severe that we are informed that blood came from the pores of his body, and this was before he was taken to the cross.
>
> The punishment of physical pain coming from the nails driven in his hands and feet was not the greatest of his suffering, excruciating as that surely was. The greater suffering was the spiritual and mental anguish coming

from the load of our transgressions which he carried. If we understood the extent of that suffering and his suffering on the cross, surely none of us would willfully be guilty of sin. We would not give way to the temptations, the gratification of unholy appetites and desires *and Satan could find no place in our hearts.*

As it is, whenever we sin, we show our ingratitude and disregard of the suffering of the Son of God by and through which we shall rise from the dead and live forever. If we really understood and could feel even to a small degree, the love and gracious willingness on the part of Jesus Christ to suffer for our sins we would be willing to repent of all our transgressions and serve him (emphasis added).[13]

Satan could find no place in our hearts if we truly understood the great suffering of our Savior in Gethsemane and on the cross at Calvary. We would not dare to do anything that would have caused our Savior additional pain and suffering. Again, we need to keep His commandments if we love Him. A grateful heart in regard to the Atonement is best shown by keeping the commandments, by taking up our cross daily, and by rising above the temptations of this world.

We are so grateful for this Church and for our Savior. We echo Nephi's words, "Rejoice, O my heart, and cry unto the Lord, and say: O Lord, I will praise thee forever; yea, my soul will rejoice in thee, my God, and the rock of my salvation" (2 Nephi 4:30). We are so grateful for the Book of Mormon and the divine instruction it contains on our hearts.

It is our prayer that those who read our book will feel of our love for the Savior and our love for each one of you. We testify that the Book of Mormon was written for our day. It is the word of God. Prophets from that book have seen our day and knew what teachings to include about our hearts. Our hearts will be changed and softened as we study their words and try to improve. May we be patient with ourselves and with others as we try to take steps forward on this humbling and difficult journey.

It is our hope that you will take upon yourselves the yoke of Christ that your burdens may be light. We pray that you will give your heart to the Savior and Redeemer. We testify that the Lord can give you a new heart that will function infinitely better than your current one. Jesus Christ, our Savior and Redeemer, promises us this eternal blessing when He said, "A new heart also will I give you, and a new spirit will I put within you: and I will take away the stony heart out of your flesh, and I will give you an heart of flesh" (Ezekiel 36:26). Of this glorious promise, we so testify.

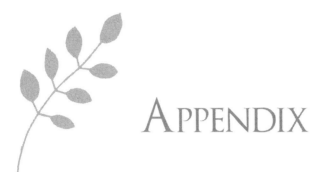

APPENDIX

HEART REFERENCES BY SUBJECT IN THE BOOK OF MORMON

SUBJECT	MENTIONS
Hard	97
Pride/Puffed up	29
People—Stir up/Lead away/Stole/Put into/Won/Gained	25
Cheer/Lift up/Glad in/Joy in/Rejoice in/Thankful	21
Satan—Rage/Stir up/Hold upon/Put into/Lead away/Possession of	20
Set upon Treasures/Riches/Vain Things	18
Thoughts/Intents/Desires/Wish/Affections	17
Sorrows/Groans/Weeps	14
Lowliness/Poor in	13
Soften	11
Broken	9
Mighty change/Changed	9
Ponder in	8
Pure	7

Said in/Says/Magnifies	7
Full purpose of	6
Prayed/Poured out	6
Satan—power over	6
Courage	5
Stabbed	5
Turn aside/against Lord	5
Foolish/Vain imaginations	4
Love	4
Murderers/Murders/Destroy	4
Pained/Grieved/Sickened	4
Planted in	4
Understand with	4
Ask in/Repent in sincerity	3
Heart of people	3
Inspired	3
Put into—Lord	3
Sobbings/Cries	3
Written in	3

HEART REFERENCES BY PROPHET

PROPHET	MENTIONS
Mormon	157
Nephi	73
Alma	56
Jacob	29
Jesus	25
Moroni	23
King Benjamin	13
Isaiah	11
Amulek	9
Samuel the Lamanite	7
Nephi, Son of Helaman	6
Abinadi	6
Ammon	6
Lehi	5
King to Ammon	3
Jarom	2
Pahoran	2
Enos, King Limhi, Amalekite to Aaron, King Lamoni, Zoramites, Helaman, Multitude with Jesus, Gidgiddoni's army, Multitude with Nephi	1

HEART REFERENCES
BY BOOK

BOOK	MENTIONS
1 Nephi	43
2 Nephi	53
Jacob	22
Enos	1
Jarom	2
Mosiah	41
Alma	139
Helaman	53
3 Nephi	38
4 Nephi	5
Mormon	17
Ether	13
Moroni	15

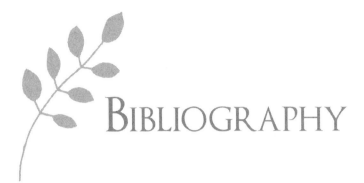

BIBLIOGRAPHY

PREFACE

1. Young, Brigham. *Teachings of Presidents of the Church: Brigham Young*. Salt Lake City: The Church of Jesus Christ of Latter-day Saints, 1997, 82–83.
2. Benson, Ezra Taft. "A Sacred Responsibility." *Ensign*, May 1986.

INTRODUCTION

1. Bednar, David A. "In the Strength of the Lord." In *Brigham Young University 2001–02 Speeches*, 2001.
2. Nelson, Russell M. "Personal Preparation for Temple Blessings." *Ensign*, May 2001.
3. Holland, Jeffrey R. "He Hath Filled the Hungry with Good Things." *Ensign*, Nov. 1997.
4. Eyring, Henry B. "The Enduring Legacy of Relief Society." *Ensign*, Nov. 2009.
5. Eyring, Henry B. "Come unto Christ," in *Brigham Young University 1989–90 Speeches*, [1989].
6. Christensen, Craig C. "A Book with a Promise." *Ensign*, May 2008.
7. Ashton, Marvin J. "The Measure of Our Hearts." *Ensign*, Nov. 1988.
8. Stevenson, Gary E. "Deeds Measure Vitality of Our Spiritual Hearts, Elder Stevenson Says." Oct. 2018. www.lds.org/church/news/deeds-measure-vitality-of-our-spiritual-hearts-elder-stevenson-says.
9. Smith, Joseph. *Teachings of Presidents of the Church: Joseph Smith*. Salt Lake City: The Church of Jesus Christ of Latter-day Saints, 2007, 72.

SECTION 1

1. Bednar, David A. "In the Strength of the Lord." In *Brigham Young University 2001–02 Speeches*, 2001.

BIBLIOGRAPHY

CHAPTER 1

1. Maxwell, Neal A. "A More Determined Discipleship." *Ensign*, Feb. 1979.
2. Smith, Joseph. *Teachings of the Presidents of the Church: Joseph Smith*. Salt Lake City: The Church of Jesus Christ of Latter-day Saints, 2007, 214.
3. The First Presidency of the Church. "The Message of the First Presidency to the Church." *The Improvement Era*, Nov. 1942.
4. Young, Brigham. *Journal of Discourses 11:14*.
5. "Stir up." *Merriam-Webster.com*. Merriam-Webster, 3 Oct. 2018.
6. Robbins, Lynn G. "Agency and Anger." *Ensign*, May 1998.
7. Hinckley, Gordon B. "The Spirit of Optimism." *The New Era*, July 2001.
8. Robbins, Lynn G. "Agency and Anger." *Ensign*, May 1998.
9. Benson, Ezra Taft. "The Book of Mormon is the Word of God." *Ensign*, Jan. 1988.
10. Faust, James E. "The Great Imitator." *Ensign*, Nov. 1987.
11. Klebingat, Jörg. "Approaching the Throne of God with Confidence." *Ensign*, Nov. 2014.
12. Benson, Ezra Taft. "Do Not Despair." *Ensign*, Nov. 1974.
13. Bible Dictionary. "Grace."

CHAPTER 2

1. Emedicinehealth. "Hardening of the Arteries (Atherosclerosis)." November 26, 2018. http://emedicinehealth.com/hardening_of_the_arteries/article_em.html.
2. Craven, Rulon G. "Temptation." *Ensign*, May 1996.
3. Teh, Michael John U. "The Power of the Word of God." *Ensign*, Mar. 2013.
4. BibleStudy.org. "Meaning of Numbers in the Bible." http://www.biblestudy.org/bibleref/meaning_of_numbers_in_bible/introduction.html.

CHAPTER 3

1. Benson, Ezra Taft. "Beware of Pride." *Ensign*, May 1989.
2. Burton, Theodore M. "A Disease Called Pride." *Ensign*, Mar. 1971.
3. Scott, Richard G. "He Lives! All Glory to His Name!" *Ensign*, May 2010.
4. Maxwell, Neal A. "Yet Thou Art There." *Ensign*, Nov. 1987.
5. Lewis, C. S. *Mere Christianity*, 1952, 122–123. © copyright CS Lewis Pte Ltd 1942, 1943, 1944, 1952. Used by Permission.
6. Kimball, Spencer W. "Becoming the Pure in Heart." *Ensign*, May 1978.
7. Maxwell, Neal A. "According to the Desire of [Our] Hearts." *Ensign*, Nov. 1996.
8. Benson, Ezra Taft. "Beware of Pride." *Ensign*, May 1989.

249

9. Kearon, Patrick. "Come unto Me with Full Purpose of Heart, and I Shall Heal You." *Ensign*, Nov. 2010.

CHAPTER 4

1. Lewis, C. S. *Mere Christianity*, 1952, 82–83. © copyright CS Lewis Pte Ltd 1942, 1943, 1944, 1952. Used by Permission.
2. Food and Agricultural Organization of the United Nations. "Help Eliminate Hunger, Food Insecurity and Malnutrition." http://www.fao.org/about/what-we-do//so1/ua/.
3. World Food Programme. "Zero Hunger." October 7, 2018. http://www1.wfp.org/zero-hunger.
4. Monson, Thomas S. "What Have I Done for Someone Today?" *Ensign*, Nov. 2009.
5. Romney, Marion G. "Welfare Agricultural Meeting." Apr. 1971, 1.
6. Romney, Marion G. "The Blessings of the Fast." *Ensign*, July 1982.
7. Nelson, Russell M. "In the Lord's Way." *Ensign*, May 1986.
8. Nibley, Hugh W. *Since Cumorah*. Salt Lake City: Deseret Book, 1970, 393–394.
9. Monson, Thomas S. "Constant Truths for Changing Times." *Ensign*, May 2005.
10. Hinckley, Gordon B. "To the Boys and to the Men." *Ensign*, Nov. 1998.
11. Young, Brigham. *Teachings of Presidents of the Church: Brigham Young*. Salt Lake City: The Church of Jesus Christ of Latter-day Saints, 1997, 237.
12. Oaks, Dallin H. "The Parable of the Sower." *Ensign*, May 2015.
13. Richards, Franklin D. "Seek Not for Riches but for Wisdom." *Ensign*, May 1976.
14. Eyring, Henry B. "The Holy Ghost as Your Companion." *Ensign*, Nov. 2015.

SECTION 2

1. Bednar, David A. "In the Strength of the Lord." In *Brigham Young University 2001–02 Speeches*, 2001.
2. Nelson, Russell M. "Revelation for the Church, Revelation for Our Lives." *Ensign*, May 2018.

CHAPTER 5

1. Benson, Ezra Taft. "A Mighty Change of Heart." *Ensign*, Oct. 1989.
2. Bednar, David A. "The Atonement and the Journey of Mortality." In *Brigham Young University 2001–02 Speeches,* 2001.
3. Oaks, Dallin H. "Miracles." *Ensign*, June 2001.

4. Clayton, L. Whitney. "Marriage: Watch and Learn." *Ensign*, May 2013.

5. Andrews, Andy. *The Noticer: Sometimes All a Person Needs is a Little Perspective*. Nashville: Thomas Nelson, 2009. ©2009–2018 Andy Andrews. Used by Permission.

6. Holland, Jeffrey R. "For Times of Trouble." In *Brigham Young University 1980 Speeches*, 6.

7. Eyring, Henry B. "Come unto Christ." In *Brigham Young University 1989–90 Speeches, [1989]*.

8. Eyring, Henry B. "We Must Raise Our Sights." *Ensign*, Sep. 2004.

9. Benson, Ezra Taft. "A Mighty Change of Heart." *Ensign*, Oct. 1989.

10. Parkin, Bonnie D. "Celebrating Covenants." *Ensign*, May 1995.

11. Renlund, Dale G. "Preserving the Heart's Mighty Change." *Ensign*, Nov. 2009.

12. Eyring, Henry B. "And Thus We See: Helping a Student in a Moment of Doubt." Address to CES Religious Educators, Temple Square Assembly Hall, Salt Lake City, UT, February 5, 1993.

13. Benson, Ezra Taft. "The Gospel Teacher and His Message." Address to Religious Educators, Salt Lake City, September 17, 1976.

14. Eyring, Henry B. "We Must Raise Our Sights." *Ensign*, Sep. 2004.

15. Benson, Ezra Taft. "Born of God." *Ensign*, Nov. 1985.

16. Kimball, Spencer W. "Be Valiant," *Conference Report*, Apr. 1951, 105.

17. Benson, Ezra Taft. "A Mighty Change of Heart." *Ensign*, Nov. 1989.

18. Eyring, Henry B. "Help Them Aim High." *Ensign*, Nov. 2012.

19. Hilbig, Keith K. "Experiencing a Change of Heart." *Ensign*, June 2008.

20. Benson, Ezra Taft. "A Mighty Change of Heart." *Ensign*, Nov. 1989.

21. Benson, Ezra Taft. "A Mighty Change of Heart." *Ensign*, Nov. 1989.

CHAPTER 6

1. Lee, Harold B. "When Your Heart Tells You Things Your Mind Does Not Know." *New Era*, Feb. 1971.

2. Guide to the Scriptures, "Ponder," scriptures.lds.org.

3. Scott, Richard G. "The Power of Scripture." *Ensign*, Nov. 2011.

4. Guide to the Scriptures, "Ponder," scriptures.lds.org.

5. Monson, Thomas S. "We Never Walk Alone." *Ensign*, Nov. 2011.

6. Christofferson, D. Todd. "The Blessings of Scripture." *Ensign*, May 2010.

7. Cook, Quentin L. "Foundations of Faith." *Ensign*, May 2017.

8. McKay, David O. *Teachings of Presidents of the Church: David O. McKay*. Salt Lake City: The Church of Jesus Christ of Latter-day Saints, 2003, 31–32.

9. Eyring, Henry B. "Serve with the Spirit." *Ensign*, Nov. 2010.

10. Eyring, Henry B. "Feed My Lambs." *Ensign*, Nov. 1997.

11. Scott, Richard G. "To Acquire Knowledge and the Strength to Use It Wisely." *Ensign*, June 2002.

12. Scott, Richard G. "To Acquire Spiritual Guidance." *Ensign*, Nov. 2009.

13. Snow, Lorenzo. *Teachings of Presidents of the Church: Lorenzo Snow.* Salt Lake City: The Church of Jesus Christ of Latter-day Saints, 2012, 76.

14. McConkie, Bruce R. "Upon This Rock." *Ensign*, May 1981.

CHAPTER 7

1. Maxwell, Neal A. "Meekness." *Ensign*, Mar. 1983.

2. Lee, Harold B. *Teachings of Presidents of the Church: Harold B. Lee.* Salt Lake City: The Church of Jesus Christ of Latter-day Saints, 2000, 197.

3. Wirthlin, Joseph B. "The Unspeakable Gift." *Ensign*, May 2003.

4. Eyring, Henry B. "The Holy Ghost as Your Companion." *Ensign*, Nov. 2015.

5. Smoot, Mary Ellen. "We are Instruments in the Hands of God." *Ensign*, Nov. 2000.

6. Maxwell, Neal A. "The Book of Mormon: A Great Answer to a Great Question." Address at the Book of Mormon Symposium at Brigham Young University, October 10, 1986. Published in *A Book of Mormon Treasury: Gospel Insights from General Authorities and Religious Educators*, Provo, UT: Religious Studies Center, Brigham Young University, 2003, 1.

7. Maxwell, Neal A. "Meekness Drenched in Destiny." In *Brigham Young University 1982–83 Speeches* [1982].

8. "Meek." *Collins English Dictionary—Complete and Unabridged*, 12ᵗʰ ed. 2014 ©2014. S.v. "meek." October 4, 2018. https://www.thefreedictionary.com/meek.

9. Soares, Ulisses. "Be Meek and Lowly of Heart." *Ensign*, Nov. 2013.

10. Maxwell, Neal A. "Meekness Drenched in Destiny." In *Brigham Young University 1982–83 Speeches,* 1982.

11. Maxwell, Neal A. "Meekness Drenched in Destiny." In *Brigham Young University 1982–83 Speeches,* 1982.

12. Smith, Joseph F. *Gospel Doctrine,* 1971, 58.

13. Maxwell, Neal A. "Meekness Drenched in Destiny." In *Brigham Young University 1982–83 Speeches,* 1982.

SECTION 3

1. Smith, Joseph. *Teachings of the Presidents of the Church: Joseph Smith.* Salt Lake City: The Church of Jesus Christ of Latter-day Saints, 2007, 172.

2. Nelson, Russell M. "The Atonement." *Ensign*, Nov. 1996.

3. Nelson, Russell M. "As We Go Forward Together." *Ensign*, Apr. 2018.

4. Faust, James E. "Who Shall Ascend into the Hill of the Lord?" *Ensign*, Aug. 2001.

5. Monson, Thomas S. "The Holy Temple—a Beacon to the World." *Ensign*, May 2011.

CHAPTER 8

1. "Broken." Hebrew "Shabar." Biblestudytools.com/lexicons/hebrew/nas/shabar.html. Retrieved October 4 2018.

2. "Contrite." Hebrew "Daka'." Biblestudytools.com/lexicons/hebrew/nas/daka.html. Retrieved October 4 2018.

3. Porter, Bruce D. "A Broken Heart and a Contrite Spirit." *Ensign*, Nov. 2007.

4. Talmage, James E. *Jesus the Christ*, 6th ed. Salt Lake City: Deseret Book Company, 1922, 669.

5. Porter, Bruce D. "A Broken Heart and a Contrite Spirit." *Ensign*, Nov. 2007.

6. Christofferson, D. Todd. "When Thou Art Converted." *Ensign*, May 2004.

7. Maxwell, Neal A. "Swallowed Up in the Will of the Father." *Ensign*, Nov. 1995.

8. Pollard, Adelaide A. "Have Thine Own Way, Lord." *Timeless Truths*. October 4 2018. https://library.timelesstruths.org/music/have_thine_own_way_lord/.

9. Marriott, Neill F. "Yielding Our Hearts to God." *Ensign*, Nov. 2015.

10. Hafen, Bruce. *The Broken Heart*. Salt Lake City: Deseret Book, 1989.

11. Gong, Gerrit W. "Becoming Perfect in Christ." *Ensign*, July 2014.

12. Smith, Joseph. *Lectures on Faith,* 1985, 58.

13. Holland, Jeffrey R. "As Doves to Our Windows." *Ensign*, May 2000.

CHAPTER 9

1. Oaks, Dallin H. *Pure in Heart*, Salt Lake City: Bookcraft, 1988, 1.

2. Featherstone, Vaughn J. "Purity of Heart." *New Era*, Aug. 1973.

3. Maxwell, Neal A. "The Seventh Commandment: A Shield." *Ensign*, Nov. 2001.

4. Pratt, Parley P. *Autobiography of Parley P. Pratt*, ed. Parley P. Pratt Jr., 1979, 297–298.

5. Hinckley, Gordon B., *Conference Report*, Oct. 1970, 66.

6. Haight, David B. "Temples and Work Therein." *Ensign*, Nov. 1990.

7. Clayton, L. Whitney. "Blessed are All the Pure in Heart." *Ensign*, Nov. 2007.

8. Browning, Elizabeth Barrett. *Aurora Leigh*, a poem. New York: Worthington co, 1890. https://lccn.loc.gov/15022886.

9. Benson, Ezra Taft. "Think on Christ." *Ensign*, Mar. 1989.

10. Packer, Boyd K. "Inspiring Music—Worthy Thoughts." *Ensign*, Jan. 1974.

11. McConkie, Bruce R. "Think on These Things." *Ensign*, Jan. 1974.

12. Clayton, L. Whitney. "Marriage: Watch and Learn." *Ensign*, May 2013.

13. Marriott, Neill F. "Pure Hearts and Clean Bodies." *New Era*, Mar. 2014, 28–29.

14. Oaks, Dallin H. "Desires." *Ensign*, May 2011.

15. Oaks, Dallin H. "The Desires of Our Hearts." In *Brigham Young University 1985–86 Speeches,* 1985.

16. Smith, Joseph. *Teachings of the Prophet Joseph Smith*, Salt Lake City: Deseret Book, 1938, 216.

17. Pratt, Parley P. *Key to the Science of Theology*, 9th ed. Salt Lake City: Deseret Book, 1965, 101.

18. McConkie, Bruce R. "Come." *Ensign*, May 1977, 117.

19. Miller, Dale E. "The Kingdom's Perfect Pathway." *Ensign*, May 1998.

20. Derrick, Royden G. "The Way to Perfection." *Ensign*, May 1989.

21. Uchtdorf, Dieter F. "Of Regrets and Resolutions." *Ensign*, Nov. 2012.

CHAPTER 10

1. Smith, Joseph. *Teachings of the Prophet Joseph Smith*, Salt Lake City: Deseret Book, 1938, 216.

2. "Full." https://en.oxforddictionaries.com/definition/full.

3. "Purpose." https://en.oxforddictionaries.com/definition/purpose.

4. Kearon, Patrick. "Come unto Me with Full Purpose of Heart, and I Shall Heal You." *Ensign*, Nov. 2010.

5. Maxwell, Neal A. "Willing to Submit." *Ensign*, May 1985.

6. Petersen, Mark E. "Where Do We Stand?" *Ensign*, May 1980.

7. Hinckley, Gordon B. "Stay the Course—Keep the Faith." *Ensign*, Nov. 1995.

8. Hinckley, Gordon B. "Stay the Course—Keep the Faith." *Ensign*, Nov. 1995.

9. McKay, David O., *Conference Report*, Oct. 1907, 62.

10. "Dwindle." Dictionary references.

11. "Dwindle."

12. "Dwindle."

13. Hunter, Howard W. "The Dauntless Spirit of Resolution," in *Brigham Young University 1991–92 Speeches,* 1992.

14. Nibley, Hugh W. "Nibley's Commentary on the Book of Mormon: Commentary on the Book of Mormon."

15. Bible Dictionary. "Repentance."

16. "Cleave." *Merriam-Webster.com*. Merriam-Webster, n.d., 19 Nov. 2018.

17. The Church of Jesus Christ of Latter-day Saints. *Handbook 2: Administering the Church*, 2010, 1.3.1.

18. Hales, Robert D. "Meeting the Challenges of Today's World." *Ensign*, Nov. 2015.

19. Pingree, Anne C. "To Look, Reach, and Come unto Christ." *Ensign*, Nov. 2006.

20. Kearon, Patrick. "Come unto Me with Full Purpose of Heart, and I Shall Heal You." *Ensign*, Nov. 2010.

21. Scott, Richard G. "Personal Strength through the Atonement of Jesus Christ." *Ensign*, Nov. 2013.

22. Cook, Gene R. *Receiving Answers to Our Prayers*, Salt Lake City: Deseret Book, 1996, 54.

CHAPTER 11

1. Hunter, Howard W. "The Great Symbol of Our Membership." *Ensign*, Oct. 1994.

2. Smith, Joseph F. *Doctrines of Salvation*, 2:127–28.

3. Smith, Joseph. *Teachings of Presidents of the Church: Joseph Smith*. Salt Lake City: The Church of Jesus Christ of Latter-day Saints, 2007, 472.

4. Bible Dictionary. "Elijah."

5. Nelson, Russell M. "A New Harvest Time." *Ensign*, May 1998.

6. Eyring, Henry B. "Hearts Bound Together." *Ensign*, May 2005.

7. Smith, Joseph. *Teachings of Presidents of the Church: Joseph Smith*. Salt Lake City: The Church of Jesus Christ of Latter-day Saints, 2007, 469.

8. Bednar, David A. "The Hearts of the Children Shall Turn." *Ensign*, Nov. 2011.

9. Hunter, Howard W. "The Great Symbol of Our Membership." *Ensign*, Oct. 1994.

10. Monson, Thomas S. "Blessings of the Temple." *Ensign*, May 2015.

11. Rector, Hartman, Jr. "Turning the Hearts." *Ensign*, May 1981.

12. Kimball, Spencer W. "President Kimball Speaks Out on Personal Journals." *New Era*, Dec. 1980.

13. Kimball, Spencer W. "Let us Move Forward and Upward." *Ensign*, May 1979.

14. Kimball, Spencer W. "The Foundations of Righteousness." *Ensign*, Nov. 1977.

15. Eyring, Henry B. "O Remember, Remember." *Ensign*, Nov. 2007.

16. Kimball, Spencer W. "Listen to the Prophets." *Ensign*, May 1978.

CHAPTER 12

1. "You Can Make the Pathway Bright," *Hymns*, no. 228.

2. Nelson, Russell M. "Joy and Spiritual Survival." *Ensign*, Nov. 2016.

3. Uchtdorf, Dieter F. "Living the Gospel Joyful." *Ensign*, Nov. 2014.

4. "Rejoice, the Lord Is King," *Hymns*, no. 66.

5. Uchtdorf, Dieter F. "Have We Not Reason to Rejoice." *Ensign*, Nov. 2007.
6. First Presidency Letter, April 14, 1969.
7. Hinckley, Gordon B. "If Thou Art Faithful." *Ensign*, Nov. 1984.
8. Hales, Robert D. "To Act for Ourselves: The Gift and Blessings of Agency." *Ensign*, May 2006.
9. Hinckley, Gordon B. "If Thou Art Faithful." *Ensign*, Nov. 1984.
10. Hinckley, Gordon B. *Teachings of Presidents of the Church: Gordon B. Hinckley*. Salt Lake City: The Church of Jesus Christ of Latter-day Saints, 2016, 70.
11. Benson, Ezra Taft. *God, Family, Country: Our Three Great Loyalties*. Salt Lake City: Deseret Book, 1974, 199.
12. Hinckley, Gordon B. "At the Summit of the Ages." *Ensign*, Nov. 1999.
13. Smith, Joseph Fielding. *The Restoration of All Things*. Salt Lake City: Deseret News Press, 1945, 199.

ACKNOWLEDGMENTS

We would like to thank Cedar Fort Publishing and Media for working with us. They improved our dream of writing this book into a much more effective and refined reality. Team members in every area have helped us to both expand our vision and personalize the scope of this work.

Derek would like to thank his beautiful wife, Elizabeth, who stole his heart seventeen years ago and continues to hold the key to his heart today. He'd also like to thank his four fantastic children—Abby, Kate, Lily, and Jack. They fill his heart with joy every single day and give his life profound meaning.

Ryan would like to thank his lovely wife, Melissa, whose arrival in his life six years ago was the answer to many years of prayers. Her love brought color, richness, and joy that were lacking for so long. He would also like to thank his fabulous children—Jaden, Finn, and Gracie. While they make writing at home a virtual impossibility, they also make life a bundle of fun!

We would both like to thank our wonderful parents, Joe and Jan. We were born of goodly parents whose examples are far better than we can effectively communicate in an acknowledgment. They have given us every advantage that selfless love can create. Both have been firm and unwavering in their discipleship of Christ. Their passion and labor in life has been to set their children's hearts on the Savior and His gospel. We are eternally grateful to have our parents to look up to throughout our journey in mortality.

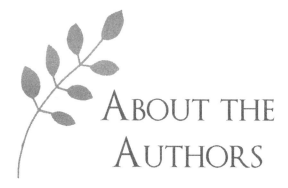

About the Authors

Ryan was born and raised in Utah Valley. He grew up mowing lawns and picking fruit for work, and playing basketball, tennis, and golf for fun. An experiment on President Ezra Taft Benson's counsel to study the Book of Mormon daily forever changed his life, and he has loved the Book of Mormon ever since.

With an educational and career background in accounting and healthcare, the highlight of his career came when he had the chance to own and operate a home health and hospice company with his brother, Derek. He loves the game of golf and any other opportunity to get outside and enjoy the beauties of the earth. He and his lovely wife, Melissa, have three children. They currently reside in Bountiful, Utah.

Derek Squire's love for the Book of Mormon started at an early age and has only grown with time. He has read the Book of Mormon dozens of times and devours any commentary or article he can find about it. He felt a strong impression to write a book about the heart in the Book of Mormon a couple of years ago, and this work is the fruition of that prompting.

Derek graduated from Brigham Young University with a master's degree in accounting and has been a CPA, nursing home administrator, and business owner of a home care company with his brother. He and his beautiful wife, Elizabeth, have four wonderful children they are raising in Bountiful, Utah.

Scan to visit

www.thebookofmormonblog.com